Fundamentals of Management in Physical Therapy

Fundamentals of Management in Physical Therapy: A Roadmap for Intention and Impact helps to strengthen the development of transferable management skills and pragmatic business knowledge for physical therapists. This book will help physical therapist students, academic faculty, clinical faculty, adjunct faculty, and clinicians learn how to manage effectively at all levels and in a variety of diverse settings within the profession of physical therapy and within health care teams/organizations. Learners have multiple opportunities to reflect upon and apply practical and relevant information to build fundamental management skills that translate across settings.

The book is a resource to help physical therapist assistants – as students and as practitioners – "manage up and across," and to strengthen their ability to leverage high performing teams and value-based care.

Jennifer E. Green-Wilson, PT, MBA, EdD, is an Associate Professor in the Healthcare Administration program (HCA) at SUNY Brockport in Brockport, New York. She is also the principal of the Institute for Business Literacy and Leadership in Rochester, New York. She is the President of the Physical Therapy Learning Institute (PTLI) and the founding Director of the LAMP Leadership Institute for the Academy of Leadership and Innovation of the American Physical Therapy Association (APTA). Previously serving as a Director on the Board of Directors of the APTA, she speaks nationally and internationally on topics related to management, business literacy, and leadership in physical therapy and healthcare.

Fundamentals of Management in Physical Therapy

A Roadmap for Intention and Impact

Edited by
Jennifer E. Green-Wilson

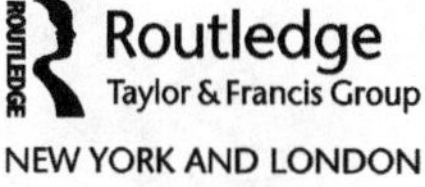

NEW YORK AND LONDON

Designed cover image: Getty Images

First published 2025
by Routledge
605 Third Avenue, New York, NY 10158

and by Routledge
4 Park Square, Milton Park, Abingdon, Oxon, OX14 4RN

Routledge is an imprint of the Taylor & Francis Group, an informa business

ISBN: 978-1-032-99891-6 (hbk)
ISBN: 978-1-638-22087-9 (pbk)
ISBN: 978-1-003-52425-0 (ebk)

DOI: 10.4324/9781003524250

Typeset in Times New Roman
by codeMantra

To my children – Ericka, Jessie, and Jeremy – for your love, for listening, for cheering me on, and for keeping me focused. To my colleagues and friends – Dr. Stacey Zeigler, Dr. Barbara A. Tschoepe, Dr. Diane Clark, Dr. Wendy Featherstone, Dr. Dave Morris, and Dr. Jeannette Anderson – for keeping me engaged in developing business literacy and management in physical therapy at the grassroots level. To my mentors – the Rev. Susan Shafer and Dr. Dianne Cooney-Miner – from the very beginning, for believing in me and encouraging me to keep going. To my dogs – Gracie, Abbey, Moose, and Midge – for staying calm (i.e., not barking), unwearied, and *being* close by (i.e., under my desk, in my office, at the lake) – hour after hour after hour. Gracie – I miss you terribly. To Mario – for your heart, patience, understanding, and heavy lifting. To my mom – Mary Lou Green – a heartfelt thank you for your love, encouragement, and support.

Contents

List of Figures *ix*
List of Tables *xi*
List of Contributors *xiii*
List of Vignette Contributors *xv*
Preface *xvii*
Acknowledgments *xxi*
Foreword *xxiii*
About the Author *xxv*

UNIT 1
Introduction 1

1 Management Essentials: Developing Your Management Style 3
JENNIFER E. GREEN-WILSON

2 Learning to Manage: Strategies for Success 31
JENNIFER E. GREEN-WILSON

3 Getting Down to the Business of Physical Therapy 61
JENNIFER E. GREEN-WILSON

UNIT 2
Introduction 87

4 Creating Culture and Why It Matters 88
JENNIFER E. GREEN-WILSON

5 **Purpose-Driven Operations Management** 111
BRIAN L. HULL

6 **Managing People (Human Resources Management)** 140
CHRIS CHIMENTI AND JENNIFER E. GREEN-WILSON

7 **Managing the Financial Bottom Line (Financial Management)** 164
KAREN M. HUGHES

8 **Marketing a Physical Therapy Practice (Marketing Management)** 195
BRANDONNE OUILLETTE RANKIN

UNIT 3
Introduction 219

9 **Entrepreneurship, Innovation, and Change** 220
CHRIS PETROSINO AND KRISTIN SCHWEIZER

10 **Business Modeling: Identifying Successful Practices and Avoiding Unsuccessful Ones** 248
JENNIFER E. GREEN-WILSON

11 **Getting Started: Planning for the Future** 268
KRISTIN SCHWEIZER AND CHRIS PETROSINO

Index *293*

Figures

1.1	An Overview of Managerial Work	7
1.2	Three Basic Skills Needed by Different Levels of Management as Proposed by Katz	7
1.3	Ten Managerial Roles by Category as Proposed by Mintzberg	8
1.4	An Example of an Organizational Chart	14
1.5	The Three Levels of Management	15
1.6	Five Competency Domains (Framework 1)	21
1.7	National Center for Healthcare Leadership Health Leadership Competency Model 3.0 (Framework 2)	23
5.1	Accuracy versus Precision	115
5.2	A Visualized Goal of Pursuing Simple Health Care Value	120
5.3	Intermountain Healthcare Low Back Pain Algorithm	127
5.4	Intermountain Healthcare Standardized Total Knee Arthroplasty Care	128
5.5	Pareto Chart Identifying Highest Volume of Patients' Primary Diagnosis	129
5.6	Plan, Do, Study, Act	132
6.1	Employee Life Cycle	143
6.2	The 9 Box Grid: A Tool for Career and Succession Planning	159
6.3	Self-Assess Your Fit	159
7.1	Revenue Cycle Schematic	178
8.1	Defining Health Care Consumer Characteristics by Generation	201
8.2	Internet Health Care Search Topics by Age Group	202
8.3	The Three Ps of Physical Therapy Practice Marketing	206
8.4	The Four Traditional Ps	209
8.5	Marketing Strategy and Plan: What's the Difference?	211
9.1	John Boyd's OODA Loop	234
11.1	SWOT Matrix	278

Figures

Tables

2.1	Your Action Plan for Setting Goals	39
2.2	Four Categories of Time Management	41
2.3	Your Action Plan for *Being* Organized	43
2.4	Your Action Plan to Practice Self-Care	49
3.1	Understanding Business Jargon	83
4.1	Four Stages for Fostering Psychological Safety at Work	104
4.2	Appraising Organizational Cultures: One Model to Consider (Bowlman and Deal's Four Frame Model)	105
5.1	DMAIC	124
5.2	The Eight Categories of Lean Management	124
5.3	Examples of Lean Activities	126
5.4	Sample Team Dashboard	131
6.1	Seven Stages of the Employee Life Cycle	143
6.2	Essential Human Resources Management Processes: Common Terms and Definitions	144
6.3	Compensation: Some Common Terms and Definitions	149
6.4	Categories of Laws for Human Resources Management	153
6.5	Description of Federal and State Employment Laws	155
7.1	Operational Definitions	173
7.2	Charges versus Price versus Cost	173
7.3	Breakeven Calculation Example	176
7.4	Revenue Cycle Management Operational Definitions	178
7.5	Key Steps in the Revenue Cycle Process	179
7.6	HCPCS Codes versus CPT Codes	183
7.7	Medically Unlikely Edits	186
7.8	Summer Off Physical Therapy Practice Financial Performance Review for the Years Ending December 31, 2023, and December 31, 2024	188
8.1	Evaluate Your Patient Experience	199
8.2	Connect Physical Therapy and Mind-Body Wellness	200
8.3	Create a Demographic Profile of Your Target Audiences	203
8.4	Define Your Business	208
8.5	Develop Your Marketing Strategy and Plan	212

9.1 A Personal SWOT Analysis 232
9.2 RACI Matrix: TMD 238
10.1 Ideas! 259
11.1 Example of Vision, Mission, and Values 272
11.2 Examples of Organizational Goals and KPIs for Each Pillar 288
11.3 Parallels between Strategic Planning and Patient/Client Management Model 289

Contributors

Chris Chimenti, PT
Senior Director of Clinical Innovation at HCR Home Care
Rochester, NY

Brian L. Hull, PT, DPT, MBA
Director of Rehabilitation for Baylor University Medical Center in Dallas, TX
Baylor Scott & White Medical Center at Waxahachie, and Baylor Scott & White Medical Center-All Saints
Fort Worth, TX

Karen M. Hughes, PT
Customer Success Manager
The Craneware Group
Edinburgh, UK, with US headquarters in Delray Beach, FL

Brandonne Ouillette Rankin
Strategic Communications Leader
Greater Boston, MA

Chris Petrosino, PT, PhD
Professor and Chair
Physical Therapy and Human Movement Sciences
Program in Physical Therapy
Sacred Heart University
Fairfield, CT

Kristin Schweizer, PT, DPT
Clinical Assistant Professor
Associate Director of Clinical Education
Program in Physical Therapy
Sacred Heart University
Fairfield, CT

Vignette Contributors

Andrew Baldwin, PT, DPT
Co-director of Clinical Education
Assistant Professor
Mary Baldwin University
Staunton, VA

Jason Berl, PT, MSPT
Director, Clinical Improvement
HCR Home Care
Rochester, NY

Patrick Buckley, PT, DPT, Pn1
Dynamic Edge PhysioTherapy
Wilton, CT

Jennifer M. Brown, PT, DPT
Board Certified Geriatric Specialist
Founder and Chief Executive Officer
Dynamic Home Therapy & NeuroFit
Berwyn, PA

Diane Clark, PT, DSc, MBA
Associate Professor Emeritus
Physical Therapy
University of Alabama at Birmingham
Birmingham, AL

Steve Foster, PT, LAT
President and Chief Executive Officer
TherapySouth
Birmingham, AL

Fred Gilbert, PT, DPT
Board Certified Orthopedic Specialist
Chief People Officer
MovementX
Washington, DC

Hilary Harris, PT, MPT
Vice President and Chief Operating Officer at Christian Hospital and Northwest HealthCare
Saint Louis, MO

Karen M. Hughes, PT
Customer Success Manager
The Craneware Group
Edinburgh, UK, with US headquarters in Delray Beach, FL

Sandra Norby, PT, DPT
Chief Executive Officer and Co-founder
Home Town Physical Therapy LLC
Des Moines, IA

Lori Pearlmutter, PT, MPH
Certified Professional in Healthcare Quality
Adjunct Faculty, Northern Arizona University, Flagstaff, AZ
Past Treasurer, APTA's Academy of Leadership and Innovation

Chris Petrosino, PT, PhD
Professor and Chair, Physical Therapy and Human Movement Sciences Program in Physical Therapy, Sacred Heart University
Fairfield, CT

Tracy Sher, PT, DPT
Certified Strength and Conditioning Specialist
Founder and Chief Executive Officer, Pelvic Guru, LLC/Pelvic Global and Global Pelvic Health Alliance Membership
Owner and Clinical Director, Sher Pelvic Health and Healing, LLC
Maitland, FL

Barb Tschoepe, PT, DPT, PhD, FAPTA
Education Consultant
PTLI Past President
Boulder, CO

Jerre van den Bent, PT
Founder and Chief Executive Officer
Therapy 2000
Dallas, TX

Ryan Wood, PT, DPT, MHA
Board Certified Orthopedic Specialist
Chief Executive Officer and Co-owner
Forefront Therapy
Chief Executive Officer and Co-founder
Forefront Community Therapy
Evansville, IN

Preface

Five unique experiences shaped my passion for integrating management skills and business literacy into physical therapy. The first experience was when I had the opportunity to create my first *real* business plan (just under a year and a half post-graduation from Physical Therapy school). The opportunity was to start my own physical therapy practice in Puerto Rico, while I was living there on an expatriate assignment. Prior to attending university, I had some business experience working different part-time jobs. I took an Introduction to Business course as an elective in the final year of the Physical Therapy program. This course exposed me to the different jargon, concepts, practices, and models that I hadn't thought about while focusing on physical therapy. Overall, this course expanded my perspective tremendously. So, when I was presented with the opportunity to start crafting my business plan, I pulled my Introduction to Business textbook off the bookshelf and started creating! The whole process of drawing up a business plan taught me how to be intentional about developing networks and different strategies, really thinking through the planning process, and being creative and innovative while looking for opportunities. I developed and used my *elevator pitch* to sell the practice idea to others. As part of this experience, I also looked at different sites, drafted floorplans, met with banks about financing (i.e., loans), and explored potential partnerships. Even though this clinic never opened officially, the entire learning experience was invaluable and opened the door to my next experience (i.e., my first management role in physical therapy).

This took place about two and a half years post-graduation (from Physical Therapy school). I was promoted to a Center Manager position in an established outpatient physical therapy clinic in a thriving suburb of Chicago, Illinois. While meeting with the CEO and the Vice President of the company (the day before I started this new management role), I found out that the previous Center Manager had been "let go," and that the clinic was "underperforming" (i.e., the clinical team was only seeing 25 patients per day, but senior management believed that the business potential for the clinic was 60 patients per day). I left this conversation feeling overwhelmed. I hadn't held an official management position before in my professional career, so I was curious about what I would be walking into the next day. Also, I wondered how we would grow this underperforming clinic to meet the goal of 60 patients per day. I decided purposefully to start this new management role by not making any changes for two weeks, and to spend time listening, observing, and connecting to what was really going on (i.e., what was working and not working). I focused specifically on developing relationships with each team member (clinical and non-clinical), getting to know the patients, and then starting to get to know our referring physicians. After these initial two weeks, I started facilitating and implementing some changes thoughtfully and strategically. Within three to four months, we hit our goal of 60 patients per day. And we kept growing. From this experience, I learned pragmatic lessons about how to self-manage and adapt, how to manage and inspire others, and how to create a culture that achieved excellence – awesome patient and provider experiences, amazing outcomes, an incredible team spirit, and strong relationships with referrers and the surrounding community.

My third experience related to the decision to earn an MBA degree after ten years of real-world experience. At this point in my career, the switch to classroom learning was meaningful because I could reflect and draw upon numerous authentic experiences (from within physical therapy) to apply these new business concepts or models, exemplary management practices, ideas and jargon to which I was exposed. I started to understand that practicing in a profession such as physical therapy requires many business-related practices and strategies in order to be successful and that not understanding the jargon, the terms, and the concepts was holding us back. It was during this time that I became passionate about how important it is for us to understand business and management for success.

The fourth experience provided me with the opportunity to teach physical therapy students about business and management. I redesigned the Business of Physical Therapy course for an entry-level physical therapy program and for five years, in my role as the Faculty Coach (aka Course Coordinator), the physical therapy students started, managed, and expanded an on-campus pro bono clinic while learning about real-world marketing, operations management, financial management and fundraising, teamwork and the importance of using management *and* leadership skills to drive change and innovation. Students reported that this experiential learning opportunity became one of their most valuable learning experiences in preparing them for clinical practice.

Finally, the fifth unique experience afforded me the chance to transform all this insight to formally investigate (as a research study) the expanded role of physical therapists and the integration of practice management knowledge and skills into professional preparation (i.e., to fulfill my dissertation required to complete my EdD degree). This research project was supported by a small research grant funded by APTA's Academy of Leadership and Innovation.

I believe that we must see the "whole picture" (the clinical *and* the non-clinical aspects) as physical therapists to thrive as providers, as a profession, and for our patients. Seeing only the clinical side limits our full potential. Health care is a business. Physical therapy is a business. Once we open (broaden) our clinical blinders to gain and use business literacy and management skills, integrated with our unique clinical expertise, at all levels of clinical practice, we will *be* the agents of change and innovation needed by health care.

Dr. Jennifer E. Green-Wilson, PT, MBA, EdD
Rochester, New York
August 5, 2024

Acknowledgments

The author would like to express sincere appreciation to the following contributors and individuals:

- Contributing authors: A huge thank you for your enthusiasm, patience, dedication, and expertise in developing the content of your chapter(s) for this first edition.
- Authors of the Foreword and management vignettes: Thank you for sharing your personal and professional stories related to your business and management journeys in physical therapy. These narratives have enriched our messages and provided demonstrated models for others to (hopefully) consider as they develop their own management and business literacy skills.
- DPT Programs with a Vision for Management and Business Literacy: Thanks to the University of Alabama at Birmingham, Mercer University, Marquette University, the University of Vermont, Misericordia University, Drexel University, and Clarkson University for their willingness to be some of the first to enthusiastically integrate business literacy and management in their teaching material.
- Dr. Nancy Farina: Thank you for your "hallway delegation" and for supporting the innovative integration of business literacy and management into our physical therapy curriculum. Your mentorship sparked the start of this journey; this spark continues to fuel my passion. We miss you.

Acknowledgments

Foreword

I love being a physical therapist. And having other physical therapists as friends and colleagues has been one of the greatest blessings of my life. We are intelligent, compassionate contributors to the communities in which we live. We make a difference to the lives of our patients and clients, and we are integral to the health of our communities. Most physical therapists make the decision to become a therapist for these very reasons. I'm also confident that most therapists are more concerned about their patients' wellbeing than the financial statements of their practice setting. It is common for therapists to view the business goals of their practice to be antithetical to providing excellent patient care. Yet we must all deal with regulations and accreditation requirements, new payment methods, quality assurance, access, patient safety and patient experience. As health care providers, we also need to be aware that the costs of health care are bankrupting individuals, corporations, and the government. Therefore, it is our responsibility, our professional duty, to assure value for the consumers of our services, and that means that we are facilitating superior outcomes while holding down costs. This is a tricky predicament. For us to participate in, *better yet lead*, the efforts to improve our health system, we must understand the fundamentals of the business environment.

As I reflect on my career, the decision to get my master's degree in business was central to understanding "the other side of the coin." I realized that keeping my private practice afloat, and later contributing to the operational viability of a health system, was as important as being an effective clinician. If your desire is to be an integral part of your work team, a positive contributor, and be relied upon to make good decisions about your practice, then your behaviors need to reflect an understanding of sound business principles.

This is where this book comes in. As the author(s) take you on this journey, following this road map, you will see that you will use the essential management resources every day, regardless of your position in the organization. These might include the following:

1. Human resources ("the people"): Understanding the expectations of human resources along with their requirements, e.g., orientation, attendance, time off, certifications, payroll, team dynamics, communication strategies, employee benefits, recruitment, culture.

2. Machine: Understanding the product and/or service to be delivered and drive efficiency, e.g., productivity, outcomes, specialty practice.
3. Material: Effective utilization of supplies, equipment, and durable medical equipment.
4. Money: Understanding finance principles, e.g., charge capture, charge collection, billing requirements, insurance authorizations, profitability, budgets, operating costs, supply costs.
5. Marketing: Participating in promoting the business, e.g., patient satisfaction, word of mouth advertising, public service events.
6. Methods: Applied procedures, e.g., documentation, patient scheduling, staff scheduling, workflow, delegation.
7. Maintenance: Preventative and planned, e.g., continuing education, licensure, credentialing, laundry, cleaning.

I wish that I had been more aware of the importance of being a good steward of the company's resources when I first started practicing. I would have paid closer attention to those things that affected both my practice and the profession. Advocating for legislative changes around direct access, insurance reform, Medicare caps, supervision requirements, and referral relationships would have been a higher priority. I could have been a better support to my fellow therapists and promoted better health for my community. So, I encourage you, the physical therapist on the path to business literacy, to embrace the importance of learning these management fundamentals and business principles and leave a legacy of elevating our profession and maximizing the health of the population.

Gail Altekruse, PT, DPT, MBA
Vice President of Operations
Parkview Southwest, Parkview Health
Northeast Indiana

About the Author

Dr. Jennifer E. Green-Wilson, PT, MBA, EdD, is an Associate Professor in the Healthcare Administration program (HCA) at SUNY Brockport in Brockport, New York. She is also the principal of the Institute for Business Literacy and Leadership in Rochester, New York. She is the President of the Physical Therapy Learning Institute (PTLI) (https://www.ptlearninginstitute.com/) and the founding Director of the LAMP Leadership Institute for the Academy of Leadership and Innovation of the American Physical Therapy Association (APTA). Previously serving as a Director on the Board of Directors of the APTA, she speaks nationally and internationally on topics related to management, business literacy, and leadership in physical therapy and health care. Dr. Green-Wilson is the primary editor and lead chapter author of *Learning to Lead in Physical Therapy* – the first textbook of its kind – targeted at DPT programs in the United States. Dr. Green-Wilson has been awarded APTA's Lucy Blair Service Award (2024), APTA Georgia's RM Barney Poole Leadership Academy Award for Excellence in Leadership and Education (2019; renamed the Jennifer Green-Wilson Award in 2023), the Rochester Hearing and Speech's James DeCaro Leadership Award (2017), and the APTA's Academy of Leadership and Innovation's LAMPLighter Leadership Award (2014). Dr. Green-Wilson holds an EdD degree in Executive Leadership from St. John Fisher University in Rochester, an MBA degree from the Rochester Institute of Technology in Rochester, and a BS degree in physical therapy from Queen's University in Kingston, Ontario, Canada.

Unit 1

Introduction

Everyone in physical therapy practice manages "something" (i.e., resources, such as time or equipment) or "someone" (i.e., patients) even if they do not have a formal role or responsibilities as "the manager." For example, you must be able to manage the process of patient care in physical therapy, from start to finish. When managing your patients (i.e., patient/client management), foundational expectations also include managing your schedule (time management), managing your stress (stress management), managing your relationships (relationship management), and managing your responses to change and conflict. Moreover, management is a critical subset of managing "the business of physical therapy." Therefore, business literacy, prevailing at all levels of clinical practice, is also an important asset in any in health care organization because it helps practitioners to interpret complex jargon and constantly moving inter-related parts. As Dr. Diane Clark states clearly in her management vignette (at the beginning of chapter 3), "Knowing how the business works makes your care better."

The good news is that you can develop your management and business literacy skills with intention and practice. Developing these skills will expand your ability to practice successfully throughout your professional career as most of these strategies are transferable to different practice environments and different roles.

Learning how to manage optimally requires the deliberate *management* of a variety of tangible and intangible resources and the first resource you need to learn how to manage is *you* – your time, your energy, your stress, your response to conflict, and your relationships. Developing solid self-management practices will prepare you for when you supervise others (and you will) or when/if you transition to your first management role. Even if you decide not to move into a formal management position, developing self-management strategies will allow you to manage the "business of your life," both personally and professionally.

The three chapters comprising unit 1 are:

- Chapter 1: "Management Essentials: Developing Your Management Style"
- Chapter 2: "Learning to Manage: Strategies for Success"
- Chapter 3: "Getting Down to the Business of Physical Therapy"

DOI: 10.4324/9781003524250-1

In chapter 1, you will discover practical aspects for starting to develop your management "style" (i.e., how to manage). Chapter 2 will help you to develop self-management strategies. Learning how to self-manage will ultimately prepare you well for managing others. Finally, in chapter 3, you will examine the reasons why business literacy is so relevant for (and needed in) health care and physical therapy. In addition, chapter 3 gives you the terminology and a basic explanation of how the world of business works to prepare you for diving more deeply into the specific areas of business management that are presented in unit 2 (chapters 4–8) and unit 3 (chapters 9–11) of this book.

1 Management Essentials

Developing Your Management Style

Jennifer E. Green-Wilson

Managing is about influencing action. It is about helping organizations and units to get things done, which means action. Sometimes, managers manage actions directly or other times, they fight fires, manage projects, and negotiate contracts.

Henry Mintzberg, writer and educator, mostly about managing organizations, developing managers, and rebalancing societies[1]

Chapter Objectives

1. Define management as a fundamental aspect of business.
2. Discuss managerial work.
3. Review differences between management and leadership.
4. Discuss practice management and evidence-informed practice management applied to the business of physical therapy.
5. Examine essential management strategies by reviewing management theories and management competency frameworks.
6. Begin to identify your management approach/management "style."

Management Vignette

Jerre van den Bent, PT

Jerre van den Bent was asked about his management experiences as the Founder and Chief Executive Officer of Therapy 2000 (https://www.t2000.com/). His real-world responses are captured in the following.

Management is about *creating order out of chaos*. Management is about having very clearly defined measurable goals and reasonable timelines. Management is about setting solid, meaningful, precise expectations for team members. Management is different from leadership. To me, leadership is about creating a *bit of chaos* because leadership is about disruption,

DOI: 10.4324/9781003524250-2

envisioning, innovation, and about setting the tone and setting the direction. To me, leadership is not as precise (i.e., not like specific goals) but about the direction – the big vision – that is *very* clear, and the core values come more from leadership (not management). Management is executing on the big vision.

My organization's culture is key for successful management practices. We believe in intrinsic motivation and hiring the right people in the right positions. My personal philosophy is that management is all about high empowerment. It's about giving people tools to be successful, setting the direction and the deliverables, and then getting out of the way and making sure that people can be successful in their own ways. Previously, I completed two LAMP Leadership courses (called C1 and C2 courses at the time) offered by the American Physical Therapy Association (APTA) Academy of Leadership and Innovation. This formal training experience was life-changing for me because it gave me words for things for which I had an intuitive sense. I learned that there was research around leadership and management. It was one of the best decisions I've ever made in my entire life. I remember when the instructor said:

> Instead of *telling* people what to do, *ask* them questions, and let *them* tell *you* what they are going to do. It's about coaching, facilitating, and cheering. When people tell you, then they own it but when you tell them what to do, they don't.[2]

Now, we also embrace the *4 Disciplines of Execution* and *Traction* (an approach very similar to *Execution*). Since we embraced these methodical ways of goal setting and goal achievement, we have been "killing it" on reaching our goals.

I've learned a lot about managing others through experience. When you have the right person in the right position, you really don't have to manage. Instead, you are coaching, you're motivating, and you're cheering. Hopefully, you're just cheering all the time because they have intrinsic motivation, they're excited and aligned in core values. You just manage that. Management comes down to having a great plan for execution, and making sure that everybody is communicating.

It is of the utmost importance that physical therapists understand what leadership is and what management is. First and foremost, you're always managing yourself. In many ways, management is about having the grandest vision for yourself but then breaking up that vision into bite-size pieces. Whether you're a new graduate who decides to go for board certification right after graduating; that's a **self-management** decision that has implications for the rest of your life. Or, whether it's about setting reasonable hours for yourself, so that you're not burning out in five years, working 80 hours a week; that's self-management. Almost all of us work in teams, so we also manage others – our colleagues, our patients, and our office staff. Probably not by title, but we're managing those around us and above us. There's a lot of leadership and management that happens intuitively that we don't even realize that we're engaging in. I discovered many years ago that *the best way to manage is to lead.* I wish I had known more about self-management when I graduated as a physical therapist. I wish that I had had more of a vocabulary and more self-awareness of what self-management is, and how it relates to both our professional and our personal lives. We make so many decisions especially early on as new grads (i.e., whether it's the first "job" out of school, whether it's earning advanced degrees and board certifications, etc.), we don't realize how empowered we are. All the decisions that we make are choices. If I think back to those early years, I don't know that I felt that empowered. I just felt like I needed a solid income, and I wanted to feel safe.

Some management advice or wisdom I'd like to share with physical therapist students is to feel empowered to lead across, up and down, and maybe even in diagonal directions from day one. Accept that very few ideas are accepted the first time that you present them. Sometimes you *really, really, really* must have the endurance and the confidence to push and try again and accept failure. **Empowerment** is all about awareness and understanding that you have options, and not always great options. You might be in a 30,000-employee organization where you're just a statistic, and where there's a structure and procedures that you must play within. But even within that structure and procedures, you still have the power and the ability to influence. You still can make choices and set a direction for yourself, even when there are limitations.

Aha!

"If you don't have the right person, leave the position open because if you hire the wrong person, that one person can impact the team and the culture."

Jerre van den Bent

Chapter Introduction

As a physical therapist, you will need to use management skills in a variety of ways especially as you transition from the classroom to clinical practice and into different roles over time. General ideas about management, managerial work, and why good management practices will help you to succeed are introduced in this chapter. You will discover important management skills that you can develop with intention and practice to improve your ability to manage. You will examine management by diving into some essential theories and strategies that can shape your overall approach and philosophy for managing yourself and others in common or unique situations. You will also discern foundational differences, and perhaps similarities or areas of overlap, between management and leadership. By the end of the chapter, you will understand practical aspects for starting to develop your management "style" (i.e., how to manage).

Activity 1.1 Nuggets of Wisdom from the Management Vignette

In the management vignette (at the beginning of this chapter), Jerre van den Bent offered a few key nuggets of wisdom about management. Review this vignette and write down two ideas or suggestions that resonate with you.

____

____

What Is Management?

Management is concerned with coordinating and guiding human, financial, and other resources (i.e., tangible, such as equipment; intangible, such as information and time) in ways to ensure that organizational and collective goals can be achieved. Clarifying *managerial work* – what managers do, the roles managers must assume to achieve their responsibilities, and the specific skills they need to be successful – has been an ongoing and evolving dialogue (debate) for many decades. In general, management matters because it helps individuals and groups to achieve their goals, ensures the optimal utilization of resources, reduces costs, organizes moving parts to ensure efficiency (i.e., streamlines workflows, avoids duplication of efforts through coordinated functions), and enables individuals within the organization to adapt and hopefully thrive in changing environments.

Management is characterized as a purposeful activity or action. Management can also be viewed as an ongoing or continuous process (i.e., the continuous handling of problems; conflict management), issues, and opportunities (i.e., innovation). Management activity is assessed by its deliberate achievement of predetermined goals or objectives. Management must effectively integrate human resources or efforts (especially in health care) while working with non-human resources to achieve outcomes. Therefore, management is viewed as a social process which highlights the importance of the "human factor" in managing; effective management requires the development of dynamic productive relationships and useful interactions among people to achieve organizational goals.

Longstanding descriptors of *managerial work* identified "the manager" as a person in a formal role who plans, organizes, commands (or directs), coordinates, and controls[3,4,5] (see figure 1.1).

Alternative frameworks supported by data and offered in the 1970s and the 1980s progressed and expanded the understanding of managerial work. One perspective (proposed by Katz) advocates for a *skills-based approach* to management; this model, in which managers are referred to as *administrators*, suggests that *technical, human, and conceptual skills* are used/needed for executing managerial work and that these three basic skills can be developed[6] (see figure 1.2).

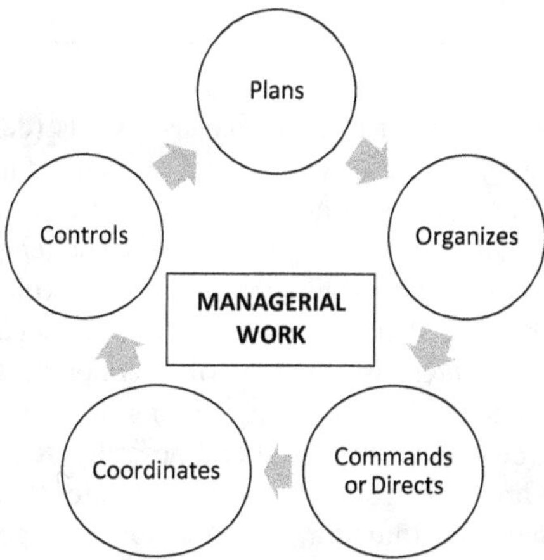

Figure 1.1 An Overview of Managerial Work

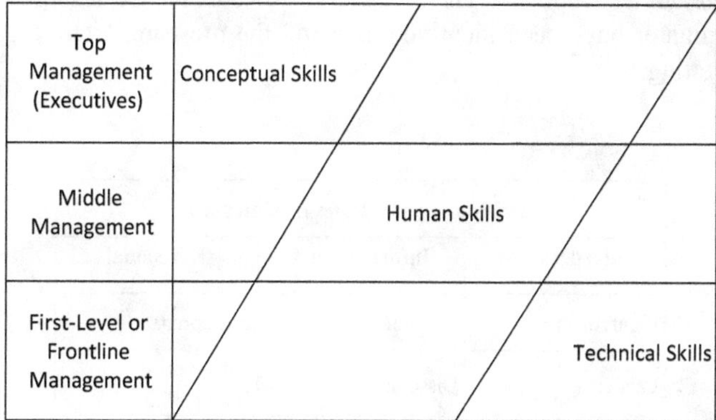

Figure 1.2 Three Basic Skills Needed by Different Levels of Management as Proposed by Katz

Box 1.1 Three Types of Administrative or Managerial Skills as Proposed by Katz

Technical Skills: allow managers to apply practical knowledge and use specific methods to achieve what they need to achieve. Technical skills are important for first-level or frontline managers and are not as significant for top (senior) management.

Human (Relationship) Skills: essential skills, needed by *all* levels of management, allow managers to work with people effectively.

Conceptual Skills: enable managers (especially top managers) to use strategic and abstract thinking, from a "big picture" perspective, to envision or predict the future.

The use (or development) of these managerial skills (described in box 1.1) could vary depending on the management level or scope of management responsibilities. From this view, frontline managers need greater technical skills to be effective in solving their day-to-day management challenges while executive managers (i.e., CEOs) would need greater conceptual skills (and less technical skills) to integrate broadly defined, futuristic, and competitive organizational strategies for the entire enterprise. It is worth mentioning that managers need to use and develop human skills at all levels or roles for managerial success. Another framework (developed by Mintzberg) describes ten managerial roles organized within three broad categories: interpersonal roles (figurehead, leader, and liaison), informational roles (monitor, disseminator, and spokesman), and decisional roles (entrepreneur, disturbance handler, resource allocator, and negotiator)[7] (see figure 1.3).

These managerial roles are regarded as transferable because they can apply to any manager in any industry. The managerial roles of leader, resource allocator, and disseminator have been identified as being the most important regardless of the work setting.[8]

Ten Managerial Roles by Category		
Interpersonal	**Informational**	**Decisional**
Figurehead	Monitor	Entrepreneur
Leader	Disseminator	Disturbance Handler
Liaison	Spokesperson	Resource Allocator
		Negotiator

Figure 1.3 Ten Managerial Roles by Category as Proposed by Mintzberg

Aha!

What Is Management?

Management creates, operates, and directs the performance of a series of inter-related functions (i.e., human resources, operations management, finance) within an organization through intentional, systematic, and coordinated efforts.

Is Management *Really* Leadership?

So far, the terms "management" and "managerial activity" or "managerial work" have been discussed. Before diving into deeper considerations about management, it is important to clarify that management is *not* leadership. Management and leadership are fundamentally different.[9] Yet even today, people use the terms "management" and "leadership" interchangeably because they do not understand the vital differences between these two concepts/terms (that sometimes appear to overlap), nor the crucial *and* complementary functions that each play. At times, people may use the term "leadership" when referring to those at the top of organizations (i.e., at the top of the "hierarchy") and use "management" when referring to those at the levels below them (i.e., middle management). Kotter suggests that the misunderstanding around these two terms is enormous and lingering confusion limits practical/useful discussions about *what* management is, *why/when* management is needed, and *how to* manage effectively.[9]

Management is and will continue to be essential, even though it is different from leadership. According to Kotter, management (not leadership) is how individuals can keep large, complex, cumbersome organizations operating reliably and efficiently.[9] Effective management is a tremendously difficult task for all organizations regardless of size and complexity; often, the complexity of management is underestimated and underappreciated.[9]

Both management and leadership are necessary domains of competence that add value to systems, such as organizations (i.e., health care systems) and teams. Neither is better than the other; they are just different. Warren Bennis, in his book *On Becoming a Leader*, identified key differences between managers and leaders; some of these differences are captured below:[10]

- The manager administers; the leader innovates.
- The manager maintains; the leader develops.
- The manager focuses on systems and structure; the leader focuses on people.
- The manager relies on control; the leader inspires trust.
- The manager asks how and when; the leader asks what and why.
- Managers have their eyes on the bottom line; leaders have their eyes on the horizon.
- The manager imitates; the leader originates.
- The manager accepts the status quo; the leader challenges it.

Aha!

"Management means to bring about, to accomplish, to have charge of or responsibility for, to conduct whereas leading is about influencing, guiding in a direction, course, action, opinion."[11]

Mini-Vignette

Effective Management Means Developing Your Leadership Skills

Management cannot be separated from leadership; you can't manage without leadership skills. You can't get things done if you can't influence; leadership is about influence. You must understand the environment that you're working in to understand the business of your practice. Whatever your practice setting (acute care or outpatient private practice), you *own* your practice as an individual physical therapist every day when you're seeing people. You are influencing all day long. Sometimes you need to negotiate or mediate (to influence) because there will be conflict. Everybody wants a "piece of the pie," whether it's money, time, power, control, or influence. You've got to be adaptable and get yourself to the table, to help make or influence change that is positive for all.

Dr. Diane Clark

Bottom Line!

It's important to recognize the difference between *management* when we talk about *leadership*. Otherwise, when we say we need more leadership, we will just try to work harder to manage. Then we end up with "over-managed and under-led" organizations.[9]

You Will Need to Manage and to Lead in Physical Therapy

Management *and* leadership skills are critical for effective clinical practice. Therefore, *all* physical therapists need to learn how to manage and how to lead. As a physical therapist, you will need to manage yourself, your relationships (i.e., patients/clients, family members), other people (i.e., team members), and a variety of resources (i.e., time, equipment) effectively even if you are not in a formal management role. Without a doubt, managing your patients (i.e., patient/client *management*) successfully will require you to use your management skills. But you will also need *to lead* at all levels of clinical practice even if you do not have formal "leadership responsibilities."[12,13] Recall from the management vignette (at the beginning of the chapter) that Jerre van den Bent stated that "the best way to manage is to lead." Moreover, like self-management, self-leadership is also critical for *all* physical therapists.[13]

There follows a list of the some of the obvious ways you will manage (use your management skills) as an individual, while managing patients and your relationships while working with others (i.e., on a team).

You will need to:

- ✓ manage yourself (self-manage, i.e., your behavior, your decisions, your communication);
- ✓ manage your stress (develop stress management skills);
- ✓ manage your time (develop time management skills);
- ✓ manage your energy (develop energy management skills);
- ✓ manage your patients (apply the patient-client management model effectively, use resources, i.e., equipment, efficiently);
- ✓ manage your motivation (develop intrinsic motivation);
- ✓ manage your performance (manage your schedule, manage your productivity, meet your financial, i.e., billing, targets, manage your documentation);
- ✓ manage your relationships (develop relationship management, i.e., interpersonal skills);
- ✓ manage conflict (develop conflict management skills, develop negotiation skills);
- ✓ manage change (develop change management skills).

Aha!

There is compelling evidence that supports the need for physical therapists "to lead" at all levels of clinical practice.[13,14,15] Fortunately, there are resources available to help you to learn how to lead. One useful resource is listed below.

Tool

Learning to Lead in Physical Therapy is available at: https://www.routledge.com/Learning-to-Lead-in-Physical-Therapy/Green-Wilson-Zeigler/p/book/9781630916589?gad_source=1&gclid=CjwKCAjw4ri0BhAvEiwA8oo6F87nrm_4hPpDsyRC7uQvSCYbCEIftgvcj9msFg6OIMkgGxdpassP0xoCJ0MQAvD_BwE

Activity 1.2 Are You Managing Your Life or Leading It?

Answer the following questions in the spaces provided.

Are you *managing* your life right now or are you *leading* it? Why do you feel this way?

____

____

Do you feel your approach is appropriate for the role and responsibilities you have right now in your life? Why or why not?

____

____

Bottom Line!

Management and leadership skills are fundamental non-clinical (i.e., non-technical) skills that are essential for all physical therapists.

Management Applied to Physical Therapy: Practice Management

Practice management is the term frequently used and applied to the general management or *administrative* practices in physical therapy and it includes all areas and responsibilities of management. Certain health care organizations/practices can support (i.e., afford) a dedicated "practice manager" (possibly a non-clinical or businessperson), yet it is common in physical therapy for "the manager" (or practice owner) to juggle dual roles as the practice manager *and* as a clinician. Ideally, when proactive and seamless practice management strategies (the non-clinical practices) are integrated within clinical practices, these management strategies can alleviate the "administrative" tasks (frequently perceived as burdensome) required for successful practice/business management.

Standard II of APTA's *Standards of Practice for Physical Therapy*[16] outlines specifics related to the *Administration of the Physical Therapy Service*. This Standard provides a baseline for shaping, integrating, and promoting effective practice management strategies in physical therapy to ensure the provision of a high-quality professional service to society.[16] Within Standard II, ten different sub-categories are delineated and include the following:[17]

A. Statement of Mission, Purposes, Goals, Objectives, and Scope of Services
B. Organizational Plan
C. Policies and Procedures
D. Administration
E. Fiscal Management
F. Improvement of Quality of Care and Performance
G. Staffing
H. Staff Development
I. Physical Setting
J. Coordination

> **Tool**
>
> The details specified in each sub-category of APTA's *Standards of Practice for Physical Therapy*[17] can be found at: https://www.apta.org/apta-and-you/leadership-and-governance/policies/standards-of-practice-pt

It is worth mentioning that, for effective administration, the APTA advocates for the physical therapist to be responsible for the clinical direction of physical therapist services and to be guided by APTA's positions, standards, guidelines, policies, and procedures.[17]

Unfortunately, the existence of *administrative burden* in physical therapy impacts all members of a clinical team, even the patients. Administrative burden includes the costs (time and resources) spent on documentation and administrative tasks associated with applying for, receiving, and participating in (publicly funded) health insurance programs. Suggestions for reducing the burden (revealed through an APTA 2022 survey) include standardizing documentation across all stakeholders; eliminating the requirements for Medicare's plan of care signature and recertification; standardizing the coverage policies across payors; standardizing the prior authorization process; and allowing unrestricted direct access per payor policies.[17]

Evidence-Informed Practice Management

The physical therapy profession recognizes the use of evidence-based practice (EBP)[18] as vital to reducing unwarranted variation in practice and providing high-quality care. Interestingly, the principles behind EBP (seen as clinical) are extending into general management practices. Evidence-based management encourages management decisions to be based on a combination of critical thinking and the best available evidence; evidence may come from scientific research, as well as internal business information (i.e., data) and professional experience. Evidence-informed "practice management" encourages management decisions to be based on the information gained from a diligent, explicit, and judicious process of using the best available evidence from multiple sources.[19]

Management: A Deeper Dive

Effective management requires understanding organizations – their purpose, how they operate, how they are supposed to operate, and what they want to accomplish. The general approach to management may be influenced by several factors, such as how the organization is organized or structured. An **organizational structure** is a system designed by management (or the owners) to delineate and guide how specific activities (i.e., "the work" to be done) are directed, aligned, and focused to achieve the organization's goals efficiently.[20] An **organizational chart** is a diagram created to convey this organizational (internal) structure visually by depicting roles, responsibilities, and relationships between individuals within an entity[21] (see figure 1.4).

The structure also determines how information flows (ideally) between the different levels or groups within the company. For example, in a centralized structure, decisions flow from the top down (i.e., a top-down management approach), while in a decentralized structure, the decision-making power is distributed among various levels of the organization (i.e., a bottom-up management approach). The approach to management will be influenced by the size of an organization and the number of managers employed. For example, as the size of a company and its workforce increases, it's likely that an organization will have different managers at different organizational levels, with a variety of titles (i.e., Director, Manager, or Supervisor) and different levels of decision-making authority. Levels of management refers to the line of division that exists between various managerial positions in an organization[22] (see figure 1.5).

Different management levels determine the *chain of command* within an organization, as well as the amount of authority and typical decision-making influence held by each management position. Managers at different levels are often classified as low-level management (i.e., frontline), middle-level management (middle management), and top-level management (i.e., executive); see box 1.2 for a brief

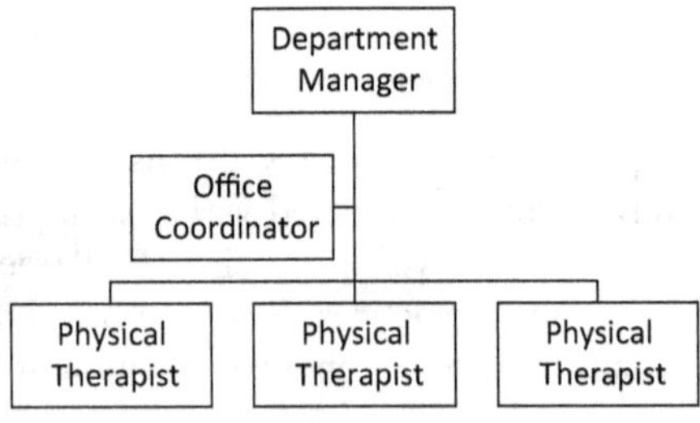

Figure 1.4 An Example of an Organizational Chart

description of these levels. It is worth mentioning that different management levels may need a different approach to management (management style) and/or the development and use of different management skills to be effective at managing at that particular level (refer back to the suggestions proposed by Katz).

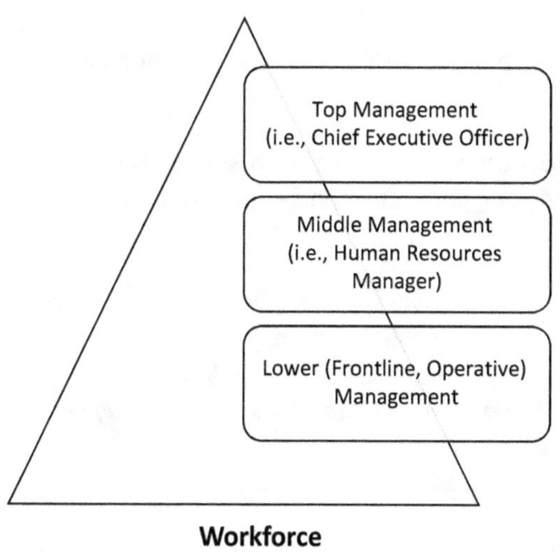

Figure 1.5 The Three Levels of Management

Box 1.2 Levels of Management

Levels of management can generally be classified into three categories. Managers at different levels perform different functions.

1. Top-level managers (i.e., executives) are responsible for controlling and overseeing the entire organization.
2. Middle-level managers are responsible for executing organizational (operational) plans which align with the company's policies and act as intermediaries between top-level and low-level management.
3. Low-level managers (i.e., frontline) focus on the execution of tasks and deliverables on a day-to-day basis. They also serve as role models for the employees they supervise.

***Top-Down or Bottom-Up Management?*[23]**

Power or authority and decision-making remains with the people at the top of an organization in a "top-down," command-and-control, or hierarchical style of management. Information may flow mostly in one direction (downward from the top) and somewhat slowly throughout the organization. Conversely, a bottom-up approach to management may engage and empower employees broadly allowing people throughout the organization across different levels to provide input and action. Recall from the management vignette (at the beginning of the chapter) that Jerre van den Bent highlighted the importance of empowerment.

Activity 1.3 Top-Down or Bottom-Up Management: Which Style Do You Prefer?

Review the scenarios below. For each scenario, circle the response that best describes your preference and explain why this is the best response for you.

Do you prefer to be told what to do (*after* a decision has been made) and told *specifically* how to do "the work"?

Yes No Sometimes It depends

___

Do you prefer to provide input (*before* a decision is made) and then participate in figuring out how to do "the work" independently?

Yes No Sometimes It depends

___

Furthermore, the general approach to management may be influenced by the extent to which an organization and its collective management team fosters organizational learning and growth. A **learning organization** is an organization that creates, acquires, and transfers knowledge, and modifies its behavior to reflect new knowledge and insights.[24] **Organizational behavior**[25] (or the behavior of organizations) is the academic study of how people interact within groups. The study of organizational behavior includes areas of research dedicated to improving job performance, increasing job satisfaction, promoting innovation, and fostering management development. Managers who apply or use the principles of organizational behavior can help their businesses to operate more effectively. Managers who use practices informed by the study of organizational behavior understand why and how people interact with one another within an organization in different situations and can influence or guide these multi-level interactions to impact how the organization *behaves* and, ultimately, how well it performs. When managers apply the key elements of organizational behavior, they will be better at streamlining efficiency, improving productivity, sparking innovation, and creating a positive workplace culture.[25]

Aha!

Organizations Can Learn!

A learning organization is an environment "where people continually expand their capacity to create the results they truly desire, where new and expansive patterns of thinking are nurtured, where collective aspiration is set free, and where people are continually learning how to learn together."[26]

Management Theories: An Overview

Applying and adapting certain elements from various management theories can be useful in different ways. In the sections that follow, select theories will be reviewed briefly to help you to learn more about management and how to practice it. These theories include classical management, bureaucratic management, scientific management, behavioral management, human relations management, X and Y management, systems management, contingency management, and chaos theory applied to management.[27]

Activity 1.4a Management Theories Can Influence How You Manage

Using distinct theories about management and organizational behavior may/can influence your approach to management.[27] As you review the following descriptions of different management theories, reflect upon how you prefer to work and in what kind of work environment you work best. Capture your reflections below.

I prefer to work (examples: independently, on a team) …

____

____

I work best when (consider time of day, alone or with people) …

____

____

I work best in an environment in which I can …

____

____

Classical Management

Classical management is recognized as an approach to management that emphasizes hierarchy, specialized roles, and centralized management.[28] This management theory proposes that an ideal workplace implements (1) a centralized structure of management; (2) labor specialization; and (3) wage incentives.[28] Top-down oversight of the workplace is provided by three distinct levels of management: first/top-level management; second/mid-level management; and third/bottom-level management (see box 1.1). Labor specialization requires an organizational structure in which large tasks/projects are broken down into specific (smaller) tasks assigned to particular (units or groups of) employees. Breaking down the scope of work is done to increase productivity by preventing multitasking and duplication. Wage incentives (i.e., income/salary and bonuses) are used as the primary way to "motivate" employees (an external or extrinsic motivational strategy). Advantages of this style of management include (1) a clear organization hierarchy; (2) an easy-to-understand division of labor; (3) increased productivity through monetary rewards; and (4) single-manager decision-making.

Bureaucratic Theory

The bureaucratic management theory, often aligned under classical management theories, suggests that management (within an organization) sets its rules, policies, and procedures according to its organizational structure. This theory describes a structure that includes a formal hierarchy or centralized administration that delegates tasks to individuals (top-down approach) throughout distinct (i.e., specialized) departments. The division of labor is clear and "the work" is broken down into well-defined tasks and activities that are subsequently "managed."

Scientific Management Theory

The scientific management theory is an evidence-based method for improving efficiency in the workforce. This management theory promotes the need for understanding organizations from *within* and uses scientific methods to assess work processes. Managers observe their workplaces, test different methods of completing tasks, and analyze the effect of the changes. When implemented correctly, organizations can improve their level of task completion (productivity) to increase their value.

Behavioral Management Theory

Behavioral management means that managers need to understand human beings' or workers' needs within an organization to be effective at managing. This theory suggests that managers cannot separate the person (human being) from "the worker" (i.e., they are one and the same). A successful workplace therefore ensures that the management approaches used are the best option(s) for the company *and* the workers/employees (not just for the owners and management). It is worth highlighting that this theory has impacted learning organizations.

Human Relations Management Theory

This theory suggests that employee productivity and motivation can be increased through positive social interactions/connections in the workplace and from acknowledging "the worker" as a unique individual. Therefore, by improving the working conditions and by using certain management approaches (i.e., empowerment, participation, positive treatment, civility), productivity will increase. Utilizing this management approach (theory) allows employees to develop their own understanding of how they "fit" (i.e., their roles, responsibilities, and ability to influence others) within their organization.

X & Y Management Theory[29]

In this theory, the "X" and the "Y" designations represent two different perceptions of human behavior at work.[29] Theory X assumes that employees lack motivation and will avoid responsibility. Therefore, managers must increase their level of supervision to get employees to do their work. In contrast, Theory Y assumes that employees are ambitious, intrinsically or self-motivated, and driven to complete their work, and therefore managers need to supervise their employees minimally. Note how these two different perspectives of "the employee" (and their perceived levels of motivation) influence the management approach or style used to manage them.

Systems Management Theory[30]

The systems management theory proposes that a business (like the human body) consists of multiple components or systems that work harmoniously together so that the larger system can function optimally. According to this theory, the success of an organization depends on emphasizing its employees and factors such as synergy, interdependence, and interrelations between the various subsystems. Managers evaluate patterns and actions within departments and workgroups within their company to determine the preferred management approach to facilitate and support collaborative (versus siloed) work.

Contingency Management Theory[1]

The contingency management theory suggests that "one style of management does *not* fit all situations all of the time." Situational factors (internal/within the company and/or external/outside the company) require managers to adapt their approach to management and/or be flexible depending on the changing environment. Moreover, situational/internal factors (i.e., size of an organization, technology used) may influence the organization structure directly and uniquely.

Chaos Theory Applied to Management[31,32]

Chaos theory provides a lens through which managers can try to understand how the complicated and various internal and external factors interact and influence the behavior of an organization. This theory views organizations/businesses as complex, dynamic, non-linear, co-creative systems that are far from a state of equilibrium. It emphasizes unpredictability in occurrences and behaviors and that small changes in conditions can lead to significant and unpredictable outcomes. Further, it suggests that future performance cannot be predicted by past or present events and actions. In a state of chaos, organizations behave in ways which are simultaneously both unpredictable or chaotic and patterned or orderly. Chaos theory suggests that systems (i.e., organizations) have the capacity to self-organize, creating order from apparent chaos.

Aha!

Chaos?

Recall from the management vignette (at the beginning of the chapter) that Jerre van den Bent described management as *creating order out of chaos* and leadership as creating a *bit of chaos*. Managers can apply the chaos theory by using decentralized decision-making (bottom-up management) and employee empowerment. By giving individuals autonomy to make decisions within defined boundaries, organizations can tap into the self-organizing capabilities of their workforce.[32]

Activity 1.4b Management Theories: Which Ideas Resonate With You?

Answer the following questions in the space provided:

Identify and rank a few of the ideas just described in the management theories that resonate with you and/or align best with your individual preferences (i.e., how you prefer to work) in order to start to identify your preferred management style or philosophy.

____

____

Discuss *why* you picked one theory (over another) as your top choice.

____

____

Identify and describe a few aspects from the other theories that *don't* align well with your preferences and explain why they don't align.

____

____

You Can Develop Your Own Management Style!

You can start to develop your own management approach or management style when you practice, use, or apply different management skills and philosophies (informed by different management theories) in various situations or encounters. Fortunately, in addition to an abundance of management theories, there are also contemporary management frameworks that outline competencies (knowledge, skills, abilities, and behaviors) for effective management in health care. Using these frameworks as a guide will increase your understanding of management. Two different frameworks are presented in this section to provide you with examples of the competencies (i.e., skills) needed for management success in physical therapy.

In the Competency Directory found in the *Leadership Competencies for Health Services Managers* (Framework 1),[33] the competencies are categorized into five critical domains (groups) (see figure 1.6).

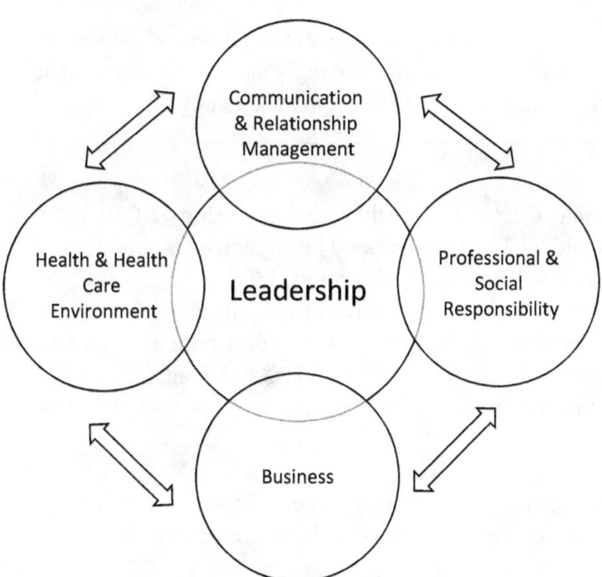

Figure 1.6 Five Competency Domains (Framework 1)

Each domain is defined as follows:

- Leadership: Inspiring excellence within individuals and organizations, creating a shared vision, and managing change to perform successfully (i.e., achieve an organization's strategic goals/plans).[33] It is worth noting that the domain of *Leadership* intersects with the other four domains.
- Communication and Relationship Management: Communicating clearly and concisely with stakeholders (internal and external), establishing/maintaining relationships, and facilitating productive interactions with individuals and groups.
- Professional and Social Responsibility: Aligning behavior (personal and organizational) with ethical and professional standards and demonstrating responsibility to the patient and community, a service orientation, and a commitment to growth and lifelong learning.
- Health and the Health Care Environment: Understanding the health care system and its environment(s) (i.e., practice settings) in which health care managers and health professionals function.
- Business: Being able to use/apply business principles (i.e., systems thinking) to the health care environment.

According to this framework, health care managers should demonstrate competence in all five domains.

Tool

The *Leadership Competencies for Health Services Managers* framework can be found at: https://www.ache.org/-/media/ache/about-ache/leadership_competencies_healthcare_services_managers.pdf

The National Center for Healthcare Leadership (NCHL) Health Leadership Competency Model 3.0 (Framework 2) is organized around four "action" domains and three "enabling" domains[34] (see figure 1.7).

This validated framework is derived from current evidence in leadership development and performance research.[34] It is worth noting that the "action" domains (Boundary Spanning, Execution, Relations, and Transformation) contain competencies relevant to the work of management; these "action" domains are defined below:[34]

- Boundary Spanning: Optimizing relationships between management (spans of control) and the departments, organizations, communities, and/or broader networks within which it operates.
- Execution: Translating vision and strategy into actions to support optimal organizational performance.

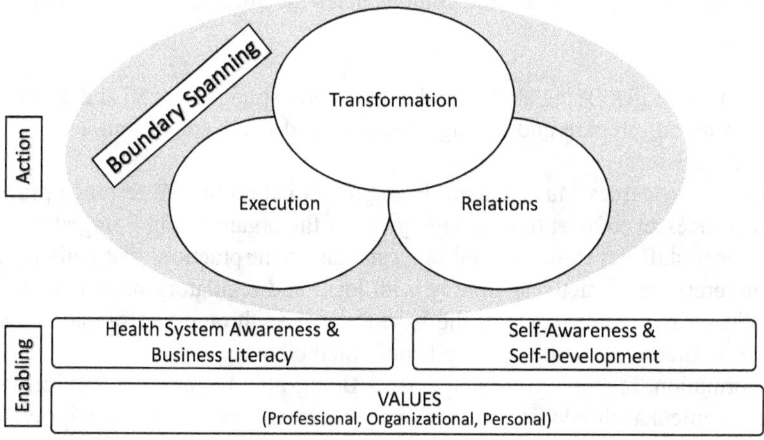

Figure 1.7 National Center for Healthcare Leadership Health Leadership Competency Model 3.0 (Framework 2)

- Relations: Managing through example and actions (role modeling), to create an organizational climate that values employees (i.e., from all backgrounds), offers an energizing and healthy work environment, and encourages continuous development for everyone.
- Transformation: Creating and implementing persuasive, inclusive change processes that support improvement of health quality, efficiency, and access.

The "enabling" domains (Health System Awareness & Business Literacy, Self-Awareness & Self-Development, and Values) encompass core professional knowledge and self-awareness competencies that strengthen (are foundational for) the effectiveness of the "action" domains.[34] The enabling domains are defined below:[34]

- Values: Understanding and utilizing values (personal, professional, and organizational) to guide decision-making.
- Health System Awareness & Business Literacy: Understanding the health system's current business/operating models and the dynamic contexts/environments within which they operate (i.e., community, workforce, financial, legal, regulatory).
- Self-Awareness & Self-Development: Habits adopted and actions taken to continuously improve self-knowledge, interpersonal effectiveness, health and wellbeing.

Collectively the NCHL model includes 28 core competencies, each with accompanying behavioral descriptions at multiple levels of proficiency. It is interesting to note that within the Health System Awareness & Business Literacy "enabling" domain, Financial Skills, Human Resources Management, and Information

Technology Management are the competencies included and these are defined in the following:

- Financial Skills: Being able to understand and explain financial and accounting information, prepare and manage budgets, and make sound long-term investment decisions.
- Human Resources Management: Being able to align human resource practices and processes to meet the strategic goals of the organization. Being able to implement staff development and other management practices that embody contemporary best practices, comply with legal and regulatory requirements, and optimize the performance of the workforce (i.e., through performance assessments, alternative compensation/benefit methods).
- Information Technology Management: Being able to leverage administrative and clinical technologies to support process and performance improvement while actively promoting and continuously seeking enhanced technological capabilities.

Tool

The NCHL Health Leadership Competency Model 3.0 can be found at: https://www.nchl.org/research/

Note that both frameworks identify either a domain of *business* or a domain of *business literacy*. See chapter 3 for a discussion about why it is important for you to develop business literacy and a greater awareness of the business of health care.

Your Management Style (How You Manage) Will Impact Engagement, Motivation, and Job Satisfaction

The approach used "to manage" people contributes to engagement, motivation, and job satisfaction, either directly or indirectly and positively or negatively. **Employee engagement** represents the level of enthusiasm and dedication that individuals (workers or employees) feel towards their jobs.[35] Engaged employees are more likely to be higher performing and (more) productive. Individuals are more likely to be engaged if they feel that they are adding value, are valued, can apply their skills to the best of their ability and if they have a clear understanding of how their contributions impact the team/company. **Job satisfaction** measures employee contentedness at work (i.e., feelings of enjoyment or fulfillment) that people derive from their work/practice.[36] Job satisfaction tends to increase when employees have good relationships and good communication with their immediate supervisor.[37,38,39] Moreover, job satisfaction may increase when an employee understands what motivates them (i.e., intrinsic or self-motivation) and then is able to align their motivators to their work contributions.

Aha!

An engaged employee knows what their role is and what their job entails. An engaged employee wants to do their work and does it. They are loyal to their employer and motivated to work towards the success of their organization.

Burnout, Job Dissatisfaction, and the Provider Experience

The management approach used within health care practice settings can ultimately influence the **provider experience**. Moreover, there is a well-established link between provider experience and patient outcomes.[40] Studies that investigate burnout among the health care workforce (i.e., providers and staff) have shown how the presence of burnout negatively impacts patient care (patient experience) and outcomes.[41] For example, research demonstrates that (physician) burnout is associated with an increased risk of patient safety and poorer quality of care,[42] dissatisfied physicians are more likely to prescribe inappropriate medications,[43] and patient safety is threatened by nurse dissatisfaction.[44] **Burnout** is defined as a syndrome resulting from chronic workplace stress that has *not* been *managed* successfully. Therefore, managing in ways that help to reduce the prevalence of burnout, minimize workplace stress, and improve the provider experience should be a priority for all health care organizations and practices.

The Perils of Micromanagement[45]

No one likes to be micromanaged. Yet micromanagement does exist. Micromanagement means that the manager or supervisor maintains constant or excessive supervision/oversight of individuals and teams or team members by watching each person's actions closely and providing frequent input/criticism related to their performance.[46] A person who micromanages is very "hands-on" (sometimes to the extreme), gives very prescriptive directions about how they want tasks completed, and always wants to know who is doing what, where, when, and how. Micromanagement can produce short-term results because very clear directions are given; however, over time this approach impacts employee and company morale negatively. Micromanagers typically struggle with letting go (i.e., they aren't effective at delegating), which causes individuals and teams to become demotivated and less confident in their own abilities. Eventually, individuals and team members become frustrated and resentful if their work is undermined at every stage, and they have no autonomy over how to get things done.[45,46] Micromanagement wastes time, reduces job satisfaction, lowers creativity and efficiency, and reduces employee motivation. Often micromanagement occurs when the individual who is micromanaging uses management approaches or strategies, such as "command and control," fears losing power (somehow), does not fully trust others, or lacks awareness of contemporary ways to motivate, empower, and engage individuals and teams.

Activity 1.5 Do You Tend to Micromanage?

Believe it or not, you will be supervising or managing early on in your career, each time you work with a patient/client, or alongside a physical therapist student, physical therapist assistant, or volunteer. The ability to recognize whether you tend to micromanage others (i.e., team members) requires you to self-assess your own behavior. Answer the following questions to start to detect if you tend to micromanage others. Review the list of characteristics of a micromanager (below) and choose (circle) the response that best describes you.

I resist giving (delegating) tasks/work to other people (i.e., I want to hold onto it).

Yes No Sometimes It depends

I am overly involved in what others (i.e., team members) are working on.

Yes No Sometimes It depends

I discourage independent decision-making because I prefer to make the decisions.

Yes No Sometimes It depends

I am rarely satisfied with work completed by other people.

Yes No Sometimes It depends

I feel that if a task/work is to be done right, I should do it myself.

Yes No Sometimes It depends

I re-do the tasks/work done by others (after they have completed it).

Yes No Sometimes It depends

What have you discovered?
Do you tend to micromanage others?

Yes No Sometimes It depends

Or do you tend to adopt a more hands-off approach?

Yes No Sometimes It depends

In contrast, someone who is a **macromanager** will define broad tasks for their direct reports/team members to accomplish and then will leave them alone to do their work.[46] Macromanagers have confidence that the team can complete the tasks without being continually reminded of the process or the specific "to do" list. A macromanager uses a more *hands-off* approach and lets their employees do their jobs with minimal direct supervision.

Aha!

Delegation Tip!

Delegate "what" needs to be done, give authority to make decisions, and leave out the "how." Let others determine how they are going to complete the "what."

Early on in your career, you will use your management skills to manage yourself as an individual, your patients, and your relationships. You will also use your management skills when/if you move into a more formal supervisory role that requires you to manage the performance of others. Additionally, you will need to use your management skills to manage organizational systems and structures as/if you move into different management roles. Further, you will use your management skills if/when you decide to own your own practice as a business owner.

Bottom Line!

Developing your management skills starts with developing **self-management**. The importance of self-management was emphasized in Jerre van den Bent's management vignette (at the beginning of this chapter) and is discussed in-depth in chapter 2.

Suggested Readings

Green-Wilson J, Zeigler S. *Learning to Lead in Physical Therapy*. Slack, Inc.; 2020.

McChesney C, Covey S, Huling J. *The 4 Disciplines of Execution: Achieving Your Wildly Important Goals*. Free Press; 2012.

Wickman G. *Traction: Get a Grip on Your Business*. Virtual CEO; 2012.

References

1. Mintzberg, H. *Managing*. Berrett-Koehler Publishers; 2009.
2. Green-Wilson J. LAMP Leadership Program ("C2"). Paper presented at the APTA Academy of Leadership & Innovation; Pittsburgh, PA; 2009.
3. Schafer DS. Three perspectives on physical therapist managerial work. *Phys Ther*. 2002; 82: 228–236.
4. Fayol H. *Administration industrielle et generale*. Dunod; 1916.
5. Fayol H. *General and Industrial Management*. Pitman; 1949.
6. Katz R. *Skills of an Effective Administrator. Harvard Business Review*; 1955.
7. Mintzberg H. Managerial work: Analysis from observation. *Manage Sci*. 1971; 18(2): B97–B110.
8. Pavett CM, Lau AW. Managerial work: The influence of hierarchical level and functional specialty. *Academy of Management Journal*. 1983; 26(1): 170–177. https://www.jstor.org/stable/256144
9. Kotter JP. Management is (still) not leadership. Published January 9, 2013. https://hbr.org/2013/01/management-is-still-not-leadership
10. Bennis W. *On Becoming a Leader*. 4th ed. Basic Books; 2009.
11. Bennis W. *Learning to Lead: A Workbook on Becoming a Leader*. Basic Books; 2003.
12. Green-Wilson J, Zeigler S. *Learning to Lead in Physical Therapy*. Slack Inc.; 2020.
13. Green-Wilson J, Tschoepe BA, Zeigler SL, Sebelski CA, Clark D. Self-leadership is critical for *all* physical therapists, *Phys Ther*. 2022; 102(6): 1–9. doi:10.1093/ptj/pzac029
14. Tschoepe BA, Clark D, Zeigler S, Green-Wilson J, Sebelski CA. The need for a leadership competency framework for physical therapists: A perspective in action. *J Phys Ther Educ*. Published online November 4, 2020. doi:10.1097/JTE.0000000000000164
15. Sebelski C, Green-Wilson J, Zeigler S, Clark D, Tschoepe B. Leadership competencies for physical therapists: A Delphi determination. *J Phys Ther Educ*. 2020; 34(2): 96–104.
16. American Physical Therapy Association. Standards of Practice for Physical Therapy. September 20, 2019. https://www.apta.org/apta-and-you/leadership-and-governance/policies/standards-of-practice-pt
17. American Physical Therapy Association. The impact of administrative burden on physical therapist services. March 7, 2023. https://www.apta.org/advocacy/issues/administrative-burden/infographic
18. CEBMa. What is evidence-based management? Accessed March 14, 2024. https://cebma.org/resources/frequently-asked-questions/what-is-evidence-based-management/
19. Janati A, Hasanpoor E, Hajebrahimi S, Sadeghi-Bazargani H, Khezri A. An evidence-based framework for evidence-based management in healthcare organizations: A Delphi study. *Ethiop J Health Sci*. 2018 May; 28(3): 305–314. doi:10.4314/ejhs.v28i3.8
20. Kenton W. Organizational structure for companies with examples and benefits. Investopedia. Updated February 25, 2024. Accessed May 11, 2024. https://www.investopedia.com/terms/o/organizational-structure.asp#:~:text=An%20organizational%20structure%20is%20a,between%20levels%20within%20the%20company
21. Chen J. Organizational chart types, meaning, and how it works. Investopedia. Updated March 26, 2024. Accessed May 11, 2024. https://www.investopedia.com/terms/o/organizational-chart.asp#:~:text=An%20organizational%20chart%20is%20a,way%20to%20visualize%20a%20bureaucracy

22. The 3 different levels of management. SpriggHR. Accessed May 11, 2024. https://sprigghr.com/blog/hr-professionals/3-different-levels-of-management/
23. Cooks-Campbell A. Top-down vs. bottom-up management: What is the best fit? BetterUp. Updated September 7, 2021. Accessed May 11, 2024. https://www.betterup.com/blog/top-down-vs-bottom-up-management-approach#:~:text=Often%20referred%20to%20as%20command,and%20only%20in%20one%20direction
24. Garvin DA. Building a learning organization. *Harv Bus Rev*. 1993; 71(4): 78–91. https://pubmed.ncbi.nlm.nih.gov/10127041/
25. Kopp CM. What is organizational behavior (OB), and why is it important? Investopedia. Updated May 3, 2024. Accessed May 11, 2024. https://www.investopedia.com/terms/o/organizational-behavior.asp
26. Senge PM. *The Fifth Discipline: The Art and Practice of the Learning Organization*. The Crown Publishing Group; 2006, p. 1.
27. Smith C, Babich C, Lubrick M. Classical management theories. In *Leadership and Management in Learning Organizations*. Accessed May 11, 2024. https://ecampusontario.pressbooks.pub/educationleadershipmanagement/chapter/2-1-classical-management-theories/#:~:text='%20Understanding%20organizations%20comes%20from%20understanding,theory%2C%20and%20human%20relations%20theory
28. Q&A: What is the classical management theory? Indeed. Published December 12, 2019. Updated September 9, 2022. Accessed May 11, 2024. https://www.indeed.com/career-advice/career-development/classical-management-theory#:~:text=The%20classical%20management%20theory%20emphasizes,wage%20increases%20to%20motivate%20employees
29. Miller A. Top 8 organizational behavior theories. Noodle.com. Published October 31, 2022. Accessed May 11, 2024. https://resources.noodle.com/articles/top-8-organizational-behavior-theories/
30. Skochelak, SE, Hammoud, MM Lomis, KD, et al. Health Systems Science. 2nd ed. Elsevier; 2023.
31. Gordon, J. Chaos theory of management – explained. Updated April 22, 2024. Accessed May 11, 2024. https://thebusinessprofessor.com/en_US/management-leadership-organizational-behavior/chaos-theory-of-management
32. Peters T. *Thriving on Chaos: Handbook for a Management Revolution*. Harper Perennial; 1988.
33. International Hospital Federation. Leadership competencies for health services managers. 2015. Accessed May 11, 2024. https://www.ache.org/-/media/ache/about-ache/leadership_competencies_healthcare_services_managers.pdf
34. Health leadership competency model 3.0. National Center for Healthcare Leadership; August 2018. https://www.nchl.org/research/
35. What is employee engagement and how do you improve it? Gallup. Accessed May 23, 2024. https://www.gallup.com/workplace/285674/improve-employee-engagement-workplace.aspx
36. Montuori P, Sorrentino M, Sarnacchiaro P, Di Duca F, Nardo A, Ferrante B, D'Angelo D, Di Sarno S, Pennino F, Masucci A, Triassi M, Nardone A. Job satisfaction: Knowledge, attitudes, and practices analysis in a well-educated population. *Int J Environ Res Public Health*. 2022; 19(21): 14214. doi:10.3390/ijerph192114214
37. Grasso AJ. Management style, job satisfaction, and service effectiveness. *Adm Soc Work*. 1994; 18(4): 89–105. doi:10.1300/J147v18n04_05

38. Lucas MD. Management style and staff nurse job satisfaction. *J Prof Nurs*. 1991 March–April; 7(2): 119–125. doi:10.1016/8755-7223(91)90096-4
39. Rad AM, Yarmohammadian MH. A study of relationship between managers' leadership style and employees' job satisfaction. *Leadersh Health Serv*. 2006; 19(2–3): 11–28. https://doi.org/10.1108/13660750610665008
40. Bodenheimer T, Sinsky C. From triple to quadruple aim: Care of the patient requires care of the provider. *Ann Fam Med.* 2014 Nov.–Dec.; 12(6): 573–576. doi:10.1370/afm.1713
41. Burn-out an "occupational phenomenon." World Health Organization. Accessed May 11, 2024. https://www.who.int/standards/classifications/frequently-asked-questions/burn-out-an-occupational-phenomenon#:~:text=%E2%80%9CBurn%2Dout%20is%20a%20syndrome,related%20to%20one's%20job%3B%20and
42. Panagioti M, Geraghty K, Johnson J, Zhou A, Panagopoulou E, Chew-Graham C, Peters D, Hodkinson A, Riley R, Esmail, A. Association between physician burnout and patient safety, professionalism, and patient satisfaction: A systematic review and meta-analysis. *JAMA Internl Med.* 2018; 178(10): 1317–1331.
43. Williams ES, Skinner AC. Outcomes of physician job satisfaction: A narrative review, implications, and directions for future research. *Health Care Manage Rev*. 2003; 28(2): 119–139. doi:10.1097/00004010–200304000-00004
44. McHugh MD, Kutney-Lee A, Cimiotti JP, Sloane DM, Aiken LH. Nurses' widespread job dissatisfaction, burnout, and frustration with health benefits signal problems for patient care. *Health Affairs*. 2011; 30(2): 202–210.
45. Indeed Editorial Team. What is a micromanager? Definition and signs. Indeed. Updated October 23, 2022. https://ca.indeed.com/career-advice/career-development/micromanager-signs
46. Kagan J. What is a micromanager? Impact, signs, and ways to reform. Investopedia. Updated July 11, 2021. https://www.investopedia.com/terms/m/micro-manager.asp

2 Learning to Manage

Strategies for Success

Jennifer E. Green-Wilson

Managing yourself with discipline and integrity is not just about personal growth – it's about setting the standard and becoming a living example of the management skills you wish to inspire in others.

Stacey L. Zeigler, PT, DPT, MS

Chapter Objectives

1. Examine strategies to increase your ability to self-manage.
2. Develop action plans to improve your time management, organizational skills, and ability to prioritize and focus.
3. Develop action plans to improve your self-care practices by managing stress and your energy (self-renewal).
4. Examine the need to develop your ability to manage change.
5. Identify the importance of managing relationships and networks for effective management.
6. Examine the need to develop your ability to manage conflict.
7. Understand the need to manage risk.

Management Vignette

Dr. Andrew Baldwin's Reflections as a First-Time Manager

I moved into my first management role after practicing for three years as a lead clinician in an outpatient setting. I was approached by the rehab program manager at a local skilled nursing facility where I practiced as needed on the side who was leaving; he asked me about becoming the manager. I hadn't been seeking a management position; it was more that they approached me, and it piqued my interest. It seemed like a good time to advance my career, even though I had my doubts. I questioned myself: "Am I ready for this?" My move into management stemmed more from the relationships I had with

DOI: 10.4324/9781003524250-3

other physical therapists in the community than from me seeking a management role. In hindsight, I probably wasn't "qualified" at the time but the encouragement I received from this colleague pushed me in that direction.

In my first management position, I showed up with no training and I just did the work. *Basically, I learned on the fly*. I worked alongside a colleague (not in a management role) who had handled some of the logistical tasks previously; she helped me to learn the "ins and outs" of the computer system, the schedules, and many other daily management tasks.

Past leadership experiences in Physical Therapy school through athletics and physical therapy-related activities, and my personal "style" helped me to succeed in management. Establishing the day-to-day operations, or the logistics of being a manager, was an easy transition. I was used to a full schedule where I had patients from the beginning to the end of each day. I found it easy to establish priorities and manage the logistics even though I was in an unfamiliar setting. But the transition to the manager's schedule of "to dos" required me to carve out time "to manage." Even though I had a baseline understanding of what to do and how to do things, now I had to manage others and guide them through the process. I devoted about 25% of my time and energy to managing the people on my team and it probably wasn't enough. That 25% of time devoted to managing was above and beyond my "normal" hours. That's where I always struggled.

I faced several challenges as a manager. One of the biggest challenges was meeting the needs of all the staff in different ways and understanding that there's no "one size fits all" approach to management when considering different personality types. Owing to my inexperience, I thought that the "people aspect" of management would be the easier part of management because I felt that I could "read the room" well, but I quickly realized that expecting to please everyone all the time was not possible. Another challenge was that, as the manager, I wanted to have all the answers; I wanted to prove myself to my team. But I had to accept early on that I needed to lean on others quite a bit. An additional challenge was that I had less experience when I started as the manager than someone who had worked at that facility for several years. This was a difficult situation because I had to figure out how to approach this person in a way to encourage collaboration yet understand the position that this other person was in (i.e., I needed to be empathetic). I also struggled with how to delegate tasks where delegation did not mean I was trying to do less work. I probably got worse at delegating as I learned more and gained confidence; I even stopped delegating for different reasons as new staff came in. I discovered that it was challenging to know when to "let go," to let others run with their ideas to see what they could add to the team. My last challenge was that I had to learn how to give time to myself. I made sure that everyone else got what they needed (i.e., time off) but I gave too much to others at my own expense (i.e., I wouldn't take time off).

I have a few "secrets for success" for physical therapists *learning how to manage* and as they transition into a formal management role. Learn how to "let go" (i.e., to delegate) and have faith in the team. It takes time to develop that mindset and create a common goal; understand that most people will rise to the occasion. But if you constantly expect them not to do as well as you'd like then they probably won't. Recognize that you won't know it all and shouldn't know it all. Your main role as a manager is to get the team to work together to achieve your goals and know your own limitations. Celebrate others and their successes – individually and collectively. Find out what motivates them even if it's not your style and understand that everyone's a bit different. Be willing to be flexible to meet the needs of the team. Recognize that not everyone loves a gift card; it might not motivate them. Step outside of your own comfort zone. Expect to pivot and juggle multiple tasks, even though there's no such thing as multitasking. You must learn to prioritize, and it helps to be ready and willing to change directions quickly. Finally, recognize that you'll make mistakes, so own it and if you own it, the team will recognize and appreciate it.

Chapter Introduction

Most likely, at some point early in your career (and earlier than you think), you will be tapped on the shoulder and asked to move into a management role/position. Successful management requires the effective management of resources and the first resource you will need to learn to manage is you – your time, your energy, your stress, and your relationships. Developing solid self-management practices will help you to prepare for your first management or supervisory role. However, if you decide not to move into a formal management role, developing self-management strategies will be invaluable in helping you to manage yourself, your patients, and your relationships. Therefore, this chapter is mainly about how you can develop self-management strategies rather than preparing you to transition to a formal management role. Yet learning how to self-manage will ultimately prepare you well for managing others.

In this chapter, we provide you with practical strategies or "secrets" for successful management in physical therapy. These "secrets" are based on real-world experiences and lessons learned. Many ideas are transferrable when/if you decide to transition to management roles in different practice settings and at different levels of management in organizations.

Strategy 1: Manage Self

Good management practices start with developing self-management. Self-management is a process whereby you make changes to your own thinking, emotions, and behavior. Self-management is a vital skill for effective management and one that you can improve with intention and practice. Self-management is closely connected to emotional intelligence, and emotional intelligence is linked directly to successful leadership and management practices. Self-management means that you know how to control, manage, and/or adapt your thoughts, emotions, and behaviors, in intentional and productive ways.[1] Developing self-management skills will guide you to know what to do and how to act in different situations in different aspects of your life.

Recall in Andrew Baldwin's management vignette (at the beginning of this chapter) that he found it challenging to learn how to adapt and modify his approach when managing others. To be effective at doing this, Andrew first needed to learn how to self-manage (by adapting his own behaviors or approach) before he could manage others. Adapting also requires you to learn how to manage change. For example, adapting occurs after an individual reassesses, reframes/reorients, and accepts something new in a positive or proactive way to re-engage in the original interaction.

Activity 2.1 Managing Yourself

Take a few moments to reflect upon your habits or tendencies towards self-management by answering the questions listed below (circle the best response for each question).

Have you stayed up late to watch *one more* episode of your favorite TV show, even though you know you have a busy schedule the next day and should get some sleep?

Yes No Sometimes

Have you missed a deadline because you kept procrastinating and pushing off/ignoring the assignment/project deadline for too long?

Yes No Sometimes

Have you ruminated through a period of indecision about some task or responsibility that could have been solved easily by deciding sooner?

Yes No Sometimes

Have you remained "stuck" in a previous plan long after the plan had become outdated and needed to change?

Yes No Sometimes

Do you set unrealistic goals (i.e., the number of things you can get done within a finite period)?

Yes No Sometimes

Have you ever become frustrated with one of your team members for not completing some portion of your team's project (on time or ever)?

Yes No Sometimes

What insights did you gain about yourself?

___

Describe a situation: I am effective at self-management when …

___

Describe a situation: I am not effective at self-management when …

___

Self-Managed Teams

Teams can also develop their collective ability to self-manage and this is critical for managing effective performance within organizations.[2] A self-managed work team is a small group of team members who take full responsibility for delivering a service (or product) through peer collaboration without direct guidance from management.[2] Most **self-managed teams** have autonomy over their processes and roles within the boundaries of what team members agree is needed (ideally through shared decision-making) to achieve their agreed upon team outcomes. These teams develop effective shared decision-making practices by staying focused on shared outcomes and can innovate well because they are comfortable with each other and share their ideas freely.[2] Moreover, self-managed teams provide unique opportunities for team members to expand their own skills by allowing individuals to experiment with and develop new capabilities through rotating roles on the team and through peer mentorship (i.e., learning from each other as team members).

Aha!

Self-Managed Teams in Health Care

Clinical microsystems are described as small groups of health professionals who work together on a regular basis to provide care to discrete populations of patients.[3] Imagine how well it could work when these clinical microsystems function as self-managed teams. Consider how this might change clinical practice in a positive way. If everyone on the team knows how to self-manage, then teams can become better at self-managing too.

Mini-Vignette

Community-Based Nursing: An Example of Self-Directed Teams

In Denmark, it's part of the culture that every single community has a (designated) community-based nursing group; these groups go from house to house within that community to check on older adults who need assistance, check medications, or provide basic support for day-to-day living. For a long time, the nursing groups noticed that their nurses were not getting paid well, they were burning out, and they were leaving the nursing profession because they had no flexibility. The nursing community implemented these self-managed team-based groups. One nursing group is responsible for that community and they're responsible for taking care of all the people who live in that neighborhood. They're also responsible for knowing all the community "influencers" from a policy, business, and community health standpoint. Their payment is based on patient outcomes, but they're encouraged to have legitimate relationships with people in the community and to be a part of the community. In the United States, one *hopeful vision for the future* is that rather than continuing to practice as groups siloed inside the walls (of an organization and throughout the medical system), as physical therapists, we are part of communities and have an impact on community health. If we stay in our siloes within the (traditional) medical system, physical therapists are always going to be health professionals who just treat pain versus if we can get into the community, we can create deep relationships and take care of that community, we can be more of an actual change agent.

Dr. Fred Gilbert

Strategy 2: Manage Your Time (Develop Time Management Skills)[4]

Time management is the process of organizing and planning how to divide your time between different activities and responsibilities – personally and professionally.[5] Time management means that you coordinate and organize your tasks, activities, and responsibilities to maximize the efficiency and effectiveness of your efforts. The purpose of time management is to enable you to get more and better work done in less time. However, managing time becomes more complicated when you are not just managing yourself but also need to manage the workflow and workload (productivity) of others. Recall from the management vignette (at the beginning of this chapter) that Andrew Baldwin stated that managing his time while managing others was one of his significant challenges as a new manager.

As a physical therapist learning how to manage yourself and/or as a new manager learning how to manage others, there are a few ways in which you can manage time effectively – individually and collectively. These practices include learning how to do the following:

- plan proactively by setting and prioritizing goals;
- focus (i.e., not multitask);
- avoid procrastination; and
- delegate.

These practices are discussed below.

Plan Proactively by Setting and Prioritizing Goals

Successful "time managers" aim for distinct objectives by planning and then prioritizing (by focusing on) specific goals to tackle (i.e., what, when, and why). Planning and goal setting are foundational management practices (planning and developing SMART goals will be discussed in chapters 6 and 11). According to the "goal-setting theory,"[6] goals affect behavior, performance, and focus to mobilize energy that leads to higher levels of effort overall. Prioritizing goals, a step that is often missed, is one that is extremely helpful for effective time management because it helps you to focus clearly on the most critical tasks at the right time, and to avoid getting bogged down in or distracted by less important work. Prioritizing goals means that you rank your SMART goals based on importance, urgency, and possibly by due dates.

Activity 2.2 You and Goal Setting

In activities 2.4, 2.6, and 2.9, you will craft your own action plans to help you to develop better time management skills, organizational habits, and better self-care strategies. You will capture your "to dos" in the tables provided (tables 2.1, 2.3, and 2.4). Take a few moments now to reflect upon your goal-setting habits by answering a few brief questions (circle the best response for each question listed below).

Do you set goals regularly?

Yes No Sometimes (It depends)

Do you tend to set daily goals or weekly goals?

Daily Weekly It depends

How often do you revisit your goals?

Daily Weekly It depends Not at all

When you set goals, do you typically set SMART goals? (See chapters 6 and 11 for discussions about SMART goals.)

Yes No Sometimes (It depends)

Describe how you set goals (the process or approach you use).

____

____

Do you prioritize your goals?

Yes No Sometimes (It depends)

Describe how you prioritize your goals (the process or approach you use).

____

____

Setting goals and then identifying the goals that are to be prioritized are critical steps that should be done together, but often they are not. Once you establish your goals (i.e., know what you need to do), it is important to establish priorities. A priority is a responsibility, concern, interest, or desire that comes before all others. Self-managing your priorities means that you put tasks or work in a particular order so that you (and/or your team) become more efficient. Setting priorities will help to ensure that you get to the most important tasks and projects, even as other demands on your time continue to emerge.

Activity 2.3 How to Prioritize (One Method to Practice)

In the space provided, make a list of all the things (i.e., activities and tasks) you need "to do" today. Next, review your list and put the letter A next to any activity/task that *must* be completed today (by the end of the day). Then put the letter B next to any activity/task that "it would be nice to complete today but is not absolutely necessary." Finally, put a letter C next to any of the remaining tasks that can wait to be done another day.

____

____

____

____

____

Now, review your list of "A" items and rank or prioritize these using numbers 1, 2, 3, and so on, by deciding that "this is the *one* task/activity that I *must* do *today*." This process will reveal priority #1 as A.1, priority #2 as A.2, and so on. Repeat this process with your "B" list. Don't worry about ranking your "C" list because you probably won't get to these things today (or indeed ever)!

Activity 2.4 Your Action Plan for Setting Goals

Table 2.1 Your Action Plan for Setting Goals

Instructions: Identify one thing you can START doing, one thing you can STOP doing, and one thing you can CONTINUE doing to IMPROVE your ability to **set goals**. *For each action, identify why these actions will IMPROVE your goal setting.*	
I will START:	(List one thing)
This action will improve my ability to set goals because:	(Identify why)
I will STOP:	
This action will improve my ability to set goals because:	

I will CONTINUE:	
(Identify an activity you are doing now that seems to be helpful or makes you productive/efficient at setting goals.)	
This action will improve my ability to set goals because:	

Effective time management requires you to be organized. If you're organized, you will be able to plan, prioritize, and execute essential and important activities effectively and efficiently. Developing and using organizational "systems" will help you to manage or focus your time, physical space, energy, and thinking better to improve your performance and goal achievement. It's helpful to start by assessing your existing approach.

Tool

Time Management Framework

Another useful framework for prioritizing your time, activities, and tasks is the FranklinCovey Time Matrix®.[7,8] This framework helps you to focus on improving the balance between your personal (life), your professional (i.e., work) responsibilities, and your goals by categorizing each task, responsibility, and aspects of your life (personal, professional) based on two different dimensions:

- Urgency: Tasks or responsibilities requiring immediate attention (focus) or action.
- Importance: Tasks or responsibilities with high significance or value to goals (personal and professional).

Four different categories (identified by Stephen R. Covey as quadrants) are created when these (adapted) dimensions are combined and include the following:[8]

Category 1: Essential (i.e., important) and critical (i.e., urgent)
Category 2: Essential but not critical
Category 3: Not essential but critical
Category 4: Not essential and not critical

Review the same list of "to dos" you created in Activity 2.3. Add other "important" goals or responsibilities to this list (if they are missing). Make sure this list includes personal goals as well as professional goals (i.e., the goals you need to accomplish as a doctor of physical therapy student). Now try to place these items into the four different categories listed in table 2.2.

Table 2.2 Four Categories of Time Management

Category 1: Essential and critical	*Category 2: Essential and not critical*
Example: due dates or deadlines	Examples: relationships, fitness, self-care
Category 3: Not essential but critical	*Category 4: Not essential and not critical*
Examples: emails (some), interruptions	Examples: time-wasters, i.e., scrolling through social media

Adapted from the FranklinCovey Time Matrix®.

In the space below, reflect upon how you defined your responsibilities or activities as either "essential (important) or not essential" and "critical (urgent) or not urgent."

____

____

____

____

Aha!

Prioritizing Matters!

Prioritizing your work or professional schedule is not enough. It is helpful to remember to *schedule your "life" priorities* (i.e., those items from your list in category 2).[7,8]

Tool

Go to https://www.franklincovey.com/blog/manage-your-time-and-energy-effectively/ for more information about how to use the original Time Matrix.[9]

It is worth mentioning that in Covey's four quadrant model, quadrant 2 is flagged as an area on which to focus or prioritize. According to Covey, you add quality to your life when you spend more time in quadrant 2. In this quadrant, activities that are "important" are listed but because these are also "not urgent," it may be easy to put these "important but not urgent" "to dos" on the back burner. To focus on these significant activities, you must be proactive to carve out time (and energy) to achieve them.

Aha!

Your Style of Organization: Are You a Filer or a Piler?

Your environment needs to be organized as well as your thinking. Individuals may tend to organize either by *filing* or *piling*. Filers like everything sorted and out of sight, while pilers prefer papers and "stuff" right at their fingertips. "Filers" use file folders, file drawers, or electronic folders to store electronic or hard copy documents. Everything has a distinct label, place (i.e., different "binders" or certain books sit on different shelves for methodical reasons), and possibly is color-coded (i.e., certain colors represent specific categories). In contrast, "pilers" may put hard copy documents into stacks and piles using open bins or trays, while electronic folders may have "stuff" all over the place (not organized). These approaches are different, but both can be helpful. Therefore, it is important for you to become self-aware of your own natural tendencies and then use them to your advantage.

Activity 2.5 You and Organization

Self-assess your effectiveness at organizing, focusing, and balancing your time to get the important things done and done well.

On a scale of 1–5, with 1 being "not very organized" and 5 being "super organized," self-assess your ability to organize yourself.

1 2 3 4 5

Next, take a few moments to describe how you tend to organize yourself (i.e., do you plan? Do you set goals? If you set goals, do you prioritize your goals?).

____

____

Identify Your Tools or Systems

Different tools (i.e., systems) or practices can help you to become (even more) organized. Using the right one(s) may take some trial and error or practice. Review the following list and check off the tools/systems or practices that you use currently.

- ☐ Planner or calendar (electronic or hardcopy)
- ☐ To-do list(s) (daily, weekly)
- ☐ Note-taking (using an app or hard copy/paper)
- ☐ Smartphone reminder(s)
- ☐ Filing or "piling" system, or some combination
- ☐ Desk organizer(s)
- ☐ Noise-canceling headphones (to reduce distractions; increase focus)
- ☐ Agendas (i.e., for meetings)

On a scale of 1–5, with 1 being "easily distracted" and 5 being "very focused," self-assess your ability to focus yourself to organize and manage your time.

1 2 3 4 5

Activity 2.6

Table 2.3 Your Action Plan for *Being* Organized

Instructions: Identify one thing you can START doing, one thing you can STOP doing, and one thing you can CONTINUE doing to IMPROVE your ability to **be organized**. *For each action, identify why these actions will IMPROVE your organization:*	
I will START:	
This action will improve my ability to be organized because:	
I will STOP:	
This action will improve my ability to be organized because:	
I will CONTINUE:	
(Identify an activity you are doing now that helps you to be organized)	
This action will improve my ability to be organized because:	

Develop Focus (Develop Your Ability to Focus)

Being busy isn't the same as being effective. Time management means shifting from activities to results. It requires focus. Often, the busier that people are, the less they achieve. Focusing your attention means you are selectively aware, or you are concentrating on something to the exclusion of other things. Focus is a key ingredient needed to tackle complex challenges (i.e., writing a paper or starting/finishing a (new) project). Daniel Goleman, in his book *Focus: The Hidden Driver of Excellence*, claims that "the more our focus gets disrupted, the worse we do,"[10] and that "we learn best with focused attention."[10] In his book, Goleman discusses "triple focus" or the combination of (1) inner focus; (2) other focus; and (3) outer focus, where "inner focus" refers to self-awareness, "other focus" refers to concepts such as empathy, and "outer focus" refers to the system in which a person exists or functions.[10] Moreover, Goleman suggests that people who manage others need to practice a balanced "triple focus" approach to be effective in their management of others.

Activity 2.7 Discover What Happens When You Focus

Identify a time when you *really* focused on something. Describe what happened to your performance (output) when you focused.

____

____

Describe what happens to your performance (output) when you multitask or switch back and forth from one activity to another.

____

____

Aha!

Apply the 30-Minute Rule

Here is a practical way to self-discipline or self-manage your ability to focus while limiting your multitasking habits. Focus on a single task (one that you have prioritized as important) for 30 minutes. Turn off social media and all other notifications, put your cell phone out of sight, and close the windows on your computer that aren't related to the task at hand. When you complete your 30 minutes, take a quick break, and then continue the same task or switch to another task for 30 minutes. Practice devoting 30 minutes at the beginning and end of your day for checking emails instead of checking them obsessively multiple times throughout the day.

The Myth of Multitasking

Do you tend to multitask? Multitasking could mean that you have music or the television on in the background while you are writing a paper, bouncing back and forth between emails and working on a presentation that you're trying to finish. It could also mean that you scroll through social media every few minutes while reading a rather dull document or research study. Using technology (i.e., virtual meetings) makes it easy to do multiple things at once and some think that multitasking makes them more productive. Yet the human brain is incapable of completing more than one cognitive task at a time.[11] Studies have shown that people almost always take longer to complete a task and make more errors when switching between tasks than when they focus on one task at a time.[12] Continual switching saps attention from full, concentrated engagement.[10]

Aha!

Practice Mindfulness to Improve Focus

Mindfulness[13] is awareness of your internal states and surroundings. Mindfulness is the quality or state of being conscious or aware of something; it is a mental state achieved by focusing your awareness on the present moment, while calmly acknowledging and accepting your feelings, thoughts, and bodily sensations. Mindfulness is the basic human ability to be fully present, aware of where you are and what you're doing, and not overly reactive or overwhelmed by what's going on around you.[14] Mindfulness can help people to avoid destructive or automatic habits and responses by learning to observe their thoughts, emotions, and experiences – in the moment – without judging or reacting to them.

Break the Habit of Procrastination[15]

Do you tend to procrastinate by evading one of your top priorities? Procrastination means you avoid, postpone, or delay something that needs to be done. It is an active process because you *choose* to do something else instead of the task that you *know* you should be doing. By procrastinating (instead of focusing), you may cause yourself unnecessary stress or feelings of anxiety or guilt. Procrastination can also lead to reduced productivity or not achieving specific goals. You can break your habit of procrastinating by developing the habit of self-motivation (i.e., your intrinsic motivation). **Self-motivation** is the ability to take initiative to start and finish tasks you know should be completed. When you're self-motivated, you anticipate (think ahead) and make a "project" plan to work on significant assignments and priority goals.

Aha!

Stop Procrastinating!

The following suggestions identify a few practical ways in which you can break the habit of procrastination:

- Create a "project" plan (i.e., list times or dates for major tasks or deliverables – steps to be completed). A plan helps you to gain clarity about what you need to concentrate on or do and by when.
- Break large tasks down into smaller ones, and then pick one (small) task to tackle right away. This approach changes an overwhelming "to do" list into tasks that are more manageable.
- Limit distractions. Change your environment to improve your focus. Put things out of reach (i.e., your cell phone) until the task is done (see also the 30-Minute Rule outlined earlier in this chapter).

Bottom Line!

Time management means personal management, life management, and management of yourself.

Brian Tracy, Canadian/American motivational speaker

Delegate and Let Go

Delegation refers to the transfer of responsibility for specific tasks from one person to another.[16] Delegation occurs when a manager or supervisor assigns specific tasks to specific individuals or team members. By delegating tasks to team members, managers will clear time (and energy) so that they can focus on other/different priority goals and activities. Delegation is a fundamental management skill, yet it can be hard to practice. Recall (from the management vignette at the beginning of the chapter) that Andrew Baldwin found it challenging as a new manager to delegate work to others. Managers may hesitate to delegate to others because they:[16]

- think it will take longer to explain the task to someone else rather than just completing it;
- want to feel valuable to their team by doing work that is perceived as important;
- enjoy working on certain tasks or projects;
- feel guilty about giving more work or something else to someone else;

- lack confidence or trust in members of the team to whom they would delegate; and
- believe no one else can do the task the right way (except themselves).

But choosing not to delegate can overload your own schedule, curb your own productivity, and limit the capacity of the team. Choosing to delegate provides opportunities for your team members to engage in different ways, learn new skills, and become a higher performing team.

Aha!

How to Delegate

Here are a few tips to help you learn how to delegate:

Tip 1: Know what to delegate and what not to delegate. Not every task can or should be delegated.
Tip 2: Align the strengths, specific skills, interests, and professional development goals of each team member with the specific tasks that can be delegated.
Tip 3: As you delegate, discuss, describe, and clarify the desired outcome(s). Focus on what the desired end goal is, why the task is important, and review the timeline.
Tip 4: Provide the right resources (i.e., support), training, and level of authority (i.e., decision-making) to help your team members to complete the work as autonomously as possible. Identify any gaps or resources (i.e., training) needed to complete the task.
Tip 5: Avoid the "delegation dump," where *dumping* is having someone do something that you just don't want to do (i.e., forsaking some responsibility).

Caution: Don't micromanage the work that's delegated. Review chapter 1 in which micromanagement and its negative effects on engagement, motivation, and performance were discussed.

Strategy 3: Manage Your Energy, Not Just Your Time

In *The Power of Full Engagement: Managing Energy, Not Time, Is the Key to High Performance and Personal Renewal*, **energy** (not time) was identified as the most important organizational resource.[17] This means that when you manage yourself (i.e., self-manage) and others, you must act as the supervisor and guardian of your own energy, the energy of others, and organizational energy. The authors claim that full engagement requires individuals and teams to draw on four distinct but connected sources of energy: physical, emotional, mental, and spiritual. In another book, *The Seven Habits of Highly Effective People*, Habit 7, "Sharpen the Saw," is described as a practice used to increase motivation, energy, and work/life balance by making time for renewing activities.[18] Developing and practicing this habit helps you to develop a way to balance self-renewal in the physical, social/emotional, mental, and spiritual areas of your life.

Activity 2.8 Managing Your Energy

Describe what "fully energized" means to you.

____

____

Describe when you feel most energized and reflect upon why.

____

____

Identify two ways (i.e., things that you do intentionally) in which you regain energy or refuel. Examples could include swimming, listening to music, reading a book, hiking in the woods, or sleeping in.

____

____

Aha!

Refuelling Matters!

According to Covey, Habit 7, "Sharpen the Saw," helps you to preserve and enhance the greatest resource you have which is *you*![18] Self-renewal can be a way to refuel.

Activity 2.9 Your Action Plan to Practice Self-Care

There are many ways to practice self-care but it's important for you to engage in ways that care for you. Some examples include engaging in physical activity or fitness and healthy eating habits, attending social events (especially for extroverts), sleeping (i.e., taking a nap), unplugging or taking a break from work (i.e., turn off your computer or setting the boundary to not check your emails before you go to bed). Recall that practicing mindfulness can help you to focus, manage stress, and regain energy.

Table 2.4 Your Action Plan to Practice Self-Care

Instructions: Identify one thing you can START doing, one thing you can STOP doing, and one thing you can CONTINUE doing to IMPROVE your ability to practice self-care. For each action, identify why these actions will IMPROVE your self-care habits.	
I will START:	
This action will improve my self-care practices because:	
I will STOP:	
This action will improve my self-care practices because:	
I will CONTINUE:	
(Identify an activity you are doing now that seems to help you to practice self-care)	
This action will improve my self-care practices because:	

Bottom Line!

Work hard, play hard, and don't forget to rest hard too!

Develop Energy Management Practices

Thriving as an individual starts with nurturing the self first. **Self-care** is described as your ability to care for *you* through awareness, self-control, and self-reliance to achieve, maintain, or promote your optimal health and wellbeing.[19] Practicing self-care is not selfish! If you don't practice self-care, you may erode your capacity to self-manage or limit your ability to focus, engage, perform, and contribute. Good self-care means an improved mood, reduced anxiety, a good relationship with yourself and good relationships with others. Self-care is any activity that you do deliberately to take care of your mental, emotional (social/spiritual), and physical health.

Manage Your Stress

Stress management can take many forms, from maintaining a healthy diet and exercise regimen to proactively engaging in activities such as mindful meditation or journaling about certain experiences. Proactively managing workplace stressors can help you to remain calm while you are at work. Handling stress before it becomes an issue allows you to focus on your goals to make steady progress towards goal achievement. Managing stress helps you to self-manage your emotions and maintain a professional demeanor in the workplace.

Activity 2.10 What Are Your Stress Triggers?

A trigger is a stimulus or something that elicits a reaction or a response. Certain situations or interactions may trigger your stress in different ways. Reflect on the following questions.

What *triggers* your stress? The "what" could be a person, a situation, an event or an interaction.

____

____

Describe *what happens* when you feel stressed? (Consider physiological response(s), actions and feelings)

____

____

Describe *how* you manage your stress now.

____

____

Overall, how effective are you at managing your stress?

Very capable *Somewhat capable* *It depends* *Not at all*

Bottom Line!

Successful self-care and energy management take practice and intention.

Strategy 4: Manage Change (Develop Change Management Skills)

Learning how to manage change is an essential management practice and you can develop change management skills. Change is needed for many reasons, especially in health care, and you can gain benefits from change. Self-change means personal change. You grow and learn new things every time something changes or when you make changes intentionally as an individual. Personal growth, or self-improvement, refers to when you guide your own development as you strive to reach your goals or your own potential. By making changes in how you think and in what you do, you can leverage your passions, strengths, and abilities in different ways. Moreover, you can gain insights from changes that do not end up where you want to be. Believe it or not, you can learn valuable lessons from changes that resulted in failure in some way.

Activity 2.11 You and Change

Identify a change you want to make.

Why is this change important to you?

____

____

How often do you change your daily routine? Why or why not?

____

____

What motivates you to pursue something new?

____

____

Identify a time when you had to change something, for example your weekly schedule, your mode of transportation or your workout regime.

What was easy about making this change? Why?

____

____

What was difficult about making this change? Why?

____

____

Managing change is a process and can occur in different ways.[20] Planned change occurs when deliberate decision-making, planning, and goal setting by an individual (and organizations) cause changes to happen. Developmental change occurs when you recognize a need to make improvements to an existing situation or level of performance. In this case, whatever needs to change must be refined in some way to make it better. Making incremental changes may help individuals to feel like they are still in control during the process of change. Finally, deep change is the more difficult type of change to make, and it can occur at the personal level (and at the organizational level). Deep change tends to be meaningful, significant in scope, multifaceted, and usually irreversible. For deep change to occur, individuals need to be open, vulnerable, and able to surrender control (i.e., take on risk).

Change requires taking risks. Change can be uncomfortable for many reasons and this discomfort can fuel resistance, sometimes unintentionally. Letting go of habits, routines, and even memories may cause resistance to change. **Resistance to change** is the act of opposing or struggling with anything that alters the status quo. There are many reasons why resistance to change exists. One of the most common reasons for resistance is fear of the unknown (and possibly fear of failure). Individuals will only take active steps towards the unknown if they feel that the risks of maintaining the status quo are greater than the risks of moving forwards. People may also fear that they lack the skills or ability to perform effectively in a new way. Nonetheless, you can gain confidence when you experience change. Confidence is the feeling of self-assurance resulting from when you achieve new abilities. Gaining confidence will fuel your capacity to take on (more) risk and keep changing your behaviors or habits. In managing change, it is important to understand that resistance to change exists and that the process of change may trigger emotional or other reactions.

The good news is you can build readiness for change (i.e., to overcome resistance to change). Readiness is a state of mind about the need for change. Individual readiness for change involves connecting your beliefs, perceptions, and intentions regarding the need for change and the awareness of your ability to make the change successfully. **Change readiness** means that all the obstacles that prevent you from changing have been removed, so the only thing left for you to do is change!

Activity 2.12 Are You Ready to Make a Change?

Write down a personal behavior change you want to make but have not made yet. Examples may include exercise more, lose weight, sleep longer, practice yoga, or eat more healthily.

____

Why have you not changed your behavior yet?

___

Throughout this chapter, you have been encouraged to create action plans for making personal changes to improve your goal setting, priority setting, organization, time management, and energy management. Review your action plans and the changes that you want to make.

What difference will these changes make? Why?

___

___

Bottom Line!

Effective self-management requires you to initiate personal change proactively.

Strategy 5: Manage Relationships and Networks (Relationship Management)

Working in health care requires people to work with people. Therefore, developing relationship management skills will help you to engage better with others. There are a few ways to start building better relationships intentionally and to strengthen your networking skills. One place to start is by developing your "people skills" (also referred to as self-leadership skills) in order to strengthen your ability to manage relationships, communicate, collaborate, and manage conflict. It may be helpful to identify your relationship needs explicitly (i.e., within your department, outside your department, within your professional networks) or those relationships that you *really* need to "count on" to enhance your ability to be effective day-to-day and in the long term.[21] Finally, you may want/need to add relationship building to your goals (i.e., the "essential but not critical" category (see table 2.2) to make relationship building visible as a proactive activity which you need to "schedule." By doing so, you will invest quality time and energy in shaping strong relationships and networks.

Moreover, relationships and being socially connected (i.e., to colleagues at work – in-person or virtually) can improve your performance and wellbeing.[22] Gallup found that the manager (alone) can account for up to 70% of team engagement (i.e., relationships, management "style").[22] Therefore, building and sustaining healthy relationships is a critical part of learning how to manage effectively as well as making work enjoyable.[23] Boundary-spanning relationship skills means that individuals and managers develop and work across typical work boundaries (i.e., horizontal, vertical, stakeholder, demographic, and geographic).[24] By spanning boundaries, individuals and managers can expand and build invaluable networks of relationships within and outside of departments and organizations.[24] This approach to intentional relationship management can break down siloes within organizations/departments and, by doing so, can increase collaboration between different groups.[24]

There are some practices to consider using (i.e., "to dos and not to dos") while building your relationships to make the interactions healthier, authentic, or more productive. These practices are listed below:

- Manage (set) boundaries to prevent (some) relationships or social interactions from monopolizing your time and energy or becoming unhealthy or toxic.
- Stay positive and avoid engaging in negativity, gossip, or "office politics."
- If you're experiencing conflict with someone in your group, talk directly to them about the problem to try to diffuse the situation or resolve the conflict.
- Gossiping with other colleagues, instead of talking directly to the person with whom you have the conflict, may exacerbate the situation, and create mistrust or animosity.

Strategy 6: Manage Conflict (Develop Conflict Management Skills)

Perceptions of conflict vary. To start this discussion, it is important to understand how you perceive conflict by answering the following questions.

Activity 2.13 Your Perception of Conflict

How do you perceive conflict? Is it mostly negative, mostly positive, or both? Why?

____

____

Describe an example of a conflict which you perceived as mostly negative.

____

____

Describe an example of a conflict which you perceived as mostly positive.

____

____

Like change management, learning how to manage conflict is an essential management practice and conflict management skills can be developed. Conflict is inevitable when interacting and engaging with others. Yet conflict may offer you opportunities to make significant and transformational changes in your relationships when you engage in conflict productively. Therefore, learning to frame conflict in a positive way and considering conflict as inevitable are two strategies you can use to manage conflict differently. Transforming conflict requires you to have an awareness of self, an awareness of others, and to value both equally. Simply agreeing on, or seeing things the same way, is not the same as making room for understanding how other people view situations, or how they express their values.[20]

Aha!

Your current perspective on conflict will influence your actions but a new perspective can be learned and cultivated through engagement and practice.

Conflict management is the process of limiting the negative aspects of conflict while increasing the positive aspects of conflict. Moreover, because conflict is rooted within human interactions, managing conflict effectively may *never* completely resolve it. Therefore, learning how to live with conflict and participating in it constructively may be a more realistic goal than truly resolving conflict by managing it.

Conflict can be positive! Conflict can improve the quality of decisions, release tensions that may be overt or covert, stimulate creative thinking and innovation, spark interest, and hopefully encourage self-reflection and self-improvement.[20] Conflict may be transformational because it encourages growth, change, learning, and a deeper understanding of self and others. In some cases, conflict may strengthen your relationships by building greater confidence in your ability to work with and through differences and by building greater trust within the relationship itself.

Aha!

The Good News about Conflict

Conflict management can be an opportunity for you to establish strong relationships.

Frameworks have been developed to help individuals to understand (i.e., self-assess) how they respond to conflict. Two practical frameworks are the Thomas-Kilmann Conflict Mode Instrument (TKI) and the Kraybill Conflict Style Inventory (Style Matters).[25,26] These frameworks present similar but different "conflict management styles." By gaining an awareness of how you tend to approach and react to conflict (through self-assessment), you can learn how to respond or adapt better (though self-management) to different conflict situations. According to these frameworks, different styles can be effective, and the most effective style (at certain times) may depend upon the situation.

Activity 2.14

How Did You Approach Your Last Conflict?

The last time you faced a conflict situation, how did you approach it? Describe it in the space below.

____

____

Was your approach or style an effective one? Why or why not?

____

If you could do it over again, how would you change your approach to this conflict situation and why?

____

Developing effective ways for communicating and negotiating during conflicts are specific skills you can practice managing yourself and others through conflict. Any form of conflict resolution does not occur without some form of communication taking place. Effective communication requires you to use verbal communication, non-verbal communication, and listening skills applied to relationships built upon trust. Negotiating involves discussing, debating (respectfully), and reaching a mutually satisfactory agreement in situations when some interests are shared while others are the opposite. Negotiation tends to be that back-and-forth process of communication aimed at reaching agreement with others.

You may become discouraged in a long-term conflict situation when the situation seems "stuck" or when there seems to be no possibility for change. The "ups and downs" experienced in a long-term conflict situation may be challenging in different ways and it may seem easier just to avoid it. But avoiding conflict (or trying to) in the long term may worsen the situation and/or the relationship. Continue to stay engaged by staying committed, being supportive, and resilient.

Bottom Line!

How you respond to conflict and how you understand how others tend to respond to conflict is important for learning how to manage conflict successfully.

Tool

See Patterson K, Grenny J, McMillan R, Switzler A. *Crucial Conversations: Tools for Talking When Stakes Are High.* McGraw-Hill; 2012.

Strategy 7: Protect Yourself: Manage Sources of Risk

Throughout your professional preparation (DPT education), you will learn numerous strategies to provide safe (risk-free), high-quality care for your patients. And so, another fundamental management skill you will need to learn is **risk management**. Managing risk means that you are aware of any potential risks or hazards and set about creating an environment to ensure the safest possible outcomes (i.e., high-quality care) for your patients, yourself, your team members, and your practice/organization (i.e., limit malpractice claims). Risk management requires you to be proactive rather than reactive to prevent or reduce the likelihood that something will happen. Improper treatment, equipment hazards or malfunctions, and HIPAA violations are examples of risks for your patients. Physical injury, psychological strain (i.e., burnout), and workplace violence are common risks that managers need to prevent for health care employees.

There are many ways to protect yourself and others. In all cases, it is important for you to ensure that you have an appropriate level of professional liability coverage (i.e., malpractice insurance). You can manage risk through implementing risk reduction strategies, including good communication practices (i.e., ask questions when you aren't sure about something), comprehensive documentation, supervising patients closely during treatment sessions, and by adhering to your scope of practice (i.e., as documented by the state licensing authority in the state in which you are practicing). Moreover, it is important to educate yourself on employment laws for yourself (as an "employee") or when managing others; these laws are discussed briefly in chapter 6.

Bottom Line!

Managing self allows you to maximize your productivity, improve your workplace performance, and efficiently achieve professional goals. Improving your self-management skills can help you to increase your employability and manage your career path better.[27]

Managing Change and Hopes for the Future

We asked several colleagues about their hopes for the future to underscore the importance of managing change and to (hopefully) stimulate a few positive and thought-provoking ideas. These hopes are captured in the responses that follow.

Activity 2.15 Reflective Journal Entry: Managing Change and Hopes for the Future

As you read these "hopes" or opportunities for change, identify (in the space provided) one or two novel ideas that inspire or resonate with you and describe why.

____

____

____

Response 1: Karen M. Hughes, PT

I hope to see therapists embrace technology more. Digital health can make therapists' lives easier and it can help us progress/monitor issues related to prevention. We need to be involved more in developing digital health apps by providing input into software development.

Response 2: Dr. Barb Tschoepe

I have never "discharged" my clients who have chronic neuromuscular disease. When they're having a bad month, they still reach out to me. I've been following some of my clients for 15 and 20 years. Each time we reconnect, I prepare them to self-manage while I monitor and support them. I hope we support care in different ways (i.e., by nurturing long-term relationships) and figure out to get paid for doing so.

Suggested Readings

Covey SR. *The 7 Habits of Highly Effective People: Powerful Lessons in Personal Change.* Free Press; 2004.

Goleman D. *Focus: The Hidden Driver of Excellence.* Harper; 2015.

Green-Wilson JE, Zeigler S. *Learning to Lead in Physical Therapy.* SLACK, Inc.; 2020.
  a. Chapter 8: "Leading Through Conflict"
  b. Chapter 9: "Leading Change"

Patterson K, Grenny J, McMillan R, Switzler A. *Crucial Conversations: Tools for Talking When Stakes Are High.* McGraw Hill; 2012.

References

1. Munro, I. Why self-management is key to success and how to improve yours. BetterUp. February 15, 2021. Accessed June 6, 2024. https://www.betterup.com/blog/what-is-self-management-and-how-can-you-improve-it

2. Perry E. What are self-managed teams (and how can you create them)? BetterUp. April 28, 2021. Accessed June 6, 2024. https://www.betterup.com/blog/self-managed-teams
3. Likosky DS. Clinical microsystems: A critical framework for crossing the quality chasm. *J Extra Corpor Technol.* 2014; 46(1): 33–37.
4. Herrity J. Self-management skills: Definition, examples and tips. Indeed. Updated February 3, 2023. Accessed June 6, 2024. https://www.indeed.com/career-advice/career-development/self-management-skills
5. Mind Tools. What is time management? Accessed June 6, 2024. https://www.mindtools.com/arb6j5a/what-is-time-management
6. Locke EA, Latham GP. *A Theory of Goal Setting & Task Performance.* Prentice-Hall, Inc.; 1990.
7. Franklin Planner. Understanding the time matrix. August 22, 2016. Accessed June 6, 2024. https://blog.franklinplanner.com/understanding-the-time-matrix/
8. Merrill RR, Merrill AR. *Connections: Quadrant II Time Management.* Institute for Principle; 1989.
9. Franklin Covey. Manage your time and energy effectively. Accessed June 6, 2024. https://www.franklincovey.com/blog/manage-your-time-and-energy-effectively/
10. Goleman D. *Focus: The Hidden Driver of Excellence.* Harper; 2015, pp. 14 and 16.
11. NeuroLeadership Institute. The myth of multitasking. February 9, 2023. Accessed June 6, 2024. https://neuroleadership.com/your-brain-at-work/the-myth-of-multitasking
12. Madore KP, Wagner AD. Multicosts of multitasking. *Cerebrum.* 2019 April 1: cer-04–19.
13. American Psychological Association. Mindfulness. Accessed June 6, 2024. https://www.apa.org/topics/mindfulness
14. Mindful. What is mindfulness? July 8, 2020. Accessed June 6, 2024. https://www.mindful.org/what-is-mindfulness/
15. MindTools. How to stop procrastinating. Accessed June 6, 2024. https://www.mindtools.com/a5plzk8/how-to-stop-procrastinating
16. Landry L. How to delegate effectively: 9 tips for managers. Harvard Business School. January 14, 2020. https://online.hbs.edu/blog/post/how-to-delegate-effectively
17. Loehr J, Schwartz T. *The Power of Full Engagement: Managing Energy, Not Time, Is the Key to High Performance and Personal Renewal.* Free Press; 2003.
18. Franklin Covey. Habit 7: Sharpen the saw. Accessed June 13, 2024. https://www.franklincovey.com/the-7-habits/habit-7/
19. Martínez N, Connelly CD, Pérez A, Calero P. Self-care: A concept analysis. *Int J Nurs Sci.* 2021; 8(4): 418–425. doi:10.1016/j.ijnss.2021.08.007
20. Green-Wilson JE, Zeigler S. *Learning to Lead in Physical Therapy.* SLACK, Inc.; 2020.
21. Ibarra H, Hunter M. How leaders create and use networks. *Harvard Business Review.* January 2007. https://hbr.org/2007/01/how-leaders-create-and-use-networks
22. Mental Health Foundation. Top tips on building and maintaining healthy relationships. Accessed June 13, 2024. https://www.mentalhealth.org.uk/our-work/public-engagement/healthy-relationships/top-tips-building-and-maintaining-healthy-relationships
23. Gettysburg College. One-third of your life is spent at work. Accessed June 13, 2024. https://www.gettysburg.edu/news/stories?id=79db7b34-630c-4f49-ad32-4ab9ea48e72b&pageTitle=1%2F3+of+your+life+is+spent+at+work
24. Center for Creative Leadership. Boundary spanning leadership enables breaking down silos. Accessed June 13, 2024. https://www.ccl.org/leadership-solutions/leadership-topics/boundary-spanning/

25. Thomas-Kilmann Conflict Mode Instrument (TKI®). Accessed October 10, 2018. http://www.cpp.com/en-US/Products-and-Services/TKI
26. Style Matters: The Kraybill Conflict Style Inventory. Accessed July 22, 2024. https://www.riverhouseepress.com/index.php/en/homeen
27. Herrity J. Self-management skills: Definition, examples and tips. Indeed. February 3, 2023. https://www.indeed.com/career-advice/career-development/self-management-skills

3 Getting Down to the Business of Physical Therapy

Jennifer E. Green-Wilson

People don't buy what you do; they buy why you do it.

Simon Sinek, English-born American author and inspirational speaker on business leadership[1]

Chapter Objectives

1. Discuss the need for business literacy in physical therapy.
2. Describe business.
3. Identify the fundamentals of business.
4. Discuss why business needs management.
5. Examine the business of health care.
6. Examine the business of physical therapy.

Management Vignette

Dr. Diane Clark

There are a couple of things that intersect when considering the realities that *health care is a business* and *physical therapy is a business*. One is that physical therapists want to make things better; we want to *help people* because "we are people persons." Most of us get into the physical therapy profession because we like working with people; we like the "one-on-one" interactions with our patients. It seems that the "business side" has *always* had this negative connotation. We perceive that the "business side" projects negative perceptions about us as health professionals. However, I don't think we've approached it in the right way. After moving from Canada (and the Canadian health care system) to the United States, I worked for several for-profit companies in various administrative positions. It became even more apparent to me that patient care and business are intertwined; there's

DOI: 10.4324/9781003524250-4

no separating patient care from business. After I completed my MBA degree at Georgetown University, I gained valuable perspectives about marketing, finance, and strategy that weren't so negative. *Knowing how the business works makes your care better*. Without a doubt, you make better patient care decisions knowing how business works.

You must embrace it (the business) and understand how the business shapes your environment. You must understand what's going on and the forces at work. You will still need referrals even if you own your own practice (i.e., out-of-network) and decide to do things your own way (i.e., cash-based practice). You still need to understand how the business affects your referrals and to whom you can refer. Sometimes the business seems to be encroaching on how we must practice (i.e., what we do) but it forces us to be creative. We aren't the only health profession who is feeling the crunch! We're all in it together! If you don't have a voice at the table (i.e., with the capitated payment programs), no one is going to throw money at us. You must be an advocate for your patient(s) and to be an effective advocate you must understand what's *really* going on.

It is also important for physical therapists to learn about management and how to manage. *Management is absolutely a subset of business*. You must manage up, you must manage down, *and* you must manage yourself. It's critical to understand the fundamentals of business in multiple ways – what's going on *above* (you) and what needs to happen *below* (you). When I think of management, I automatically think of productivity. Productivity is often the "big elephant in the room." You must know how productivity is being calculated, otherwise how can you comment or provide feedback to the system whether (or not) the productivity calculation is fair? Productivity is about collecting the data it should collect because if you *just* count numbers, then you're missing the qualitative side to your productivity and how that's valued. You must make a case that productivity is more than just the numbers. There are other factors that have value to both your patient, to the department, and to the system. At a minimum, you must understand how productivity relates to business because with productivity comes reimbursement and with reimbursement comes payment. You need to understand that salaries and benefits (i.e., even your own paycheck) are based on your productivity. Everybody (i.e., you, the technician, the manager, the front office staff) must get paid! You must understand and accept that you might need to see an additional patient on a particular day. Or perhaps you can't spend a full hour "one-on-one" with a patient. You need to be flexible and adapt to what's going on within (and outside of) the business. Learning how to *manage across* – working in an interdisciplinary team that is patient-centered – helps you to become more productive. So, it's critical for you to develop your team-based skills and learn how to manage your relationships well.

Aha!

Patient care and business are intertwined; there's no separating patient care from business.

Dr. Diane Clark

Chapter Introduction

All physical therapists need business literacy. There are clear reasons why it is critical for you to develop a fundamental understanding of how the business of health care and the business of physical therapy works. Perhaps you already have some experience in business, perhaps you've taken a business course at some point in your career, or perhaps you are learning about these topics for the first time. This chapter introduces you to business and the reasons why the topic of business is so relevant to health care and physical therapy. This chapter also gives you the terminology and a basic explanation of how the world of business works to prepare you for diving more deeply into the specific areas of business management that are presented in unit 2 (chapters 4–8) and unit 3 (chapters 9–11) in this book. Developing business literacy will help you to understand how you fit into the overall big picture of clinical practice and how you can improve your ability to demonstrate your own value as a physical therapist. Recall from the management vignette (at the beginning of this chapter) when Dr. Diane Clark stated that knowing how the business works makes your care better.

Why All Physical Therapists Need to Develop Business Literacy

The evolving and ever-changing complexities of the health care industry demand that all physical therapists develop business literacy. It is no longer adequate for the dedicated or assigned "practice manager" or health care administrator ("the businessperson or the non-clinical" team) to be the only person to understand the nuances of the industry or the health care organization's business goals. Now more than ever it is imperative for business literacy and business awareness to cascade throughout the entire health care organization if the enterprise is to succeed.[2]

Business literacy means that individuals have "the ability to speak and read the language of business."[3] Specifically, business literacy means individuals have "the knowledge and understanding of the financial, accounting, marketing and operational functions, including human resource management, of an organization."[2] Business literacy is an important asset to any successful enterprise but it is particularly true in health care whose seemingly complex (and confusing) jargon, history, and constantly moving parts make it challenging for everyone. The call for establishing business literacy at all levels of clinical practice is relevant and urgent so that the resources (i.e., energy and time) needed to enhance patient and provider experiences can be focused on moving towards efficient value-based patient-centered care. But making this shift work in health care cannot be accomplished if only a few people in formal management roles can truly manage.

Aha!

Knowing how the business works makes your care better.

Dr. Diane Clark

Reasons Why *All* Physical Therapists Need Business Skills

Here is a list of the reasons why all physical therapists need business skills:

- You need to manage your patients *efficiently*. To do so, you need to know how the organization/business works or operates so you can be proficient, resourceful, and productive.
- You need to manage your patients *effectively* to achieve positive clinical outcomes (i.e., positive patient experiences) while contributing to the achievement of the established key performance indicators.
- You need to manage your patients cost-effectively by being an efficient fiscal steward of the organization's resources.
- You need financial literacy to understand how you contribute to and add value to the financial bottom line. This means you need an understanding of payment/reimbursement practices (i.e., coding, billing) and the revenue cycle management process.
- You need to contribute to continuously improving how the organization works to ensure the delivery of high-quality physical therapy services.
- You need to know how your compensation packages are calculated.
- You need to understand how you contribute to and fit within an organization's culture.
- You need to know business terminology (or business jargon) so you can advocate for your patients and your communities.
- You need to know yourself, how to innovate, create, and contribute to entrepreneurial or intrapreneurial initiatives.
- You need to know how to "sell" yourself (i.e., selling is a process of building relationships).
- Your need to understand how the market drivers influence the business of health care and physical therapy.
- By understanding how the business works, you can make better decisions, especially when change is needed.

Mini-Vignette

Why All Physical Therapists Need to Develop Business Literacy

We interviewed a number of physical therapy practice owners to capture their perspectives (responses) when answering the question, "Why do all physical therapists need to understand the business of physical therapy?" As you review responses 1–4, identify in the space provided below a few key ideas or reasons why it is important for you to develop business literacy as a physical therapist student.

___

___

___

___

Response 1: Dr. Ryan Wood, PT, DPT, MHA

Physical therapy *is* a business and if we want to thrive as an autonomous profession, if we want to grow income, if we want to be competitive in recruitment for future talent, we must realize that it's a business. We must be paid for the services that we are providing or for providing high-level, doctoral-level, expert services. It is critical, even as staff, to understand how much liability insurance costs, how much it costs to provide care, how much marketing really costs, even something as simple as having a Gmail account (i.e., did you know it's nearly $200 per email address for each person on the team to have an email address?). You don't have to know all the minute details if you're an employee but it's important to understand (and respect) that there are expenses incurred to run the business (and keep it running) or to understand how you get salary raises or how you can give back to the community (and why that matters). Understanding the business allows you to trust your employer better because you don't feel they are taking advantage of you; ultimately, you'll have greater satisfaction in your work.

Response 2: Dr. Fred Gilbert, PT, DPT

We have this idea in health care that we're just delivering services. All we do as a physical therapist is deliver services "one-on-one" with patients. But at the end of the day, we must talk about financing the business. You can't keep a private practice open; you can't keep a hospital running; you can't run a robust non-profit group or clinic if you don't have ways to keep the engine running. Thinking only about the clinical side is not enough; there's so much more that drives the business side. Productivity is such a nasty word, but we must talk about knowing your metrics, understanding what drives business, and understanding the different components that play into a successful practice and how you can influence these components to create good patient *and* provider experiences. Everyone needs a base-level understanding of the business so that you can have conversations, individually and collectively, around how to create those better experiences on both sides. As a clinician (as an integral part of "the team"), you need to understand the basics – how a business operates so that you can speak the same language as the people who run the business and *contribute* to these conversations to help that business to thrive. Otherwise you're never going to agree on a lot of important things that need to be discussed and managed (and the business might suffer as a result).

Response 3: Dr. Sandra Norby, PT, DPT

I recently had crucial conversations with a new graduate employee; these conversations affirmed why physical therapists need to understand the business of physical therapy. *All* staff (including new graduate physical therapists) see what is being billed for their visits but if they don't understand the process of contract negotiations (with health insurance providers), final contracted or average payments per visit and what it costs (i.e., expenses) to provide the setting in which they practice as physical therapists, they might *assume* that they should be paid better based on the revenue billed. New graduates may see a charge for one thing, but don't understand that our contracted rate (what we get paid) is less and that we expect some "write offs." I'm transparent with sharing information, which is both good and bad, but at least my employees know how many visits they're seeing.

For job satisfaction, it is important to understand what your market value is with regards to delivering professional services, especially within a business model that may still accept health insurance reimbursement. You need to understand what it means when the practice relies heavily on Medicare and Medicaid (i.e., in pediatrics), and understand how important it is to advocate for payment, which ultimately then helps your patients to get access to care.

Response 4: Dr. Barbara Tschoepe, PT, DPT, PhD, FAPTA

We must understand and appreciate that health care is a business ("the why"). You've chosen a field to support a business. But you've done it with an added excitement that you're making an impact on individuals' lives or on their communities' lives. You have opportunities that very few other businesses have. Going into this field thinking "I just want to help people and not worry about the business," is not enough. This naivete puts the profession in a (vulnerable) place of being responsive to *other people* who have the business mindset, who *will* direct where health care will go. Instead, *we* as the health professionals need to come up with the solutions for the future. We need to be the creative ones. We need to be the innovators. We need to look at all the new potential business models that are out there. We need to figure out how *to lead* these initiatives because the research (the evidence) is on our side. If we promote health, wellness, and mobility, we're going to have less pathology and we'll have less chronic disease.

Bottom Line!

It is *every* employee's responsibility to make the business succeed, but without the right knowledge base, employees aren't going to know which questions to ask, which marketplace or regulatory changes have meaning, and how they can best contribute.

What Is Business?

The term **business** refers to organizations or enterprising entities participating in activities related to producing, delivering, and/or exchanging goods, services, or something of value.[4] Businesses operate for commercial, industrial, or professional reasons – as for-profit or non-profit entities. Apple and Walmart are examples of commercial or for-profit businesses, while Habitat for Humanity, Red Cross, and United Way are examples of non-profit ones. There are many ways to form, describe, or categorize a business – by size, industry, type, structure, etc. These descriptors define "the business" formally, how it operates (i.e., legally and day-to-day), and what it does, accomplishes, or sells (i.e., goods or services exchanged).

Business is essential to a country's economy because businesses provide goods, services, and employment or opportunities to "earn a living." Businesses enable people (i.e., consumers) to access the goods and services that consumers want and need. Businesses contribute tax money to the government, which provides funding for many services (such as health care) provided by federal, state, and local governments.

Aha!

Health Care Is Financed by Business Activity

Health care in the United States is paid for by business activity. Business provides the wages, private health insurance (i.e., as an employment benefit), and the taxes that pay directly for or subsidize public health insurance (government) programs, such as Medicare and Medicaid.

Activity 3.1 What Businesses Do You Know?

Most likely you have interacted with numerous businesses for different reasons – either as a customer or consumer looking to purchase something (i.e., clothes) or seeking to experience "something," such as food (i.e., Starbuck's) or fun (i.e., Disney). You may have been an employee or a volunteer for a business.

Describe three different businesses with which you interact on a regular basis by answering the following questions.

Identify three different businesses with which you interact on a regular basis.

____

____

____

Why do you interact with them and how often?

____

____

In what ways are these three businesses the same?

____

____

____

In what ways are these three businesses different?

____

____

____

Business Fundamentals

A **market** exists whenever individuals and organizations become involved in buying, selling, or trading something of value. A market is a place where parties (i.e., buyers and sellers) get together to facilitate the exchange of goods and services.[5] A market may be physical where people meet face-to-face (i.e., a retail store or outlet), or virtual where there is no physical presence or contact between buyers and sellers (i.e., an online market, such as Amazon).[5] **Organizations** are open systems, which means that they affect and are affected by environments.[6] An organization is a social unit of people that is distinct, structured, and *managed* to pursue collective goals; all organizations have a "management structure." Management structures determine the relationships between different activities ("functions") and its members (i.e., employees), and subdivides and assigns roles, responsibilities, and decision-making authority to carry out different tasks at different levels.

The basic concepts and strategies needed to run an organization are referred to as **business fundamentals**. By fully comprehending how a business operates, you will have a better idea of how the different functions within a business relate to each other and how (and why) your activities and decisions impact the organization. Throughout this book, we discuss different business fundamentals and provide a variety of tools and approaches that may be used by physical therapists to achieve business success. We also provide examples of approaches or strategies that typically do *not* yield good results. By doing so, we hope to help you to develop your list of "what to do" and "what not to do" in learning how to manage the business side of your (clinical) practice effectively.

Activity 3.2 Assess Your Business Literacy

Like physical therapy, business has its own language or jargon. Employees, or team members, who can't speak the *language of business* can't help their companies to bridge the gap between ambition and performance. Take a few moments to briefly assess your (basic) business literacy by circling the best response for each sample statement listed below.

I can explain how an organization generates revenue.

Not at all *Somewhat* *Absolutely*

I can explain how an organization's operations are conducted (i.e., what they do day-to-day).

Not at all *Somewhat* *Absolutely*

I can identify relevant business drivers and how each driver impacts the business.

Not at all *Somewhat* *Absolutely*

I can explain the dynamic contexts (such as community, competitive, legal, and health policy) within which health systems operate.

Not at all *Somewhat* *Absolutely*

I can explain how marketing, public relations, and sales (functions) contribute to the financial success of an organization.

Not at all *Somewhat* *Absolutely*

I can explain financial and accounting information.

Not at all *Somewhat* *Absolutely*

I can explain how productivity is measured.

Not at all *Somewhat* *Absolutely*

I can prepare and manage a budget.

Not at all *Somewhat* *Absolutely*

I can explain the components of the human resources management (i.e., recruitment and selection, retention, job design and work systems (i.e., workflow), performance management, learning and development, and succession planning).

Not at all *Somewhat* *Absolutely*

I can explain basic employment law.

Not at all *Somewhat* *Absolutely*

I can explain the key components of a job description.

Not at all *Somewhat* *Absolutely*

I can explain (basic) compensation structures.

Not at all *Somewhat* *Absolutely*

I can explain employee benefits as a component of total compensation.

Not at all *Somewhat* *Absolutely*

Aha!

Creating and keeping a customer is *the purpose* of business.

Theodore Levitt[7]

Why a Business Needs Customers

A customer is a person (an individual) or a business that purchases another company's goods or services for their own use.[8] Customers are critical because they drive revenue; without revenue generated from customers, a business cannot maintain its existence. Typically, businesses compete with other companies to attract customers through creative advertising/marketing efforts, lower prices, or by developing unique products/services and experiences that customers seek out.

Aha!

Is It Customer or Consumer?

The terms "customer" and "consumer" may be used interchangeably, yet there is a slight difference between them. To clarify: **consumers** are defined as individuals (or businesses) that *consume* or use the goods and services, whereas **customers** are the *purchasers* (as a consumer or customer) within the economy that buy the goods and services.

Successful businesses must develop "systems" to ensure that their customers have a consistent and positive experience each time they interact with the business. To develop these systems, successful businesses must invest time and resources to understand their customers thoroughly. **Consumer behavior** is the study of individuals, groups, or organizations and all the activities associated with the purchase, use, and disposal of goods and services. By studying consumer behavior, businesses can launch effective strategies, such as marketing campaigns, to connect with and attract their customers. Grouping customers according to their demographic characteristics (i.e., age, race, gender, ethnicity, income level, and geographic location) is common; developing different customer profiles may help businesses to expand their understanding of their ideal or "target" customers (markets). Ultimately, gathering, analyzing, and using information helps companies to deepen existing customer relationships and reach untapped (potential) or newer consumer groups. This topic will be discussed further in chapter 8.

Activity 3.3 You as a Consumer: How Do You Make "Buying Decisions"?

Now it's your turn to discover factors that may influence your *buying behavior* as a consumer. Think of a certain product category (i.e., sporting goods) or service category (i.e., delivery services). Answer the following questions.

Think of a specific product or service category. What is the first brand that comes to mind, and why?

____

Regarding your product or service category, do you usually plan ahead (before purchasing) or decide (to purchase) only at the time of purchase?

____

Dick's Sporting Goods or Amazon Prime could be examples of a specific product or service within each category.

Now answer the next set of questions.

What do you do when buying something for the first time? Describe how you "shop"?

____

____

Who or what influences your purchase decision?

____

____

Think of a recent purchase. Insert the name of your product or service in the space provided:

____

What made you choose this particular product or service?

____

____

How likely is it that you would recommend this product or service to others and why?

____

____

What would you likely use as an alternative if this product or service was no longer available?

___

___

Look at the following questions.

What is the name of your favorite store or online shopping site? How often do you visit it?

___

How much time do you spend on average at this store/shopping site?

___

How often do you buy something when you visit your favorite store or online shopping site?

___

Activity 3.4 The Patient as the Consumer

Health care consumers and physical therapy patients "shop" and make their buying decisions in unique ways because of the complex nature surrounding the business of health care. Consider a new physical therapy patient when answering the following questions.

Describe how the new patient typically "shops"? How does "the patient" make their buying decisions?

___

___

Does the patient "shop" because of a need or a want (or does it depend)? Explain.

___

___

Describe how "shopping" as a patient is different from shopping as a non-patient (general consumer). Explain why patient buying behavior is different. (What factors influence this buying decision?)

____

____

Bottom Line!

Studying consumer behavior helps businesses to understand why people buy and use goods and services and how consumers' emotions, attitudes, and preferences affect their buying behavior. Understanding customers enables businesses to implement "systems" to generate positive customer experiences (i.e., patient experience), create effective marketing campaigns, deliver products and services that address needs and wants, and retain customers for repeat business.

Why Business Needs Management

Recall from chapter 1 when management was discussed in detail. In this chapter, it is important to understand why business needs management. Business management is the act of overseeing the organization by coordinating and ensuring the proper execution of various business activities. This requires managing different aspects (i.e., resources) of the business separately and collectively. Business management is a crucial part of an organization's success; management is required in all types of organizations (for-profit or non-profit) within all industries (i.e., health care), and when collective effort needs to be directed towards a shared purpose. Business managers are responsible for ensuring that the day-to-day operations run smoothly and that a business remains operational, profitable, and sustainable.

Bottom Line!

All businesses involve an array of different managerial tasks. When these are coordinated properly, and there is a strong management system in place, an organization can be extremely efficient in creating value through the production of its products, services, and overall workflow.

The Business of Health Care

Health care is a business. This statement may seem harsh or difficult to accept fully as a future health professional. You may still want to perceive health care mainly as a service (i.e., patient interaction) or as the *provision of care* needed to help another person to maintain or regain their health. You may *resist* accepting the notion that health care is a business. Yet the "service side" of health care cannot exist, or be cost-effective, if the very complex "business side" is not managed; both sides must co-exist to support each other. Recall Dr. Diane Clark's comment (from the management vignette at the beginning of the chapter) that "patient care and business are intertwined." The business side in health care must constantly coordinate and monitor numerous activities (i.e., workflow), sometimes "behind the scenes," to impact the many "bottom lines" that must be achieved at the end of each day. Cumulatively, these "bottom lines" directly affect the quality of patient care/outcomes (i.e., patient experience), provider experiences, revenues generated, compensation packages, and cost of services provided.

Activity 3.5 Health Care Is a Business: What Does This Mean to You?

Reflect on the following the statements listed in the below box.

> Health care is a business.
> Physical therapy is a business.

Journal your response(s) or reaction(s) to these statements. Describe what you are thinking, feeling, and how you are reacting. Are you resisting or accepting or both?

____

____

____

Recall when Dr. Diane Clark (in the management vignette at the beginning of the chapter) stated, "We perceive that the 'business side' projects negative perceptions about us as health professionals." Do you agree or disagree with this statement? Why?

____

____

Brainstorm the different "bottom lines" in the business of health care that need to be managed (i.e., in addition to the financial bottom line).

____

____

Activity 3.6 Physical Therapy Is a Business: Why Do We Resist?

Read and reflect on Dr. Barb Tschoepe's response (shown below) after she was asked the question: "When we talk about the business of physical therapy, there's usually resistance. Why do you think we resist this reality?"

> There are many reasons why we resist the notion (*and acceptance*) that physical therapy is a business. Some resistance stems from the lack of knowledge when entering this field without fully understanding or appreciating the responsibilities you have as a physical therapist practicing at a clinical doctoral level. It's the lack of understanding that physical therapy is more than just helping people. When the profession moved from the master's degree to the doctoral degree, we were hoping this would help physical therapists develop a sense of ownership and responsibility to "level the playing field" between us and other health professionals. I was hoping that when we earned the DPT degree, the prevalent "employee mentality" would be gone; we would no longer be (or want to be) "just employees." Rather, we would become more like our colleagues in accounting, law, medicine – disciplines that have established collaborative or contractual relationships with each other (i.e., as professional associates) to provide our unique expertise (and not just our technical or "hands-on" clinical skills).

As you reflect upon Dr. Barb Tschoepe's response, describe the reason(s) why physical therapists resist the business of physical therapy.

____

____

What does it mean to you that physical therapy is more than "just helping people"?

____

Health care in the United States is a formidable business or industry. The United States spends more on health care than any other country in the world. National Health Expenditures (NHE) data shows that NHE increased to $4.5 trillion in 2022 ($13,493 per person) and accounted for 17.3% of US gross domestic product (GDP).[9] Moreover, in 2022, Medicare spending increased to $944.3 billion (21% of total NHE); Medicaid increased to $805.7 billion (18% of total NHE); private health insurance increased to $1,289.8 billion (29% of total NHE) and out-of-pocket spending rose to $471.4 billion (11% of total NHE). Under the current law, the Centers for Medicare and Medicaid Services project that NHE will expand at an average annual rate of 5.6% (for the period 2025–2031), resulting in an increase in health spending as a share of GDP to 19.6% (in 2031).[9,10] From 2025–2031, Medicare, as a proportion of health expenditure among the major payors, is forecast to increase by an average annual rate of 7.8% per year, Medicaid by 5.6%, private health insurance by 5.2% (average), and out-of-pocket spending by 4.1% (average).[10]

Although numerous resources are invested in health care, its "return on investment" and sustainability continue to be challenged. The US health care system is described as being average in quality, high in cost, and unequal in access.[11] A survey of the health care systems of 11 developed countries found the US health care system to be the most expensive and worst-performing in terms of health access, efficiency, and equity.[12] Specifically, the United States ranked 11th (bottom) in health care access and quality within this pool of 11 countries.[12] Consequently, there is an urgent and ongoing call for health care reform (change), improvement, and innovation. High costs limit Americans from accessing quality health care. Factors contributing to the rise in health care costs include the cost of new technologies and prescription drugs; the rise of chronic diseases/health problems, including obesity; aging populations and increased longevity; and high administrative costs. Like most businesses, the challenge in health care is to find that critical equilibrium of providing the highest quality of service at the lowest cost.

Health care involves many parties or stakeholders attempting to work together despite sometimes, competing goals. Moreover, change within health care is a constant phenomenon. Finding the right balance in health care, as it evolves continuously, to provide the highest quality service at the lowest cost – efficiently and effectively – is a daunting, complex mix of challenges with ever-emerging consequences. Four specific trends are introduced briefly in this chapter to illustrate how these evolving drivers or changes in health care ultimately influence business and subsequently management practices. These trends include (1) the evolution of the Triple Aim to the Quintuple Aim for optimizing health system performance; (2) the shift from volume-based care to value-based care; (3) the changing role of the health care consumer; and (4) the evolving impact of technology. Additional drivers are discussed in chapter 8.

Trend 1: Evolution of the Triple Aim to the Quintuple Aim for optimizing health system performance

The Triple Aim framework, developed by the Institute for Healthcare Improvement, described an approach to enhance the business of health care by optimizing health system performance.[13] This original three-pronged approach promoted the development and implementation of new strategies simultaneously to: (1) enhance the patient experience of care (including quality and satisfaction); (2) improve the health of populations (not just one person at a time); and (3) reduce the per capita cost of health care.[13] From a business perspective, making progress in these specific areas meant that management had to deploy different and more nimble management strategies. Moreover, the presence of persistent burnout (experienced), and dissatisfaction (reported) by members of the health care workforce/team (i.e., physicians, nurses, physical therapists, staff, etc.) called for management to improve the provider experience (not just patient experience). This action (or need) changed the original Triple Aim framework to the Quadruple Aim.[14] Moreover, adding this fourth goal called for management to improve the "work life" (i.e., provider experience) to ensure positive workforce engagement as critical for *improving population health* also (which is now explicitly part of the Quintuple Aim).[15]

Trend 2: Shift from Volume-Based Care to Value-Based Care

The shift from a volume-based care model (i.e., fee-for-service payment models) to one focused on the value of care received by patients is another significant trend impacting the business of health care. This shift is in response to rising costs and ongoing legislative mandates (i.e., Affordable Care Act, Medicare Reform). **Value** is defined as "the outcomes that patients experience relative to the cost of delivering those outcomes."[16] Value-based health care is defined as "health care that delivers the best possible outcomes to patients for the lowest possible cost."[17] Value-based care is an industry-wide strategy to improve population health and reduce the total cost of care. This shift requires two simultaneous transformations in health care:[18]

- *Care model transformation*: Redesign care delivery model(s) to focus on prevention, primary care, chronic disease management, and high-quality, low-cost episodes of specialty care.
- *Payment transformation*: Redesign payment/reimbursement model(s) to focus on paying for the quality and appropriateness of care.[18]

Trend 3: The Changing Role of the Health Care Consumer

The role of the health care consumer is changing. **Consumer-directed health care** is based on the notion that health care services are *overutilized*, and that giving financial incentives to patients will reduce the use of services that are perceived as marginal or as having no value.[19] Incentives may also encourage patients to seek out lower-cost providers of care (i.e., primary care instead of specialty care or alternative care). Typical consumer-driven health care models combine a high-deductible health insurance plan (i.e., $3,500 per annum per person) with a health reimbursement account to cover part of the out-of-pocket health care expenses (such as co-pays). Given that consumer-driven health plans are continuing to grow in popularity in the country, it is important to realize that the intent of these plans is to increase patient control, market competition, quality, and lower health care costs. These changes will (hopefully) improve patient health (outcomes) due to improved service ("patient experiences"), improved patient autonomy and self-management of regimens, and better overall health awareness. Moreover, due to improved access to information and technology, health care consumers who are "connected" are demanding seamless and more personalized or individualized experiences. These demands push the health care industry to enhance convenience while simplifying access to prescriptions, medical reimbursement, primary care, and reimagined patient experiences.[20]

Trend 4: The Evolving Impact of Technology

In addition to consumer-driven health care trends, technology has been changing the delivery and management of health care, and the ways in which patients engage in their health care. The use of telemedicine, which accelerated during the COVID-19 pandemic, provided support and access for patients in underserved parts of the country or health care deserts across the United States. Automation and strategic use of artificial intelligence has the potential to decrease administrative overhead costs (for providers and health systems) and streamline processes both before and after care.[20,21] Technology deployed in certain ways can provide patients with self-service options for routine actions such as scheduling and managing appointments, requesting referrals, refilling prescriptions, reviewing bills, and making payments. A 2022 US survey found that 81% of respondents believed that the ability to schedule health care appointments online would make the scheduling process much easier, while more than three-quarters of Americans want the ability to use technology when managing their health care experience. This means that patients will use their smartphones to make or reschedule appointments or to get clarification on test results when it is convenient for them.[22]

While there are numerous other market drivers or macro- and micro-trends relentlessly influencing the health care industry, hopefully by now you are starting to understand that the ever-evolving and constantly changing complex business of health care demands a fundamental understanding of how things "work" from a business perspective, and innovation and creativity to manage, address, and continue to solve many of its deeply rooted challenges. Executing effective health care reform requires greater business literacy at all levels of clinical practice to make sustainable change happen.

Bottom Line!

Value is defined by people who choose to pay (for something). Value is not determined by the managers who established the price.

Simon Sinek[1]

The Business of Physical Therapy

Physical therapy is a business, and the business or industry of physical therapy is competitive.[23,24] Generalist and specialist providers address a wide range of consumer needs (i.e., orthopedic, sports-related, pediatric, cardiovascular, neurological, and geriatric, etc.); over 240,820 physical therapists and 104,000 physical therapist assistants are employed in the United States.[25,26] The size of the physical therapy market is estimated at $56 billion and is expected to grow annually by approximately 3% (through 2024).[27] Market drivers for physical therapy indicate that the market (demand) will continue to grow. Some of the market drivers include: the aging American population; people's increasing desire to live an active lifestyle longer in life; ongoing sports injuries; joint replacement surgeries; rising obesity levels; outpatient and rehabilitation services' compelling care benefits (i.e., "economic value") and cost advantages; and easier patient access to treatment (i.e., direct access).[27]

The market demand for physical therapy in the United States is met by a "fragmented collection of providers,"[27] including diverse health systems (all sizes), an estimated 18,000 outpatient physical therapy clinics, and a few national companies.[27,28] This industry consists predominantly of small- to medium-sized regional providers (with annual revenue of slightly over $1 million per clinic), and with the 50 largest competitors comprising less than 25% of the total market.[27,28] Physician-owned physical therapy practices comprise an estimated 10%–15% of all physical therapy clinics. Nine out of the top 12 outpatient companies are backed by private equity.[25,27] Industry consolidation is occurring through mergers and acquisitions (backed by private equity firms) as the largest players (i.e., Upstream Rehabilitation) strive to gain greater market share to improve profit margins.[27,28]

In addition to the trends discussed above, other trends impacting the business of physical therapy include the following:

- More than 80% of physical therapy clinics are using some type of electronic medical record (EMR) system/platform allowing physical therapists to document in a more cost-efficient manner.[27,28]

- Physical therapists continue to experience (sometimes arbitrary and drastic) reform-driven cuts to their payment rates (i.e., Medicare), many of which are aligned with significant regulatory changes.
- Practices are looking at alternative methods or ways to diversify revenue generation, including wellness and other cash-based programs (out-of-network), to combat the continual decline of health insurance reimbursement.
- Physical therapists can enroll in the Merit-based Incentive Payment System (MIPS) for (Medicare) physical therapy billing. (MIPS is a value-based payment model, or rather a payment adjustment system based on quality data, to impact PTs.[29] The goal of this program is to decrease the cost of care while increasing quality.)
- Integrated health systems are referring/keeping patients within their systems or provider networks making it harder for privately owned physical therapist practices to rely primarily on physician referrals.
- Direct access, social media marketing, and digital patient engagement tools are strategies used in the business of physical therapy to maintain or increase patient caseloads and subsequent revenue streams.[25,26]

Aha!

Market Trend: "Wage Compression" in Physical Therapy

Wage compression is a trend impacting business and management practices in physical therapy. Wage or salary compression occurs when there is not much difference in pay among employees regardless of the differences in their respective knowledge (i.e., degree), skills, experience, or abilities.[30] Candidate or applicant supply and demand is a leading cause of pay compression. For example, when a manager is hiring for a position with a low supply of and a high demand for qualified applicants, they might be forced to offer higher salaries to convince talent to work for them instead of their competitors.[31]

Dr. Sandra Norby offers some sage advice for new graduates to consider:

> New grads are earning an estimated $85,000 as their starting salary (national average; estimates vary from state-to-state) but then the salary cap ranges between $101,000– $110,000. Salary or wage compression is a reality. There is not a lot of movement or room to grow income based on experience. The expectation of getting a 3%–5% raise year after year over a career spanning 35 years is no longer realistic. New grads might

want to consider asking for other things (such as benefits) that aren't tied directly to monetary compensation to grow their total earnings. It's also important for new grads to bring their own value to the practice/business as well. New grads need to understand that their starting salaries are higher (driven by market forces) but that does not mean they will get a raise every year. It's important for new grads to understand that opportunities for growth may have to do with their own ability (beyond taking care of their current patients) to add their own unique value to their organization.

Physical Therapy: Estimating Its Economic Value

A report entitled "The Economic Value of Physical Therapy in the United States" published by APTA shows how improvements gained from physical therapy can lead to economic benefits.[32] This report integrates reviews of clinical research, health economics modeling, and subject matter expertise. Studying health economics allows for a rigorous and systematic examination of the problems faced in promoting health more broadly.[33] By applying economic theories of consumer, producer, and social choice, health economics aims to understand the behavior of individuals, health care providers, public and private organizations, and governments in decision-making.[32] APTA's report attempts to quantify physical therapy's potential to deliver true economic value to patients, the US health care system, and society. Eight conditions were studied in which physical therapists and physical therapist assistants can play a key role to demonstrating how physical therapy could save the health care system millions of dollars annually. It is worth mentioning that in every case studied, the use of physical therapy was associated with a net economic benefit to the health system compared with alternative types of care.

Tool

APTA's report[32] can be accessed here: https://www.valueofpt.com/

This book and its contents apply to all physical therapists. This resource will help you to develop your business literacy and a basic set of business skills. It will also prepare you for excellence in management whether you own your own business (practice) or not. Before moving on to chapter 4, take a few moments to see if you can "talk the talk" – of business – by completing activity 3.7 to test your new business knowledge. Good luck!

Activity 3.7 Matching Business Terminology with Definitions

Review the chapter keywords from chapters 1–3 (listed in column 1) and the definitions provided (listed in column 3). In column 2, "match" the appropriate definition to the appropriate keyword by placing the letter (i.e., a, b, etc.) in this column.

Table 3.1 Understanding Business Jargon

Column 1	*Column 2*	*Column 3*
Chapter Keyword	"*Match*" (Place the letter in this column to match the correct definition (column 3) to the correct keyword (column 1)	*Definitions*
1. Change readiness		a. Costs (time and resources) spent on documentation and administrative tasks associated with applying for, receiving, and participating in (publicly funded) health insurance programs.
2. Practice management		b. Process whereby you make changes to your own thinking, emotions, and behavior.
3. Business literacy		c. Coordinating and guiding human, financial, and other resources to ensure that organizational goals can be achieved.
4. Learning organization		d. Selectively aware or concentrating on "something" to the exclusion of other things.
5. Administrative burden		e. Attempt to capture how improvements gained from physical therapy can lead to fiscal benefits.
6. Self-management		f. Administrative practices in physical therapy that include all areas and responsibilities of management.
7. Economic value of physical therapy		g. State of mind; connecting beliefs, perceptions, and intentions regarding the need for change and the awareness of your ability to make the change successfully.

(*Continued*)

Table 3.1 (Continued)

Column 1	*Column 2*	*Column 3*
8. Focus		h. Create, acquire, and transfer knowledge, and modify its behavior to reflect new knowledge and insights.
9. Management		i. System designed to delineate and guide how specific activities (i.e., work) are directed, aligned, and focused to achieve the organization's goals efficiently.
10. Organizational structure		j. Having the knowledge and understanding of the financial, accounting, marketing and operational functions, including human resources. Management of an organization.

Suggested Readings

Gerber ME. *The E-Myth Physician: Why Most Medical Practices Don't Work and What to Do About It*. Harper Business; 2004.

Herzlinger R. *Who Killed Health Care?: America's $2 Trillion Medical Problem – And the Consumer-Driven Cure*. McGraw Hill; 2007.

Makary M. *The Price We Pay: What Broke American Health Care – And How to Fix It*. Bloomsbury Publishing; 2021.

References

1. Sinek S. *Start With Why: How Great Leaders Inspire Everyone to Take Action*. Portfolio; 2009.
2. Janati A, Hasanpoor E, Hajebrahimi S, Sadeghi-Bazargani H, Khezri A. An evidence-based framework for evidence-based management in healthcare organizations: A Delphi study. *Ethiop J Health Sci*. 2018 May; 28(3): 305–314. doi:10.4314/ejhs.v28i3.8
3. Berman, K. The building blocks of business literacy. *Train Dev*. 1998; 52(9): 16–18.
4. Hayes, A. What is a business? Understanding different types and company sizes. Investopedia. Updated February 29, 2024. Accessed March 14, 2024. https://www.investopedia.com/terms/b/business.asp
5. Kenton, W. Market: What it means in economics, types, and common features. Investopedia. Updated September 30, 2023. Accessed March 14, 2024. https://www.investopedia.com/terms/m/market.asp
6. Woodward, SN. Business organization. Britannica Money. November 9, 2022. Accessed March 14, 2024. https://www.britannica.com/money/business-organization
7. Levitt, T. *The Marketing Imagination*. Free Press; 1983.
8. Kenton, W. Customer: Definition and how to study their behavior for marketing. Investopedia. Updated June 14, 2023. Accessed March 14, 2024. https://www.investopedia.

com/terms/c/customer.asp#:~:text=Key%20Takeaways,to%20improve%20service%20and%20products

9. NHE fact sheet. Centers for Medicare & Medicaid Services. Updated December 13, 2023. Accessed February 29, 2024. https://www.cms.gov/data-research/statistics-trends-and-reports/national-health-expenditure-data/nhe-fact-sheet#:~:text=Historical%20NHE%2C%202022%3A,18%20percent%20of%20total%20NHE
10. National health expenditure projections 2022–2031 forecast summary. Centers for Medicare & Medicaid Services. Accessed March 14, 2024. https://www.cms.gov/files/document/nhe-projections-forecast-summary.pdf
11. Shi L, Singh DA. *Essentials of the U.S. Health Care System.* 6th ed. Jones & Bartlett Learning; 2023.
12. Schneider EC, Shah A, Doty MM, Tikkanen R, Fields K, Williams RD. Mirror, mirror 2021: Reflecting poorly: Health care in the U.S. compared to other high-income countries. The Commonwealth Fund. August 4, 2021. Accessed March 14, 2024. https://www.commonwealthfund.org/publications/fund-reports/2021/aug/mirror-mirror-2021-reflecting-poorly
13. Berwick DM, Nolan TW, Whittington J. The Triple Aim: Care, health, and cost. *Health Aff.* 2008 May/June; 27(3): 759–769. doi:10.1377/hlthaff.27.3.759
14. Triple Aim and population health. Institute for Healthcare Improvement. Accessed March 14, 2024. https://www.ihi.org/improvement-areas/triple-aim-population-health
15. Mate, K. On the Quintuple Aim: Why expand beyond the Triple Aim? Institute for Healthcare Improvement. February 4, 2022. Accessed March 14, 2024. https://www.ihi.org/insights/quintuple-aim-why-expand-beyond-triple-aim
16. Porter, ME. What is value in health care? *N Eng J Med.* 2010; 363(26): 2477–2481. doi:10.1056/NEJMp1011024
17. Lewis C, Horstman C, Blumenthal D, Abrams MK. Value-based care: What it is, and why it's needed. The Commonwealth Fund. February 7, 2023. https://www.commonwealthfund.org/publications/explainer/2023/feb/value-based-care-what-it-is-why-its-needed
18. Advisory Board. Value-based care. Accessed March 14, 2024. https://www.advisory.com/featured/value-based-care?utm_source=google&utm_medium=cpc&utm_campaign=nb&utm_content=vbc&gad_source=1&gclid=Cj0KCQjwncWvBhD_ARIsAEb2HW-zqBvysi4wCsK9oZvQ-IbzpNKrE0XH6LoyQNSZ4g4EgdM4mYbQ0bAaAtt5EALw_wcB&gclsrc=aw.ds
19. Davis K. Consumer-directed health care: Will it improve health system performance? *Health Serv Res*. 2004 Aug.; 39(4 Pt 2): 1219–1234. doi: 10.1111/j.1475–6773.2004.00284.x
20. Patient experience: Five ways to improve patient interactions. NICE. Accessed March 14, 2024. https://get.nice.com/rs/069-KVM-666/images/0146647_eBook-Five-Ways-To-Improve-Patient-Interactions-2023.pdf
21. Tollen L, Keating E, Weil A. Health affairs: How administrative spending contributes to excess US health spending. February 20, 2020. Accessed March 14, 2024. https://www.healthaffairs.org/content/forefront/administrative-spending-contributes-excess-us-health-spending
22. New data finds 69% of Americans would consider switching healthcare providers for more "appealing" services: Same-day appointments top the list. Businesswire. February 15, 2022. Accessed March 14, 2024. https://www.businesswire.com/news/home/20220215005224/en/New-Data-Finds-69-of-Americans-Would-

Consider-Switching-Healthcare-Providers-for-More-%E2%80%9CAppealing%E2%80%9D-Services-%E2%80%93-Same-Day-Appointments-Top-the-List

23. Marketdata LLC. Physical therapy practice for sale – must read industry report. Vetted Biz. Updated May 14, 2024. https://www.vettedbiz.com/physical-therapy-business-trends/
24. Physical therapists in the US: Market size (2004–2029). IBIS World. Updated January 24, 2024. https://www.ibisworld.com/industry-statistics/market-size/physical-therapists-united-states/
25. Occupational employment and wages, May 2023: 29–1123 physical therapists. US Bureau of Labor Statistics. Accessed June 1, 2024. https://www.bls.gov/oes/currenT/oes291123.htm
26. Occupational employment and wages, May 2023: 31–2021 physical therapist assistants. US Bureau of Labor Statistics. Accessed June 1, 2024. https://www.bls.gov/oes/current/oes312021.htm
27. Physical therapy market overview. Harris Williams. July 13, 2022. https://www.harriswilliams.com/our-insights/hcls-physical-therapy-market-overview
28. Physical therapy market and valuation multiples. Health Value Group. March 1, 2021. https://healthvaluegroup.com/physical-therapy-market-and-valuation-multiples/
29. MERIT-based incentive program. American Physical Therapy Association. Accessed March 14, 2024. https://www.apta.org/your-practice/payment/value-based-payment-models/quality-payment-program/merit-based-incentive-program
30. Pay compression: What it is and how to fight it. Insperity Accessed March 14, 2024. https://www.insperity.com/blog/pay-compression/
31. Shuster L. What every employer needs to know about pay compression. *Forbes*. March 17, 2023. Accessed March 14, 2024. https://www.forbes.com/sites/forbeshumanresourcescouncil/2023/03/17/what-every-employer-needs-to-know-about-pay-compression/?sh=10c52f093971
32. The economic value of physical therapy in the United States. American Physical Therapy Association. September 2023. Accessed March 3, 2024. https://www.valueofpt.com/
33. What is health economics. Johns Hopkins Bloomberg School of Health. Accessed March 14, 2024. https://publichealth.jhu.edu/academics/academic-program-finder/masters-degrees/master-of-health-science-in-global-health-economics/what-is-health-economics

Unit 2

Introduction

In this second unit, individuals learning to manage will dive more deeply to discover that management means managing multiple "moving parts" (i.e., functions) simultaneously, separately, or strategically, and in multiple directions – down, up, across, diagonally, and out. The five chapters comprising unit 2 are:

- Chapter 4: "Creating Culture and Why It Matters"
- Chapter 5: "Purpose-Driven Operations Management"
- Chapter 6: "Managing People (Human Resources Management)"
- Chapter 7: "Managing the Financial Bottom Line (Financial Management)"
- Chapter 8: "Marketing a Physical Therapy Practice (Marketing Management)"

As you submerge into learning about the "nuts and bolts" of managerial work and the different functions (such as operations management, human resources management) that must be managed to achieve efficient and effective organizational performance and successful patient/client outcomes, think about how you can add value to these processes (or functions) through applying your self-management and business literacy skills. Learning about these common organizational functions (or components of managerial work) in more detail will expand your business literacy and your understanding of the dynamic, ever-changing (sometimes behind-the-scenes) "moving parts" that must be coordinated, adapted, and realigned as needed. Remember, you can use this knowledge throughout your career in many ways to excel even if you are not in a formal management role.

DOI: 10.4324/9781003524250-5

4 Creating Culture and Why It Matters

Jennifer E. Green-Wilson

A culture is strong when people work with each other, for each other. A culture is weak when people work against each other, for themselves.

Simon Sinek, author and inspirational speaker on business leadership (posted with permission)

Chapter Objectives

1. Describe organizational culture.
2. Discuss the role of subcultures and microcultures in shaping organizational cultures.
3. Distinguish between organizational culture, organizational climate, and organization health.
4. Describe the key elements of a positive work climate/culture.
5. Examine characteristics of negative or toxic work cultures.
6. Discuss management strategies for developing and supporting positive organizational cultures.

Management Vignette

Steve Foster, PT, LAL

Foundational to our culture is our commitment to private practice and a partnership model. I originally started my private practice with a partner and we were committed to ensuring that we retained the ownership ourselves, without any outside influence. There was a lot of pressure (there still is) from physicians to form joint ventures with them or to come into their offices to provide services so they that could gain income from physical therapy. We didn't feel that was the ethical way to practice. Even when I started TherapySouth 17 years ago, we were committed to truly being a private practice regardless of the reimbursement or political situations in our profession.

DOI: 10.4324/9781003524250-6

Our culture is unique in that we were intentional about developing core values. We place our core values on a big board in all our clinics, they are on our website, and we put them in front of each other. I have a plaque that sits on my desk to remind me of our core values. We put them in front of ourselves as a constant reminder of what they are and who we are. Faith is a central part of our core values. This gives us a commonality of purpose for what we do that to some degree is bigger than just providing physical therapy services. We are always assessing if we are living up to our values. Our "service day" is an example of how we "live" our values. It's about *being in the community.* About two years ago, we set up a clinic in an underserved community to serve people who are uninsured or underinsured. When we go to this community, we help with yard work, the food pantry, and work with a private school; it's about *being* in the community.

It is challenging to maintain that same culture as you grow. When we had only one or two clinics, our culture had more of a "family feel"; we still want to think we have that but it's difficult to have a "family feel" when you've got 41 clinics in three different states. But there's a definite commonality of purpose. Leadership is important even though everyone can contribute to the culture.

As our organization has grown, our culture has certainly evolved, and in some ways, it's been strengthened because more people have contributed to it. I don't ever want to feel like I've got all the "magic answers" to culture or "for making it all happen." It's important to learn to listen – that's key. Our leadership has been good at listening to our people and adjusting our culture to what we're hearing. Things are different now within the workforce – how people look at their work/life balance and things like burnout. We must understand the mindset of the next generation of workers and try to accommodate that in what we can do.

Perseverance is one aspect of our organizational culture of which I am most proud. We've persevered when our referral sources have opened their own practices, when reimbursement has become more challenging (as it does every year), and by providing therapists with competitive salaries and good continuing education opportunities. We feel like we invest in our people even when we get paid less and less for what we do.

Organizational culture is the single most important predictor of business success. You must have alignment with(in) your leadership team and then this filters down to your staff. You must have commitment to your core values and to your culture to be able to survive when those difficult times come along. When you have cohesion throughout your culture, then you're not thinking alike to the point where everybody is just marching to the same drum. However, there is such thing as *creative conflict.* Creative conflict is when you're working through a problem and people come to things from a different vantage point and through that you can craft a *creative* answer to whatever challenge you're facing. If foundationally your culture aligns, then this process works much better.

Chapter Introduction

Understanding culture will help you to thrive purposefully within different environments (i.e., organizations). That's why it is so important for you to try to gain a perspective of the culture of an organization *before* you decide to become part of it. Culture carries *meaning*. An organization's culture offers a shared perspective of the social system – of "what is" but also "the why" behind the "what." Culture represents "the story" in which people experience the organization, and the values, symbols, and routines that reinforce this narrative. It also focuses attention on the important "things" (i.e., symbols, jargon) and the need to understand them. Culture promotes and reinforces *the way*, or the patterns of thinking and behaving that are acceptable, adapted, and reinforced over time. The purpose of this chapter is to frame a broad discussion of organizations from the lens of understanding their culture and why it matters. Through this discussion, you can learn how to apply your management (i.e., self-management) skills successfully.

What Is Organizational Culture?

People, especially those in management roles, talk about **organizational culture** and the need for changing it.[1,2] Definitions and perceptions of organizational culture may range from "It's the way we do things here"[1,2,3] to Edgar Schein's frequently referenced definition of culture, which states that culture is

> a pattern of shared basic assumptions that have been invented, discovered or developed by a given group as it learns to cope with its problems of external adaptation and internal integration … that has worked well enough to be considered valid and therefore to be taught to new members as the correct way to perceive, think and feel in relationship to those problems.[4]

Others may describe company culture in terms of an essential feature, such as being "innovative," "performance-based," "customer-friendly," or "traditional."

Each organization has a "dominant culture" or an overarching unique way in which it lives out its purpose and delivers on its brand promise to customers.[3] A strong organizational culture functions as a differentiator in the marketplace.[3] Recall from Steve Foster's management vignette (at the beginning of this chapter) when he emphasizes how important the partners' core values are to shaping the culture at TherapySouth. Managers play a role in nurturing the preferred or dominant culture through their actions (i.e., how they set priorities, offer guidance to employees, and communicate with teams) and through leading by example or modeling the ideal culture through their own behavior (i.e., how they "walk the talk"); see box 4.1 for Steve Foster's reflections on his role as the practice owner and CEO in developing and influencing the culture at TherapySouth (see too the management vignette at the beginning of the chapter).

Box 4.1 Steve Foster's Role at TherapySouth

My role as a founding partner and now as the CEO is pretty important. Creating our core values was a collective effort, but I've got to be the catalyst. People are certainly going to be watching what I do more than what I say. Basically, it's important that I lead by example. My work ethic is going to be reflected upon by the staff. If you're in management, you're certainly being watched by those that you supervise. You don't always have to be the first person in and the last person out, but you must carry your load. Working hard has never been a challenge for me. You must work (at least) as hard as your staff *and* you must be empathetic to the people you lead. You've got to *be* a leader. What they can't see is a leader who's coming in late, leaving early, and "dumping their workload" on them.

"Culture" is implied, invisible, and symbolic; it guides and shapes an organization. An organization's culture can be inferred from behaviors, conversations, words, images, clothes, artefacts, traditions/customs, artwork, decision-making practices, and other patterns noted within a defined group of people (i.e., a social system). The collective attributes of an organization's culture may include shared beliefs, values, norms of behavior, routines, traditions, sense-making, and perspectives; these shared dimensions tend to permeate throughout the organization. Culture results from the many dynamic interconnections and relationships within an organization. Organizational culture tends to drive collective interpretations, thinking, and perspectives of events that occur. The people in an organization perceive or view, understand, interpret, and make sense of the world around them in different ways or through different lenses. Managers who take time to understand these different viewpoints may gain greater insight into how/why performance happens (or not).

Activity 4.1 Can You Describe the Culture of an Organization?

Pick an organization with which you are associated. You can pick your current university or college or an organization for which you work (or have worked). Based on your experiences, try to describe its organizational culture using the following prompts.

Is the organization's culture formal or informal? Describe the behaviors (i.e., daily interactions with people), conversations, and/or methods of communication you have experienced. Is there a dress code? If so, what is it?

How are decisions made? Top-down or bottom-up, or "it depends?" Describe.

Does the organization have certain traditions/customs? If so, describe.

Does the organization "walk the talk"? Live its values? (You may need to research its values if they are not posted for you or others to observe.)

Consider the organization's brand image or branding. Does it use/emphasize certain colors, designs, images, and/or taglines?

Which words would you use to describe its culture? (i.e., friendly, reserved, chaotic, innovative, fun?) Consider why (i.e., describe what you "see" or perceive about this organization's culture).

Organizational Culture Impacts Performance

Employees and teams who align well with their company culture perform consistently higher on internal performance metrics than those who align the least.[3] Culture can improve the key performance goals of an organization.[3] To gain the benefits of a strong company culture, managers must correctly identify, assess/measure, and regularly monitor both their organization's culture and its relationship to the company's key performance metrics.

Activity 4.2 In What Work Environment Do You (Will You) Thrive the Most?

A company's culture can impact your work experience tremendously.[5] Organizational culture affects all aspects of the workplace, including your own performance and work style. Take a few moments to consider your preferred work style and in what kind of work environment you can thrive. Review the list below to identify the top three or four characteristics of your ideal work environment.

I work best in an environment that has/is (select from the following possible characteristics):

1. Freedom from control, supervision (i.e., no micromanagement), specific details and restrictive rules
2. Innovative and futuristic-oriented
3. Work that is non-routine
4. Opportunity for interaction with people
5. Safety to share ideas or viewpoints
6. Stable and predictable
7. Often allows time to change
8. Long-lasting work relationships; minimal turnover
9. Little conflict between people
10. Work that is specialized
11. Private office or work area

List your selections in the space provided. Feel free to add your own ideas to expand the list of possible characteristics.

____

____

____

____

____

Now select two or three characteristics (from the list above) that would cramp your work style or your ability to thrive (i.e., perform well).

____

____

___

___

___

When researching a company, make sure you understand its corporate culture (what it is) and whether it is an environment in which you can thrive (or one in which you won't). In box 4.2, Steve Foster offers some sage advice for physical therapist graduates when considering (assessing) different organizational cultures.

Box 4.2 Things to Consider about Organizational Culture before Joining a Team

Before joining a firm you might ask a potential employer, "What is your company culture? What are your company core values?" If they don't have an answer to those questions, then that tells you a lot. If they do, then listen to see if their response matches up with the culture that you want to work in and the core values that you may or may not share with that employer. I would suggest asking for a "working interview" and an opportunity to observe the clinic so that you can observe the patient population you'd be treating and interview or have conversations with the other therapists with whom you'd be working. It's easy to put words on a piece of paper but if you don't have an opportunity to see them in practice then you don't really know that those words are being lived.

Cultures are different and some can be fragmented. Identifying cultures can be difficult in some organizations. In a larger corporation, you may have one division that has a set of core values or a particular culture, while another division may have a different culture. They don't always match and there can be conflict between the two entities just within the same company. When larger corporations answer to Wall Street, that's a difficult situation because at the end of the day the CEO of that company answers to the stockholders. They are not answering to patients or to the individual physical therapists. In this case, the CEO is being judged on their competency, their position, and by what the stock price is today. That situation makes it difficult to put patients or employees or quality care first. I'm not saying it can't be done; I'm sure it can be done, but it leads to decisions that may be detrimental to the practice or to patients when productivity becomes the measure of that. This is when you may get into situations where burnout is greater, when people are working for these large corporations and seeing 20–25 patients a day; that's not sustainable.

Subcultures and Microcultures: Is There a Need for Alignment?

Not everyone is *the same* in an organizational culture; not everyone thinks the same, nor do people perform their work in the exact same way. Therefore, it makes sense that when groups of people operate independently or interdependently these groups may develop their own cultural variations. **Subcultures** form when "something" develops or emerges about a team or group that is distinctly different.[6,7] Location (i.e., geography), job function, age (i.e., different generations), work patterns, and management styles are some of the factors that could influence the development of subcultures. Local or regional teams may develop their own work habits or best practices in response to the conditions of the local environment. Certain job functions may produce unique subcultures based on specific work responsibilities and priorities (i.e., physical therapists may work in different ways compared to nurses in an acute care setting; hybrid or remote teams may work differently than non-remote teams). Managers who use certain management styles will foster different (team) subcultures depending on how they approach collaboration, adapt to change, set priorities, and share information. Subcultures can also emerge for less predictable reasons. For instance, a team that socializes or plays pickleball together outside of work might develop its own local subculture. Even though the existence of subcultures may seem like a potential challenge for managers, they are not always negative. Subcultures can co-exist well within a dominant culture for many positive reasons; they can make things better for the collective organization by creating a sense of purpose, a feeling of belonging, and cohesion within different subgroups of employees.[7]

Aha!

Subcultures

Managers need to be aware that subcultures exist, and that they are not always negative.

Another way to understand subcultures within organizations is by defining or viewing them as **microcultures**. From this perspective, introducing and nurturing microcultures in the workplace may be valuable. A majority (nearly 80%) of employees want to work for an organization where they feel connected to the purpose and the people.[8] Like subcultures, workplace microcultures form – formally or informally – when employees with common identities, challenges, interests, or job functions define, gather, and share their common experience(s) at work (and perhaps in life). Microcultures can also form organically with people/employees who don't work together but somehow connect on some (other deeper) level. For these reasons, microcultures may provide ways for employees to be more connected, feel included or belong better in the company's dominant culture. Worth noting, perceptions of *connectedness* drive retention; nearly three out of five employees would consider leaving their job if they didn't feel connected at work.[8] Therefore, when managers learn about and from microcultures, they might be able to connect better with their employees/team members.

Aha!

Positive and Supportive Organizational Cultures Matter

Companies with a positive and supportive organizational culture often have high workplace morale and highly engaged, motivated, and productive employees.

What Happens When Subcultures Become a Management Challenge?

Subcultures within organizations may become a challenge for managers if they evolve into a *counterculture* or a subculture whose values and standards of behavior differ substantially from (or completely opposite to) those of the dominant culture. Subcultures are dynamic, yet if members of a subset feel undervalued, misunderstood, or under constant scrutiny, they may resist doing things in certain ways. Changes in internal policies, communications, or management may trigger overt or covert resistance from subcultures. Resistance reduces alignment between the dominant culture and the subculture, causing problems in the long term, such as lower productivity levels or employee turnover.[7]

Bottom Line!

The culture of a company is the sum of the behaviors of all its people.

Michael Kouly, author, speaker, educator, strategy advisor, and CEO

What Is Organizational Climate?

Organizational climate can affect productivity, motivation, and employee behavior – positively or negatively.[2] Organizational climate is different from organizational culture, although these terms may be used interchangeably. Climate and culture are somewhat connected and may influence (feed off) each other. Unlike culture, yet like the weather, organizational climate can change frequently, briefly, or rapidly over time. Organizational climate is dynamic (not static), can be shaped by the organizational structure, and tends to reflect events, peoples' reactions, and circumstances between people on a timely basis. Organizational climate is described as "a set of measurable properties of the perceived work environment, directly or indirectly, created by individuals who live and work in this environment and that influences the motivation and behavior of these people."[9] Organizational climate refers to the perceptions, feelings, or atmosphere (tone/mood) that people sense and acquire in the organization (see box 4.3). For example, you may walk into an organization and (subconsciously or consciously) think, "This place has remarkable energy, people are friendly, and it feels positive here." Or you may walk into a place and think, "Something is going on. People are so negative and grumpy. The atmosphere feels 'toxic.'" It is worth highlighting that organizational climate is "something" that is "perceived" by employees or is dependent upon value judgments which can vary greatly from person to person.

Box 4.3 Descriptors of Organizational Climate

- *Perception(s)* of work environment.
- "Psychological atmosphere" (i.e., the *emotional feel*).
- Whether or not people (i.e., employees) *feel supported* by the organization.
- Relationship dynamic between the organization and its employees.

Activity 4.3 Describe the Climate of an Organization

Consider the organization you selected in order to complete Activity 4.1. This time, try to describe the organizational climate. Try to pick one word to describe the organization's climate (i.e., sunny or warm, stormy, gloomy or cloudy). You may also want to add to your description, after reflecting upon the following questions: does the organization's environment facilitate relationships between employees; are people encouraged to contribute to improving work processes to make things better; are people willing to help each other; do people seem happy in their jobs, and do people seem proud of their organization?

____

____

Managers: Beware of Negative or "Toxic" Work Cultures (and Work Climates)

Without proper guidance and positive influences, negative factors can shape culture in ways that can be harmful for organizations, managers, and teams/employees.[10] Factors such as poor communication, toxic or negative employee(s), managers who focus on "figures (profit) over people," managers who micromanage and a culture with a strongly entrenched resistance to change, can hinder/limit the development of an effective organizational culture.[11] When there is minimal bottom-up communication (and incomplete top-down communication), employees may not feel that "their voices" are being heard or they may feel intimidated to speak up, possibly fostering a culture of fear (i.e., lack of trust) rather than respect.[11] An unfriendly and competitive work environment may lead to decreased knowledge sharing (i.e., less transparency), siloed work, and increased company politics.[11] Phrases such as "We always do things this way," "That won't work here," and "It's not my problem" create resistance to change and disconnected work relationships that hinder future progress.

Activity 4.4 Your Experiences of a Potentially Negative or Toxic Work Culture

From the list below, identify situations in which you have experienced a toxic or negative work culture by putting an X in the corresponding box (check all that apply).

- ☐ The core values (of the company) are not well known (i.e., not posted or displayed).
- ☐ Managers expect others to "do as they say" but not "as they do."
- ☐ Gossip or workplace drama persists between (certain) employees.
- ☐ There is unfriendly competition between (certain) employees or teams/departments.
- ☐ Employees are often tardy or absent.
- ☐ Employees often work late or don't take lunches.
- ☐ There is little or no hiring from within (i.e., little room for promotion).

While not all the items listed may seem "toxic," over time, they could indicate symptoms of underlying resentment and dysfunction.

Organizational cultures can disappoint employees at certain times and in various ways. Yet certain elements have more of a negative impact on how employees perceive or rate their corporate culture. A toxic work culture is a work environment dominated by institution-centered practices (i.e., directives), policies, and ineffective management styles that perpetuate detrimental habits and conflicts among employees and team members.[12] Toxic work cultures may fuel workplace conditions or disorders, such as lack of team cohesion, increased absenteeism or tardiness, lower productivity, and high employee turnover. Five elements that have a negative impact on corporate culture include disrespectful, non-inclusive, unethical, cutthroat, and abusive behavior.[13] Each element is discussed in the following text.[13]

Activity 4.5 Discovering Elements That Can Negatively Impact Organizational Culture

As you continue to read about the elements that can impact work cultures negatively, reflect upon possible experiences you have had with one or more of these elements. In the space provided, keep good notes. We will return to your notes a bit later.

___

___

___

- A *disrespectful environment* means that there is a lack of consideration, courtesy, and dignity for others. Being or feeling disrespected at work negatively impacts an employee's overall rating of an organization's culture.
- An *inclusive environment* encourages representation of diverse groups of employees (i.e., based on gender, race, sexual identity and orientation, disability, and age) and diverse thoughts or perspectives. It includes whether (or not) people are treated fairly, made to feel welcome, and included in key decisions. Non-inclusive environments support "cliques," "in-groups," or "in crowds," indicating that some employees are being or feeling excluded or are marginalized.
- Ethical behavior is a fundamental aspect of culture that is meaningful at both the organizational and individual level. *Unethical* behavior means that people (i.e., managers) say one thing but do another; they don't "walk the talk." Descriptors of unethical cultures include "shady," "smoke and mirrors," "dishonest," "deceptive," or one reflecting "false promises" or that is superficial.
- *Cutthroat* environments exist when employees feel that their colleagues are actively undermining one another; coworkers are "throwing each other under the bus," "stabbing each other in the back," or "meeting after the meeting," "displaying passive-aggressive behavior," or "sabotaging one another."
- *Abusive* environments develop when there is sustained hostile behavior by managers towards employees or between employees (co-workers). Hostile behaviors include "bullying," "shouting," "belittling or demeaning team members," being "condescending," or "talking down to people."

Now return to your notes so that you can expand upon them and answer the following questions in the space provided.

Describe a time when you felt disrespected.

____

____

Describe a time when you did not feel included.

____

____

Describe a time in which you experienced an unethical situation – either directly or indirectly.

____

____

Describe a time or situation that you felt was "cutthroat."

____

____

Describe a time or situation that you felt was "abusive."

____

____

It's hard to discover that work cultures may not always be positive and, in fact, may be seen as negative or "toxic."

Incivility and Microaggression

Have you experienced a time when someone said something insensitive or did something that felt mean or offensive? Rudeness at work is widespread and it's increasing.[14] Porath and Pearson claim that 98% of surveyed workers reported experiencing uncivil behavior.[14] **Microaggression** is a term used for commonplace verbal, behavioral, or environmental insults, whether intentional or unintentional, that communicate hostile, derogatory, or negative attitudes, and are frequently aimed at stigmatized or culturally marginalized groups.[15] Often, microaggressive behavior can be seen as a form of bullying towards others. Many managers claim that incivility is not appropriate, but don't recognize the tangible costs associated with uncivil behavior. Among workers who have been on the receiving end of incivility:

- 48% intentionally decreased their work effort;
- 47% intentionally decreased their time spent at work;
- 38% intentionally decreased the quality of their work;
- 66% reported that their performance declined; and
- 78% reported that their commitment to the organization declined.[15]

Managers (and literally everyone throughout the organization) must actively combat microaggression by creating inclusive, welcoming, and healthy workplaces.[16] Organizational cultures that reflect inclusivity and civility can contribute positively to employee wellbeing and mental and physical health.[16]

Workplace Bullying Exists

Workplace bullying is described as recurrent mistreatment and abusive conduct that is humiliating, threatening, intimidating, or sabotaging.[17] According to the Workplace Bullying Institute, 30% of adult Americans suffer abusive conduct at work, another 19% witness it, 49% are affected by it, and 66% are aware that workplace bullying happens.Moreover, the majority of bullies are men (67%); male perpetrators seem to prefer targeting men (58%) more than women (42%), while women bullied women in 65% of cases.[18]

Bottom Line!

Individuals expect to find a work culture that demonstrates elements of a healthy culture. Individuals hope to work in a culture that is inclusive, respectful, ethical, collaborative, and free from abuse by those in positions of power (i.e., management).[10]

Management Imperative #1: Build Positive Work Cultures (and Climates)

A positive culture (one that is trusting and **psychologically safe**) emphasizes/fosters individuals' strengths which ultimately makes teams more productive and efficient. A positive work culture encourages collaboration, promotes respect, and values (acknowledges) quality of work and contributions. In these positive environments, managers trust and empower employees to work (on projects) without constantly hovering or correcting (i.e., they don't micromanage); consequently, team members connect, engage, and complete their work cooperatively. The benefits gained when positive organizational cultures are created and cultivated include better recruitment, increased retention/employee loyalty, greater job/employee satisfaction, greater collaboration, and less stress (i.e., workplace drama).[19] When employees are less stressed, employee health, employee morale, and, ultimately, work performance is improved.

Managers can (and should) influence and shape organizational cultures. Daniel Coyle, author of *The Culture Code*, proposes that cultures are created by a specific set of skills (that can be used by managers): "Build Safety" (the first skill) explores how connecting generates bonds of belonging and identity; "Share Vulnerability" (the second skill) explains how habits of mutual risk drive trusting cooperation; and "Establish Purpose" (the third skill) tells how narratives (i.e., storylines) create shared goals and values.[20] Coyle's research suggests that these three skills work together from the bottom up, first building group connection and then channeling it into action. He claims that "Culture is a set of living relationships working toward a shared goal. It's not something you are. It's something you do."[20]

Managers – at all levels throughout the organization – can (and should) help to build a positive organizational culture by encouraging positivity, emphasizing employee wellness, and fostering social connections and trusting relationships. To build positive cultures, managers can start by encouraging and promoting positivity in the workplace daily. Managers should "model the way"[21] (i.e., set a good example) by expressing gratitude, smiling genuinely, being authentic, and staying optimistic during difficult situations. Moreover, when employees feel "well" or feel their best (physically, mentally, and emotionally), they will also contribute to a positive culture. Healthy (productive) workplace relationships are essential for positive company cultures; managers can facilitate, support, and promote opportunities for employees to strengthen relationships through different and regular social interactions and exchanges.

Management Imperative #2: Create Environments That Are Psychologically Safe

The level of psychological safety at work represent an organization's climate *and* culture. When an organizational climate is characterized by interpersonal trust, respect, and a sense of belonging at work, team members feel free to collaborate and they feel safe taking risks, which ultimately enables them to drive innovation more effectively.[22] It is worth noting that in *The Speed of Trust*, Covey defines *organizational trust* as the act of developing and maintaining trust with internal stakeholders of an organization to assure alignment.[23] Teams with a high degree of psychological safety reported higher levels of performance and lower levels of interpersonal conflict.[22]

Psychological safety is the belief that you won't be punished or humiliated for speaking up with ideas, questions, concerns, or mistakes. Yet, according to a recent poll, only three out of ten employees *strongly* agreed that their opinions count at work.[22] At work, it's a shared expectation (and hope) held by members of a team that teammates will not embarrass, reject, or punish them for sharing ideas, taking risks, or soliciting feedback.[22] A psychologically safe workplace begins with a feeling of belonging. People are more willing to engage in interpersonal risk-taking behaviors (i.e., speaking up, asking questions, sharing doubts, and respectfully disagreeing) that contribute to greater organizational innovation when they feel that their work environment is psychologically safe.

Activity 4.6 When Do You Feel Psychologically Safe?

First, how do you define psychological safety or safety in a work situation?

____

____

Describe when and why you feel psychologically safe while working with other people.

____

____

Think about a team or group of people with whom you have worked recently. Assess whether you felt psychologically safe within this team and describe why (or why not).

____

____

In the scenario (above), what (conditions, behaviors, etc.) would need to stay the same or change to ensure or improve psychological safety within this group?

____

____

What do you do to promote an inclusive environment and psychological safety as a team member/team leader?

____

____

Aha!

Psychological Safety at Work

Simon Sinek wrote about "psychological safety" in the workplace in his 2014 book *Leaders Eat Last*.[24] Inspired by military organizations, where leaders literally put their lives on the line, he suggests that it's a manager's responsibility to create an environment in which their team feels psychologically safe.[24]

In *The 4 Stages of Psychological Safety: Defining the Path to Inclusion and Innovation*, employees must progress through four stages (over time) before they feel "safe" (i.e., free) to make valuable contributions and challenge the status quo.[22,25] These four stages include Inclusion Safety, Learner Safety, Contributor Safety, and Challenger Safety (see table 4.1 for a brief discussion of each stage).

Table 4.1 Four Stages for Fostering Psychological Safety at Work

Stage	*Description*
Stage 1: Inclusion Safety	Satisfies the human need to connect and belong. A person feels safe (i.e., feels accepted for who they are).
Stage 2: Learner Safety	Satisfies the need to learn and grow. A person feels safe to engage in the learning process by asking questions, giving and receiving feedback, experimenting, and making mistakes.
Stage 3: Contributor Safety	Satisfies the need to make a difference. A person feels safe to use their skills and abilities to make meaningful contributions.
Stage 4: Challenger Safety	Satisfies the need to make things better. A person feels safe to speak up and challenge the status quo when they think there's an opportunity to change or improve.

Source: Coyle D. *The Culture Code: The Secrets of Highly Successful Groups*. Bantam; 2018.

Tool

How to Assess Organizational Cultures and Climates

Bolman and Deal's Four-Frame Model is one tool that can help managers to assess and navigate complex workplace dynamics.[26] This model provides a useful framework when looking at an organization from four different perspectives to understand, analyze, and solve challenging situations in organizations. The four frames are Structural, Human Resource, Political, and Symbolic (see table 4.2 for a brief description of each frame).

Table 4.2 Appraising Organizational Cultures: One Model to Consider

Frame	*Description*
Structural	Emphasizes organizational goals, roles, technology, coordination, and control. Organizations have clearly defined parts working together towards a common goal. Each member within an organization has a clear role; individual roles are defined to contribute towards achieving objectives. Efficiency and coordination are key.
Human Resource	The organization is pictured as a "family." People are emphasized – their needs, skills, and relationships. Every member is important because everyone brings unique talents to the table. Individual strengths are aligned with organizational goals. Organizations address the intrinsic needs of their people. Relationship building and fostering strong bonds between individuals leads to a positive organizational culture where everyone feels valued and connected.
Political	The organization is like a dynamic "arena" with power plays, office politics, conflicts, and competition ("the show"). The *how* and *why* of power dynamics (i.e., invisible tugs-of-war) that happen in the workplace. (i.e., who gets the office with the window?)
Symbolic	Focuses on **culture**, symbols, rituals, stories, and ceremonies within organizations. Views organizations as "theaters full of meaning." Organizations have unique cultures that shape unique behaviors. Positive environments can help to foster success.

Source: Glaser, BR. Key Concepts in Bolman and Deal's Four-Frame Model. HRDQ. https://hrdqstore.com/blogs/hrdq-blog/concepts-four-frame-model#:~:text=This%20model%20comprises%20four%20frames,and%20textures%20in%20a%20painting. Bolman, LG and Deal, TE. *Reframing Organizations: Artistry, Choice, and Leadership*. 5th ed. Jossey-Bass; 2013.

The different frames provide unique perspectives from which to subsequently view organizations holistically (i.e., when the frames are put together). It is worth noting that the Symbolic frame focuses on understanding culture through stories and rituals, etc.

Bottom Line!

Organizations do not operate in black-and-white terms. Instead they exist in many shades of gray, thus representing the complex structures layered with human emotions intertwined with power dynamics and wrapped up in unique cultures.[26]

Management Imperative #3: Focus on (Managing) Organizational Health

Strong organizations are *healthy*. **Organizational health** improves when employees are happy with their work, work environment(s), and careers. Organizational health refers to the ability of an organization to cope with change and continue to function with a high-performance workplace culture.[26] According to McKinsey's Organizational Health Index, "healthy" companies significantly outperform their less healthy peers.[27] In *The Advantage: Why Organizational Health Trumps Everything Else in Business*, author Patrick Lencioni suggests that organizational health depends on four disciplines: (1) developing a cohesive leadership team; (2) creating strategic clarity; (3) over-communicating that clarity throughout the organization; and (4) reinforcing strategy through systems and ways of working.[28] Lencioni claims that clarity doesn't need to be complex and abstract; it can be achieved by answering six questions for any organization (see box 4.4).

Box 4.4 Questions to Answer for Clarity about Organizational Health

1. Why do we exist?
2. How will we succeed?
3. What do we do?
4. Who does what?
5. What's most important, right now?
6. How will we behave?

Source: Lencioni P. *The Advantage: Why Organizational Health Trumps Everything Else in Business.* Jossey-Bass; 2012.

Management Imperative #4: Embed Learning into Organizational Cultures

A **learning organization** is an environment "where people continually expand their capacity to create the results they desire, where new and expansive patterns of thinking are nurtured, where collective aspiration is set free, and where people are continually learning how to learn together."[29] It is an organization skilled at creating, acquiring, and transferring knowledge, and at modifying its behavior to reflect new knowledge and insights.[30] It is worth noting that, according to Schein, "[o]rganizational learning, development and planned change can only be understood when culture is considered as the main source of resistance to change."[31]

Management Imperative #5: Focus on Employee Experience

It is a priority for managers to focus on **employee experience.**[32] Creating an environment to influence how employees encounter and perceive their work is important because employee experience impacts the organization's bottom line. Employee experience is associated with favorable organizational outcomes, such as diversity, equity, and inclusion, performance, workforce productivity, ability to change quickly, overall organizational performance, innovation, and lower levels of stress and burnout.[32] Yet efforts to design and improve the employee experience will yield only limited results if they are not communicated explicitly – internally and externally.

Management Imperative #6: Organizational Cultures (and Organizational Climates) Can Change

Organizational cultures can change through purposeful action and resilience, but it can take many months or even several years.[33] Managers must communicate a clear rationale for *why* the culture should change and then implement specific strategies over time to shape and improve the culture. The Gallup organization identified cultural drivers that collectively shape how employees conduct themselves, make decisions, and accomplish their work.[34] These five drivers include: (1) Leadership and Communication; (2) Values and Rituals; (3) Work Teams and Structures; (4) Human Resources; and (5) Performance. Throughout this chapter (and throughout this book), many aspects of these drivers are discussed and emphasized. To conclude this chapter, the following "management suggestions" summarize how managers can influence their organizational culture constructively.

Suggestion 1: Managers can prevent (or limit) "office gossip" or "rumor mills" when they provide consistent, ongoing communication and clear expectations for employees (and avoid doing it themselves through self-management practices).

Suggestion 2: Managers must ensure alignment on core values to sharpen decision-making and drive mission-oriented behavior. Because culture is shared and lived through narratives or stories, managers can tell authentic stories about how the company's mission made a difference in someone's life (i.e., when a cultural value was modeled by a physical therapist during a patient interaction).

Suggestion 3: Managers can support and facilitate effective teamwork and work structures to guide *how* employees connect – who communicates with whom, how frequently, and on what topics. Managing "how" things happen broadly (not micromanaging each task) within an organization will contribute to an effective culture and a positive "employee experience."

Suggestion 4: Teams will grow (and performance will improve) when managers focus on empowering, mentoring, and coaching (not controlling or micromanaging) while providing opportunities for individual growth.

An organization's culture is its values, ethics, vision, behaviors, and work environment. An organization's culture makes it unique and can affect many factors from reputation and brand image to employee recruitment, engagement, sense of belonging or connectedness, and retention. When employees share a company's ethics, vision, and other cultural elements, it can positively affect the organizational success (i.e., financial bottom line, job satisfaction, operational efficiency). An employee who understands and takes part in a company's corporate culture will also enjoy their job more/have higher job satisfaction. It's important for you to find a culture that fits *your style of work* so that you can be successful in your future practice.

Mini-Vignette

Discovering Culture

I didn't understand what culture was! I thought culture just meant that people got along and that people are happy. Our culture now – we have so many passionate, amazing *fitness forward thinking* therapists who love the wellness sector of therapy, who are open-minded and not "I can't do that skilled maintenance; my other company didn't let us do that." We are comfortable "thinking outside the box" about what we can do and what's ethical – knowing that we are following the guidelines. Our culture is one in which people *want* to help each other and they feel empowered. I have people emailing me, thinking about Medicare cuts, and how we can help the business and our team grow. They're sending me things that they're finding on their own without being asked. They're scheduling social get-togethers outside of work or asking, what can we do for someone who's getting married, doing things so we have more time together to just have fun. To me, this is part of the culture.

Dr. Jennifer Brown, PT, DPT

Suggested Readings

Bolman LG and Deal TE. *Reframing Organizations: Artistry, Choice, and Leadership* (5th ed.). Jossey-Bass; 2013.

Coyle D. *The Culture Code: The Secrets of Highly Successful Groups*. Bantam; 2018.

Lencioni P. *The Advantage: Why Organizational Health Trumps Everything Else in Business.* Jossey-Bass; 2012.

References

1. Wilkinson D. What is an organizational culture? Oxford Review: The OR Briefings. Accessed February 27, 2024. https://oxford-review.com/what-is-an-organisational-culture/
2. Wilkinson D. The difference between organizational culture and climate and why it matters. Oxford Review: The OR Briefings. Accessed February 27, 2024. https://oxford-review.com/blog-research-difference-culture-climate/
3. What is organizational culture? And why does it matter? Gallup. Accessed February 27, 2024. https://www.gallup.com/workplace/327371/how-to-build-better-company-culture.aspx

4. Schein E. *Organizational Culture and Leadership*. Jossey-Bass; 1995.
5. Creating a healthy corporate culture (with tips). Indeed. November 2022. Updated June 4, 2023. Accessed February 27, 2024. https://uk.indeed.com/career-advice/career-development/corporate-culture
6. Leary B. What leaders need to know about organizational subcultures. Helios HR. May 26, 2023. Accessed February 27, 2024. https://www.helioshr.com/blog/what-leaders-need-to-know-about-organizational-subcultures
7. Keswani D. Understanding organizational subcultures and countercultures. Eko. April 27, 2020. Accessed February 27, 2024. https://www.ekoapp.com/blog/understanding-organizational-subcultures-and-countercultures#:~:text=Subcultures%20form%20when%20a%20group,their%20group's%20values%20and%20obligations
8. BlueBoard: *The State of Workplace Connection Report*; 2021 BlueBoard Connected Workplace Survey. https://fs.hubspotusercontent00.net/hubfs/6173605/Original%20Research%20Report/Blueboard_StateOfWorkplaceConnection-2022.pdf
9. Chiavenato, I. *Introducción a la Teoría General de la Administración*; McGraw Hill; 2019.
10. Gallup. Gallup's approach to culture building a culture that drives performance. Accessed February 27, 2024. https://www.gallup.com/workplace/354842/organizational-culture-paper.aspx
11. Maier S. The 5 worst influences on organizational culture. Stop bad habits before they turn your entire team sour. Entrepreneur. September 12, 2016. Accessed February 27, 2024. https://www.entrepreneur.com/leadership/the-5-worst-influences-on-organizational-culture/281292
12. Heinz K. Toxic work culture: 18 examples and how to improve it. Built In. December 2023. Accessed February 28, 2024. https://builtin.com/company-culture/bad-company-culture
13. Sull D, Sull C, Cipolli W, et al. Why every leader needs to worry about toxic culture. *MIT Sloan Management Review*. March 16, 2022. https://sloanreview.mit.edu/article/why-every-leader-needs-to-worry-about-toxic-culture/
14. Porath C, Pearson C. The price of incivility. *Harvard Business Review*. 2013 Jan.–Feb. https://hbr.org/2013/01/the-price-of-incivility
15. Sue DW. *Microaggressions in Everyday Life: Race, Gender, and Sexual Orientation*. Wiley; 2010.
16. Washington EF. Recognizing and responding to microaggressions at work. *Harvard Business Review*. May 10, 2022. https://hbr.org/2022/05/recognizing-and-responding-to-microaggressions-at-work
17. 2021 WBI U.S. workplace bullying survey. Workplace Bullying Institute. 2021. Accessed February 28, 2024. https://workplacebullying.org/2021-wbi-survey-infographic/
18. 2021 WBI U.S. workplace bullying survey: The national study. Workplace Bullying Institute. Accessed February 28, 2024. https://workplacebullying.org/2021-wbi-survey/
19. Kohll A. How to build a positive company culture. *Forbes*. August 14, 2018. Accessed February 28, 2024. https://www.forbes.com/sites/alankohll/2018/08/14/how-to-build-a-positive-company-culture/?sh=75fa61c649b5
20. Coyle D. *The Culture Code: The Secrets of Highly Successful Groups*. Bantam; 2018, p. xx.
21. Kouzes JM, Posner BZ. *The Leadership Challenge: How to Make Extraordinary Things Happen in Organizations*. 7th ed. Wiley; 2023.
22. What is psychological safety at work? Center for Creative Leadership. January 10, 2024. Accessed March 1, 2024. https://www.ccl.org/articles/leading-effectively-articles/what-is-psychological-safety-at-work/

23. Covey SMR. *The Speed of Trust: The One Things that Changes Everything*. Simon & Schuster; 2008.
24. Sinek S. *Leaders Eat Last: Why Some Teams Pull Together and Others Don't*. Penguin; 2017.
25. Clark TR. *The 4 Stages of Psychological Safety: Defining the Path to Inclusion and Innovation*. Berrett-Koehler Publishers; 2020.
26. Glaser, BR. Key concepts in Bolman and Deal's four-frame model. HRDQ. December 20, 2023. Accessed February 28, 2024. https://hrdqstore.com/blogs/hrdq-blog/concepts-four-frame-model#:~:text=This%20model%20comprises%20four%20frames,and%20textures%20in%20a%20painting
27. McKinsey's organizational health index. McKinsey & Company. Accessed February 28, 2024. https://www.mckinsey.com/solutions/orgsolutions/overview/organizational-health-index
28. Lencioni P. *The Advantage: Why Organizational Health Trumps Everything Else in Business*. Jossey-Bass; 2012.
29. Senge, PM *The fifth discipline: The art and practice of the learning organization*. Doubleday; 2006, p. 1.
30. Garvin, DA. Building a learning organization. *Harv Bus Rev*. 1993; 71: 78–91.
31. Schein EH and Schein, PA. *Organizational Culture and Leadership*. 5th ed. Wiley; 2016.
32. HR trends report 2023. McLean & Company. Accessed March 1, 2024. https://go.mcleanco.com/hr-trends-report-2023
33. Folz, C. How to change your organizational culture: The first step is defining what values and behaviors you're seeking. SHRM. September 22, 2016. Accessed March 1, 2024. https://www.shrm.org/hr-today/news/hr-magazine/1016/pages/how-to-change-your-organizational-culture.aspx#:~:text=Changing%20a%20culture%20can%20take,resources%20that%20may%20never%20come
34. Cultivate 5 drivers for a high-performance culture. Gallup. September 25, 2020. Accessed February 28, 2024. https://www.gallup.com/workplace/320960/cultivate-drivers-high-performance-culture.aspx

5 Purpose-Driven Operations Management

Brian L. Hull

There are no secrets to success. It is the result of preparation, hard work, and learning from failure.

Colin Powell, American politician, statesman, diplomat, and US Army officer and 65th US Secretary of State (2001–2005)[1]

Chapter Objectives

1. Understand the components of operations management.
2. Apply lean management frameworks to health care management situations.
3. Apply first principles thinking for purpose-driven operations.
4. Construct purpose-driven operations goals.
5. Develop and build best practices into operational structures and processes.
6. Organize quality monitoring to improve outcomes.
7. Support conflicting perspectives to dive into the situation using the power of diverse perspectives to progress.

Management Vignette

Hilary Harris, PT, MPT

The typical challenges facing a physical therapist in an operations management role aren't much different from managing other types of work. You need to have enough staff to meet the patients' needs through effective recruiting. You need to retain and develop those clinicians, so you have a steady and reliable team. You need to incorporate enough flexibility to meet all the patient needs while allowing therapists to have time for life outside of work.

Once you have a steady team, the therapy manager has to ensure quality care, efficient practice, and sound business operations. As a physical therapist, I make sure I spend time observing clinicians outside my profession to

DOI: 10.4324/9781003524250-7

gain a good understanding of their work. If I don't have direct experience in their work, I want to understand their key issues and challenges so we can work together to determine the best solution. I can then sit down with my team members to say, "Here are the issues I see. Are those the same issues that you see?" Then we discuss what things we cannot change, such as the budget, and work together to find feasible solutions. Getting everyone involved in the solution from the beginning has helped me to achieve the best results. However, some decisions must be made by the department leader. In such cases, I may not involve all the frontline staff, but keep the decision-making within the leadership team.

The therapy manager must ensure that the entire team is providing quality, evidence-based practice each day. We must make sure that the team is providing the best care so that we can achieve the best clinical outcomes. Sometimes this means seeing how effectively the team is implementing the evidence into everyday patient care.

The manager also must make sure that the therapy team is clearly showing the value they are creating each day to the organization. Every organization has productivity and finance requirements, but we must also focus on the value our teams add each day.

Successful clinical operations result from focusing on your team, making sure they feel included in the problem-solving, and included in daily operations. The team needs to know their input is valuable, and that you, as the manager, care for them. I then work with the team to make sure we are all demonstrating our value back to the organization. Therapy doesn't simply "get people out of bed or wrap a sprained ankle." We need to consistently demonstrate that we are improving clinical outcomes, quality of life, and helping to heal human lives.

Process improvement training, which includes learning strategies such as lean management, has been very helpful to me in my organizational role. I have also benefited from financial training. This includes budgeting and monitoring variance reports and being able to translate organizational productivity targets into clinical practice. Finally, I have benefited from implementation science training, and making sure that our teams are providing evidence-based practices.

To any physical therapy student moving into a managerial role I would say you should rely on your physical therapy training because many of the same evaluation and treatment planning skills work well in a managerial role. The department is your client now, not the patient, and so you approach operations and problem-solving in the same way. Similarly to clinical care, don't be afraid to reach out to other disciplines, whether that's your finance team, your nursing colleagues, or other professionals. Networking with other professions early on will help to alleviate potential headaches later.

Chapter Introduction

This chapter is organized into three sequential parts. Part 1 focuses on creating and utilizing operational structures and goals designed according to first principle and purpose. Without accuracy of purpose, health care dysfunction ensues. Part 2 discusses organizations that design coordinated communication tactics to reach all the organizational work levels effectively. In addition, all organization members must have shared outcome measurements that feed directly into the organization's purpose-driven goals. Part 3 takes a pragmatic approach to designing or repairing an organization's operations. This includes measuring success and using established quality improvement methods and philosophies, such as lean management, to improve continually. Finally, the chapter discusses team communication, decision-making, and conflict resolution.

What Is Operations Management?

Operations are the management functions that influence the efficient production of quality services and products to best meet customers or stakeholders' needs. Often, this is accomplished through clear direction from management to all work levels. The more effective the work structure, direction, and communication, the greater the likelihood of desired outcomes.

Operations management began as scientific management in Frederick Winslow Taylor's 1911 publication, *Shop Management*. Winslow's work emerged from what he saw as excessive inefficiency among steel mill workers. Scientific management suggested strict supervision of all tasks leading to the final product through time study and prescribed task techniques.[2] Taylor's authoritarian management model was later seen as limited due to its neglect of the social and psychological actualities of the workplace environment.[3,4]

Operations management continued to progress within the manufacturing industry throughout the 20th century, highlighted by the theoretical and analytical constructs of Six Sigma and Lean. Motorola created Six Sigma as a quality measurement that seeks 99.996% error-free products. Toyota created Lean to reduce manufacturing waste, thus increasing value for all stakeholders.[5,6] We will discuss these constructs in greater detail later in this chapter. In recent decades, digital data has been used to actively track service and product creation. Successful health care operations management creates value by efficiently delivering outcomes that matter to patients, health insurance payors, and all stakeholders. The operations manager, whether titled manager, director, or executive, oversees and facilitates this value creation.

Case study: "Metrics without Purpose"

Your 70-year-old grandfather considers himself fortunate to be a laryngeal cancer survivor. In 2017, he experienced pain on swallowing and immediately contacted his physician. After further workup, the oncologist discovered squamous cell carcinomas of the larynx. A surgeon proceeded with a larynx preservation surgery followed by postoperative radiation. Due to generalized weakness and an initial inability to take care of himself following the surgery, your grandfather spent three weeks in a post-acute care facility, followed by six weeks of home health care. Finally, newly independent and no longer requiring physical therapy, he excitedly returned to his neighborhood restaurant to enjoy his favorite meal. However, he noticed significant difficulty swallowing each bite due to post-radiation scar tissue. Fortunately, he was able to arrange an evaluation later that week with a speech-language pathologist specializing in head and neck cancer rehabilitation.

When he arrived for his evaluation, the office staff notified your grandfather that his speech therapy Medicare benefits were exhausted for the remainder of 2017. He responded, "I have never received speech therapy before; how is that possible?" The office manager told him that in 2017 Medicare only allowed $1,980 for annual physical therapy and speech-language pathology services combined (i.e., Medicare Therapy Cap).

It turns out that some of his physical therapy earlier that year was charged to Medicare Part B and had exceeded his $1,980 maximum for physical therapy and speech-language pathology services combined. Dejected, he thought, "Did I need the additional physical therapy? I was independent at home, but the therapist encouraged me to continue care 'just to make sure' I remained strong."

Was all the physical therapy care needed following his larynx preservation surgery? Did their employer incentivize the physical therapists primarily to achieve a volume-based metric? Was this type of excessive practice caused by flawed processes, lack of evidence-informed practice and variance, lack of training, lack of skill, malevolence and greed, or poor vision or lack of clarity?

Activity 5.1 Case Analysis

You are the manager of this clinic and are alerted to this issue when the family calls to complain. After you talk through the concerns with the patient and family, what next steps do you take with your department? What other actions would you consider outside your department?

____

____

____

____

Part 1: Starting with Accuracy of Purpose

While precision or minimization of unwarranted variance in health care is ideal, operations must begin with ensuring the accuracy of purpose. In health care

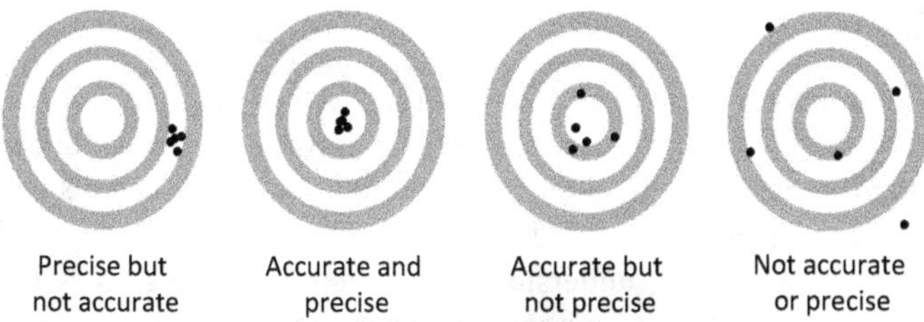

Figure 5.1 Accuracy versus Precision

Source: Compiled by the author.

operations, precision is indicated by repeatedly hitting the intended mark. These process, intervention, or outcome marks are often called metrics or **key performance indicators** (KPIs). If a well-organized and motivated organization consistently achieves its KPIs, that organization has a degree of precision. For example, one could consider the physical therapy providers in the case study as *precisely* meeting a volume-based metric. However, did these providers *accurately* meet the overall health care needs? (See figure 5.1.)

What is missing in this case study is the accuracy of purpose. The physical therapy provider could be considered precise in their potential focus on revenue capture. However, the purpose would ideally include high-quality, person-centric, equitable, and affordable care proposed by the Institute for Health Improvement's **Quintuple Aim** Initiative.[7] The clearer we are in operations about the value we are attempting to create, the more accurately we can create that value.

Activity 5.2 Improving Accuracy of Purpose

You are the newly appointed manager of the home health agency that overutilized the patient's physical and speech therapy benefits. You have received multiple complaints that your therapists are exhausting patients' annual Medicare benefits. What next steps will you take?

____

____

____

____

____

First Principle, or Our Purpose

Accuracy of purpose is achieved by starting with what Aristotle called **first principle**. All actions and outcomes result from a chain of decisions and causes extending back to the axiomatic principle or purpose. This cause is the primary purpose in operations and provides subsequent operations directives. Organizations must clearly understand *what* they are trying to achieve, build the operational structures and outcome measurements to support the work, and intentionally measure the degree of success.[8,9] Every step in the design and execution operations must focus on the organization's first principle and prime purpose.

For example, in 2002, Elon Musk founded SpaceX, the first private company to send a spacecraft to the International Space Station. Musk initially wanted to find a way to enable human beings to travel to the planet Mars. At the time, a typical launch would have cost $380,000,000, which seemed impossible to achieve. By reducing rocket construction and operation down to first principles, Musk calculated that SpaceX could build a rocket for no more than 2% of the typical total cost, leaving a 98% margin for research, development, and construction. SpaceX is now an industry leader and central National Aeronautics and Space Administration (NASA) contractor with its reusable rocket system.[10] This example shows that starting and following through with purpose at the center is essential.

How can an organization reduce its current functional or dysfunctional operations down to the first principle or the organizational purpose? Morten Hansen reminds us of the incredible success of the 1960s space race between the United States and its Cold War nemesis, the Soviet Union. The Soviet Union was "winning" the space race after launching the first successful orbiting satellite in 1957. In September 1962, US President John F. Kennedy rallied the nation by focusing not only on NASA but on the whole of the United States with a simple, concrete, and shared vision and purpose: "This nation should commit itself to achieving the goal before this decade is out, of landing a man on the Moon and returning him safely to Earth."[11] On July 20, 1969, the United States became the first country to land a man on the moon, thus propelling itself to lead the space race. This feat was only made possible through the effective creation and dissemination of a vision that was embraced by multiple industries, governmental agencies, and a nation of taxpayers ready to support the directive. This purposeful focus is also needed in health care.

If the manager knows and maintains a clear focus on the first principle they are trying to accomplish in their organization's operations, purpose-derived structures and processes will result. If the manager clearly communicates these first principles at every opportunity and decision point, all the organization members can support the shared mission, vision, and values. Furthermore, evidence shows that team members who find purpose in their work report feeling more satisfied with their lives in general and their professional lives in particular.[12,13] The purpose is the center of operations management.

Activity 5.3 Finding Your Team's Purpose

As the new manager, you find that your team is lacking purpose, direction, and cohesion. What questions should you ask the team, yourself, and the executive management team to determine your team's first principle or purpose?

____

____

____

____

Common Health Care Mishaps When Not Focusing with Accuracy of Purpose

To illustrate the importance of understanding the strong influence of purpose, let us review the ten common health care dysfunctions (listed in box 5.1) described by Elizabeth Rosenthal in her health care industry exposé, *American Sickness*:[14]

Box 5.1 Rosenthal's Economic Rules of the Dysfunctional Medical Market[13]

1. More treatment is always better. Default to the most expensive option.
2. A lifetime of treatment is preferable to a cure.
3. Amenities and marketing matter more than good care.
4. As technologies age, prices can rise rather than fall.
5. There is no free choice. Patients are stuck. And they're stuck buying American.
6. More competitors vying for business doesn't mean better prices; it can drive prices up, not down.
7. Economies of scale don't translate to lower prices. With their market power, big providers can simply demand more.
8. There is no such thing as a fixed price for a procedure or test. And the uninsured pay the highest prices of all.
9. There are no standards for billing. There's money to be made in billing for anything and everything.
10. Prices will rise to whatever the market will bear.

Activity 5.4 Finding Dysfunction

What health care dysfunctions have you experienced or read about?

____

____

____

____

Rosenthal attributes these ten dysfunctions to many health care organizations designing their primary operations around maximal reimbursement and profit with scant regard for the Quintuple Aim's goals of cost-effectively and efficiently managing the health of populations. If health care's first principle is simply to maximize insurance reimbursement, then the US health care industry has succeeded. However, I would argue that most for-profit and non-profit health care organizations have a broader purpose. To be sure, the for-profit organization is responsible for returning a profit to its shareholders, while non-profit organizations are responsible for "making money" to put back into their mission, be that for purchasing new capital supplies, building new facilities, researching, or providing charity care. However, if either type of organization attempts to obtain these margins by focusing primarily on maximum reimbursement, we find the resultant dysfunction described by Rosenthal.[14]

From a first principle perspective, I would argue that *most* health care organizations attempt to provide the highest quality care that their organization can provide using the most efficient means. The value focus can be limited by the prevalence of older Fee-for-Service or other non-value-based reimbursement models still employed by many health insurance companies. However, few health care organizations are simply interested in maximizing profit without regard for improving their patients' and customers' quality of life. Furthermore, many organizations are working to provide the highest quality of care as efficiently as possible to create high value. Such organizations may accomplish this through preventive services upstream to decrease costly surgeries, hospital stays, revolving door readmissions, and unnecessary care.

Principled Goal Setting

While mission, vision, and values are covered in greater depth in chapters 8 and 11, the operations manager must continually focus their teams on purpose. The key to operational success is to create structures, training, and goals centered on the ultimate purpose. This principled approach focuses all actions on achieving the purpose and avoiding myopically chasing siloed metrics.

Teams will benefit from a more tangible direction for achieving the organization's mission, vision, and values. Once the organization has understood its first principle and purpose, which translates into its vision, it can create its **"Man on the Moon Statement"** (MOTM). Kantabutra et al. recommend that the MOTM statement:[15]

1. is brief (so that it can be remembered and repeated easily);
2. contains a prime goal to be achieved;
3. is not a one-time, specific goal that can be met, and then discarded;
4. provides a source of motivation for employees to do their best by including a degree of difficulty or stretch (e.g., to achieve a national/international status); and
5. offers a long-term perspective for the organization and indicates the future environment in which it will function.

Activity 5.5 Creating Your MOTM Statement

Here is an example of a MOTM statement for a fictitious company.
The Movement Specialists will be recognized as a top three Texas rehabilitation provider by 2030.
Now it's your turn.

You were hired by the owner of a sports medicine clinic to "turn things around." You find a disengaged and unfocused clinical and administrative team, high turnover, and mediocre quality of care. Discuss how you will create an MOTM statement to guide the team in purpose-driven operations.

____

____

____

____

Every team member should innately understand the organization's first principle and purpose. The simpler, the better. All operations and structural design that follow will build on this purpose as the lens through which to design it.

Aha!

"Truth is ever to be found in simplicity, and not in the multiplicity and confusion of things."[15]

Sir Isaac Newton, English mathematician, physicist, astronomer, alchemist, theologian, and author

Your job as a manager is to radically simplify and reduce operations, cultures, and behaviors down to the simple goals and truths. So, keep the goals and directives simple and obvious. Perhaps consider a visual representation (see figure 5.2).

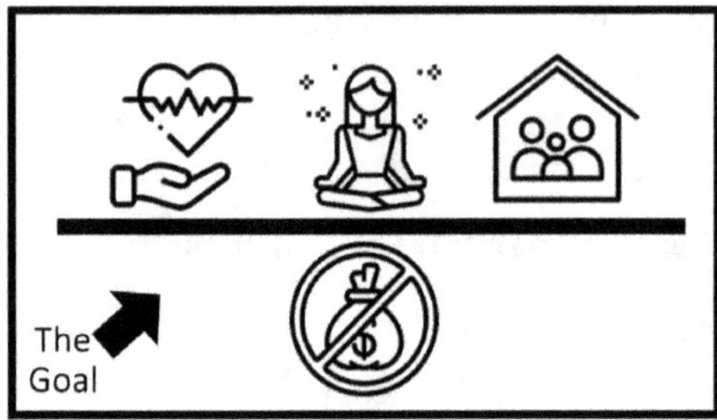

Figure 5.2 A Visualized Goal of Pursuing Simple Health Care Value

Source: Compiled by the author.

Bottom Line!

All team members must understand the first principle and purpose that the organization is working towards so that each individual can accurately and precisely accomplish the purpose-driven goals.

Part 2: Operationalizing the First Principle MOTM

After identifying your organization's accurate purpose, based on your first principle, the next step is ensuring that all team members understand the operational goals and know how to contribute to the organization's success. Organizations must design coordinated internal communication tactics to reach all the organizational work levels effectively. The purpose manifested as the MOTM statement and subsequent operational goals must be written and disseminated in language and content that connects with all team members. Additionally, each team member should have and understand goals specific to their work responsibilities. Finally, all organization members must have shared outcome measurements that directly feed into the organization's purpose-driven goals.

Successful organizations use validated outcome measurements to measure the achievement of their purposeful goals. For instance, if an organization's goal is to improve the health of their community, decreasing mortality and hospital (re)admissions may be appropriate KPIs to pursue. These goals align well with Michael Porter's recommendation to pursue goals that matter to patients.[16,17] However, an organization pursuing the maximum number or type of specific charge codes or diagnostic codes regardless of efficient clinical outcomes may mislead best efforts and organizational expertise. Value-quantifying calculations can be considered to prevent an organization or team from chasing narrow KPIs. Hull and Thut recommend combining Porter's recommendation into a Therapy Value Quotient for the physical therapy industry. Having a simple quotient for therapists to focus their efforts on improving, therapy cohorts can increase value while improving the outcomes that matter to patients.[18,19] While determining which KPIs to utilize, the organization should start with the purpose or MOTM and decide upon the most effective and valid tools to measure success. These measurements may include mortality, length of hospital stay, readmission to hospital, functional outcome, pain, return to work, quality of life, and financial metrics for efficiency and profitability. A balance focused on overall value created for all stakeholders is essential.

Activity 5.6 What Is Your Value Equation?

You are the manager of a pediatric outpatient clinic. Your health care organization wants to refocus the care it provides to high-value care calculated by outcomes achieved divided by cost. What value-focused outcomes will you choose to be divided by cost of care?

____

____

____

____

Evidence-Informed Systems and Structures

In addition to setting individual and shared operational goals for all work levels, successful organizations build evidence-informed processes (EIP) and interventions into workflows and electronic health records. Unless organizations hardwire these EIPs, the literature states that clinical practice will lag by as many as 17 years behind current best practices.[20] The organization's management team must build structures, resources, and expectations to ensure that best practices are put in place.[21]

While successful organizations build best practices into operational structures and processes, organizational policy creation is a separate consideration. Policies should address compliance considerations such as those in the hand hygiene example (box 5.2).

Box 5.2 Hospital or Clinic Sample Policy and Procedure

Hand Hygiene Policy and Procedure

Purpose:

Requires health care personnel to perform hand hygiene in accordance with Centers for Disease Control and Prevention (CDC) recommendations.

Policy Statement:

All members of the health care team will follow guidance from the CDC regarding hand hygiene.

Application:

This policy applies to all health care workers.

Exceptions:

None.

Procedure:

Health care personnel should use an alcohol-based hand rub or wash with soap and water for the following clinical indications:

- immediately before touching a patient;
- before performing an aseptic task (e.g., placing an indwelling device) or handling invasive medical devices;
- before moving from work on a soiled body site to a clean body site on the same patient;
- after touching a patient or the patient's immediate environment;
- after contact with blood, body fluids, or contaminated surfaces; and
- immediately after glove removal.

Source: Centers for Disease Control and Prevention. Hand Hygiene Guidance | Hand Hygiene | CDC. Hand Hygiene in Healthcare Settings. Published April 28, 2023. Accessed September 6, 2023. https://www.cdc.gov/handhygiene/providers/guideline.html

Policies and procedures are generally not as prescriptive as those outlined in the hand hygiene example and should allow reasonable variance to adapt to specific procedures and patient needs. Clinical operations often employ policies and procedures for basic compliance and guidance. Instead of policies and procedures, health care clinics and departments will generally rely more heavily on structured and documented competency training and check-off systems covering all essential work requirements. With these basic requirements in place, the operations manager must then focus on individual team member engagement towards the MOTM purpose.

Once all team members have received their operational directives and guidelines as to how they will measure success towards accomplishing goals, the manager and supervisor team should set up regular structured rounding sessions with each member weekly or monthly, depending on the amount of environmental change. The Studer Group popularized a hospital engagement tactic called **rounding for outcomes.**[22,23] Studer stresses the importance of monthly rounding with all employees to discuss the organizational goals and how each member contributes to its success.[22,23] The operation manager's goal should be a consistent understanding among all employees of that first principle or purpose and the employee-specific goals that contribute to that direction, as well as a desire and motivation for all team members to work towards those goals. This employee engagement will not only ensure that all team members focus their efforts on helping the organization to meet its goals but can improve job satisfaction, organizational commitment, performance, and decrease turnover.[24,25]

Monitoring and Improving Outcomes and Quality

While policies, procedures, and competencies create limits and compliance, and rounding helps to connect all team members to the shared goals, the operations manager must also focus on monitoring and improving outcomes and quality.

Lean and **Six Sigma** strategies are often used in tandem to monitor and improve clinic operations. Both methodologies attempt to optimize operations and increase value for patients and stakeholders and are commonly used together as Lean Six Sigma or the more common term *lean management.*[5,6]

Motorola originally designed the Six Sigma methodology to identify and remove manufacturing defects and variations and subsequently creating precise and reliable products. These strategies can also help to decrease unwarranted variation and care delivery failure in health care settings. Lean Six Sigma methodology typically consists of five phases known as DMAIC (define, measure, analyze, improve, and control) as shown in table 5.1.[26]

Table 5.1 DMAIC

1. **D**efine	Identify all stakeholder needs, including patients, the community, affiliated health care providers, and investors.
2. **M**easure	Using validated and purposeful outcome measurement tools to monitor overall patient outcomes and operational excellence.
3. **A**nalyze	Using Electronic Health Record (EHR) and operational data to identify areas to improve quality and efficiency.
4. **I**mprove	Iteratively improving processes for consistent, high-quality outcomes.
5. **C**ontrol	Creating policies, resources, protocols, and care pathways to maximize the likelihood of success.

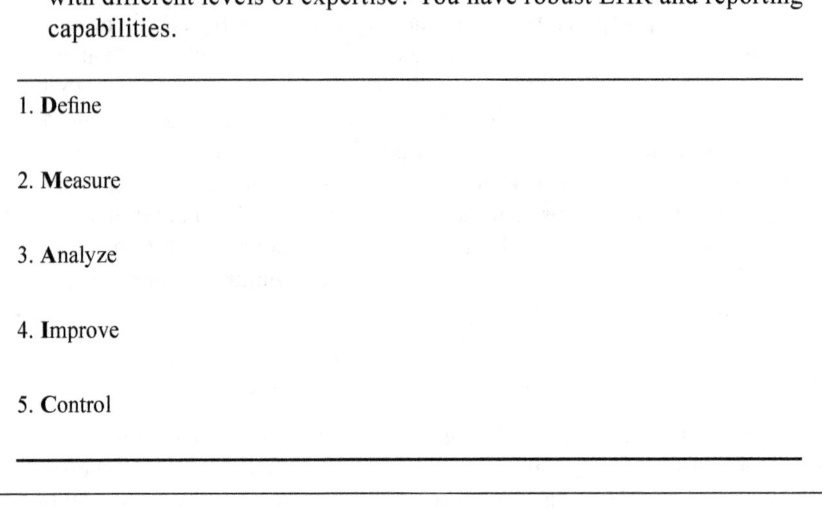

Activity 5.7 Applying Six Sigma

You are the manager of an inpatient rehabilitation facility treating a high volume of patients with spinal cord injuries, traumatic brain injuries, and stroke. What will you focus on for each category (listed below) to decrease variation in practice between different providers with different levels of expertise? You have robust EHR and reporting capabilities.

1. **D**efine

2. **M**easure

3. **A**nalyze

4. **I**mprove

5. **C**ontrol

Table 5.2 The Eight Categories of Lean Management

1. Reduce waiting	Waiting for patient care rooms or equipment.
2. Minimize inventory	Maintaining excessive inventory that may increase costs and risk expiring. There is a healthy balance here to ensure organizations are also prepared for long-tail events such as pandemics.[27]
3. Eradicate defects to improve quality of care	Reducing medical and treatment errors, infections, and hospital readmissions. This is especially important as payors transition to value-based payment models.
4. Transportation	Improving the flow and efficiency of patient care, including the supplies and personnel needed for care.

(*Continued*)

Table 5.2 (Continued)

5. Prevent injuries and save time by reducing motion	Decreasing unnecessary patient transfers and clinician bending and lifting.
6. Minimizing health care overproduction	Decreasing unnecessary procedures and treatments. Duplication of testing and extended hospital stays.
7. Remove waste from over-processing	Unnecessary paperwork and processes that do not add value or contribute to high-quality care.
8. Understand how health care waste leads to untapped human potential	When workers' time is consumed by any of the above, they cannot use it to leverage their creativity and talents for work that promotes patient care and optimized operations.

Lean methodology focuses on decreasing waste and improving value. Toyota created this quality improvement methodology to improve automotive manufacturing. These methods have also been found to be a helpful framework to analyze health care waste. Current health waste is estimated to comprise 25% of all health care expenditure or up to $935 billion annually.[28] To address this waste, Lean focuses on eight categories (see table 5.2).[5]

Activity 5.8 Applying Lean

You are the manager of a skilled nursing facility and are working with facility management to address challenges with patient transport, providing unneeded care, staff back injury, excessive bedrest, and supply expense. What will you focus on for each category below? Discuss why.

1. Reduce waiting

2. Minimize inventory

3. Eradicate defects to improve quality of care

4. Transportation

5. Prevent injuries and save time by reducing motion

6. Minimizing health care overproduction

7. Remove waste from over-processing

8. Understand how health care waste leads to untapped human potential

Table 5.3 Examples of Lean Activities

Lean Activity Type	*Activity Examples*
Lean assessment activities to identify waste and improvement opportunities	Spaghetti diagrams, Gemba walks, RCA, value stream mapping
Lean improvement activities to suggest ways to improve processes and reduce waste	5S event (Sort, Straighten, Shine, Standardize, Sustain), leveled production based on demand, standard work (ensuring best practices), stop the line

While an organization must build operational structures and a culture dedicated to the lean management principles of decreasing variance, eliminating waste, improving process flow, adding value, and continuously attempting to improve, Lean activities must also be used in daily operations management quality improvement work.

Within lean management, Lean activities include several value-assessing and improvement activities. For example, spaghetti diagrams trace patient and process flow. Observing overall flow allows participants to identify ways to improve efficiency and decrease waste. Gemba walks give senior managers regular opportunities to discuss frontline work and ideas for improvement. Furthermore, **root cause analysis** (RCA), which will be discussed in greater depth later in the chapter, brings together all process contributors to objectively determine what caused an error and what can be corrected or changed to prevent similar errors. Organizational leaders and managers should choose the Lean activity or other quality improvement tool that works best for each application (see table 5.3).

Built-in Quality, Efficiency, and Value

Health care operations management has rapidly progressed since 2000 when *To Err Is Human: Building a Safer Health System* estimated that 44,000–98,000 deaths are caused annually in the United States as a result of medical error.[29] This level of medical error, combined with the earlier mentioned $1 trillion of US health care waste, indicates a need to build quality, efficiency, and value into our processes.[27] When attempting to mitigate health care waste, the manager must keep their first principle or purpose at the center of their operations. As previously mentioned, focusing myopically on individual measurements, such as classic productivity calculated by total charge codes entered per hour worked, can not only leave out quality and value measurement but also lead to unnecessary patient expenditure, overproduction, and potentially unethical behavior.[30]

Fortunately, we have many examples of success in preventing needless health care harm and waste while improving population health. Many of these improvements focus on decreasing unwarranted variance to focus on EIP protocols. Atul Gawande popularized such protocols by highlighting a five-point checklist implemented by the Johns Hopkins Hospital in 2001, significantly decreasing central line infections in the intensive care unit and preventing an estimated 43 infections and eight deaths over the course of 27 months.[31] The same publication describes a similar program in Michigan that decreased infections by 66% within three months and saved more than 1,500 lives within 18 months.[31]

Organizations must build consistent and reliable EIP into their clinical pathways to accomplish these significant operations improvements. Intermountain Healthcare has accomplished this by introducing low back pain classification and treatment interventions. The easy-to-follow algorithm guides the clinician to EIP interventions based on symptom evaluation (see figure 5.3).[32,33]

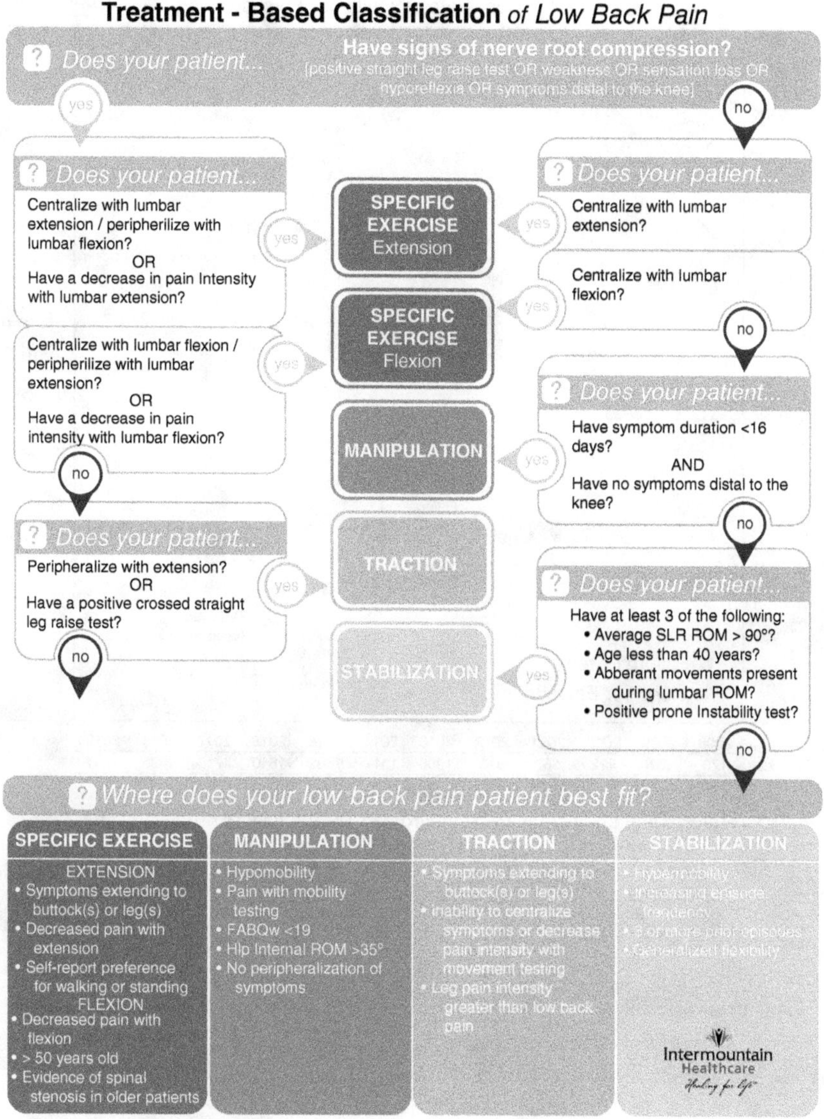

Treatment - Based Classification of Low Back Pain
? Does your patient...
Have signs of nerve root compression?
[positive straight leg raise test OR weakness OR sensation loss OR hyporeflexia OR symptoms distal to the knee]
yes
no
? Does your patient...
Centralize with lumbar extension / peripherilize with lumbar flexion?
OR
Have a decrease in pain Intensity with lumbar extension?
yes
Centralize with lumbar flexion / peripherilize with lumbar extension?
OR
Have a decrease in pain intensity with lumbar flexion?
yes
no
? Does your patient...
Peripheralize with extension?
OR
Have a positive crossed straight leg raise test?
yes
no
SPECIFIC EXERCISE Extension
SPECIFIC EXERCISE Flexion
MANIPULATION
TRACTION
STABILIZATION
? Does your patient...
Centralize with lumbar extension?
yes
Centralize with lumbar flexion?
yes
no
? Does your patient...
Have symptom duration <16 days?
AND
Have no symptoms distal to the knee?
yes
no
? Does your patient...
Have at least 3 of the following:
• Average SLR ROM > 90°?
• Age less than 40 years?
• Abberant movements present during lumbar ROM?
• Positive prone Instability test?
yes
no
? Where does your low back pain patient best fit?
SPECIFIC EXERCISE
EXTENSION
• Symptoms extending to buttock(s) or leg(s)
• Decreased pain with extension
• Self-report preference for walking or standing
FLEXION
• Decreased pain with flexion
• > 50 years old
• Evidence of spinal stenosis in older patients
MANIPULATION
• Hypomobility
• Pain with mobility testing
• FABQw <19
• Hip Internal ROM >35°
• No peripheralization of symptoms
TRACTION
• Symptoms extending to buttock(s) or leg(s)
• inability to centralize symptoms or decrease pain intensity with movement testing
• Leg pain intensity greater than low back pain
STABILIZATION
• Hypermobility
• Increasing episode frequency
• 3 or more prior episodes
• Generalized flexibility
Intermountain Healthcare
Healing for life

Figure 5.3 Intermountain Healthcare Low Back Pain Algorithm

Intermountain also demonstrated the attributes of lean management improvement activities by successfully building standardized care processes to decrease total knee arthroplasty treatment failure rates. In figure 5.4, the diagram illustrates how patient failure to progress rates decreased as the organization standardized best practice care while failing to increase therapy utilization. Improved outcomes accomplished by similar staffing expenses create value.[34,35]

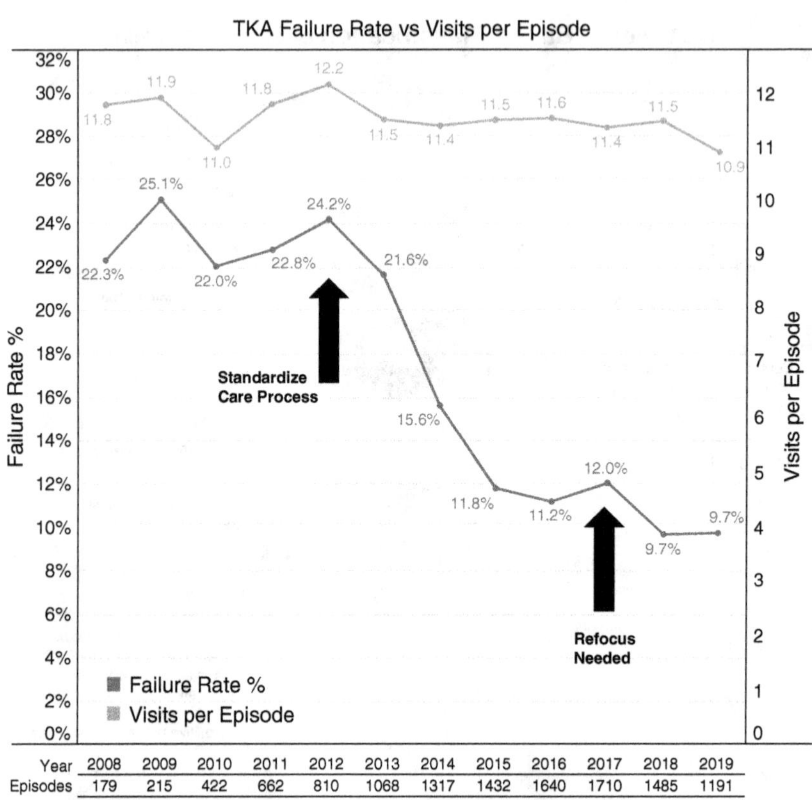

Figure 5.4 Intermountain Healthcare Standardized Total Knee Arthroplasty Care

Bottom Line!

Organizations and teams must build EIP and quality improvement monitoring into daily workflow and processes and utilize them to pursue high-value care.

Part 3: Improving Your Operations

Where does one start as a new department, service line, or manager? The operations manager must start by clearly identifying the organization's purpose and first principle. Next, they should determine how each organization member can contribute to that purpose. Then, the manager must ensure that all members are measuring success in the same way. Depending on the organization's current health, management teams may consider having intentional conversations with all team members on purpose and even consider conducting the MOTM development exercise. Finally, continue measuring success and use established quality improvement methods and philosophies such as lean management to improve continually.

Once organizations have created processes and structures designed to promote best practices and meet the organization's purpose, outcomes data collection is crucial. Hoyer advises interprofessional organizations to share an outcomes measurement language.[36] Interprofessional work and collaboration can flourish when all team members are measuring success with the same outcomes. With complex environments treating diverse populations and conducting various invasive and non-invasive interventions, successful organizations rely on **Pareto charts** to start their journey with the high volume and high-risk cohorts to realize the greatest benefit (see figure 5.5). Initial efforts can utilize the shared and meaningful outcome measurement to maximize quality for those populations.

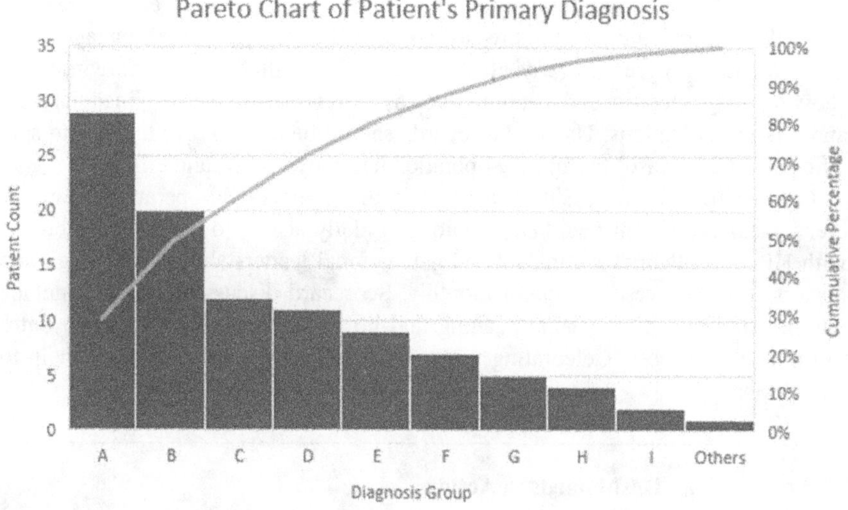

Figure 5.5 Pareto Chart Identifying Highest Volume of Patients' Primary Diagnosis

Note: In this example, a clinic wants to determine its highest frequency referral diagnosis to prioritize the next quality improvement project focus. After graphing the total volume of prior years' diagnosis group, the clinic manager determines that Diagnosis Groups A and B have the highest volumes and will be the best place to start to have the largest impact.

As the organization begins to analyze the high-volume and high-risk populations, attention should focus on identifying best practices and benchmarked results to compare. If an organization is missing the benchmarked outcomes with specific populations, it is essential to focus on flaws in the systems and processes using one of the Six Sigma and Lean analytical tools, such as RCA. While improving quality and decreasing *unwarranted practice variance*, which cannot be explained by the severity of illness or patient characteristics, managers should also focus on meeting regulatory compliance requirements. A simple and effective way of accomplishing this is by standardizing care, using EIP practice guidelines, employing consistent outcome measurement tools, auditing charts, and observing care. These activities not only ensure quality care but also encourage overall professional development.

Scorecards and Dashboards

It is essential to keep teams focused on how well the organization progresses toward its purpose-driven goals. Having a centralized tool to monitor the organization's outcomes can help. Kaplan and Norton created the Balanced Scorecard concept in 1992. The creators aimed to employ one document where leaders could see current outcome measurements on all the organization's goals and KPIs.[37] Since then, organizations in all industries have embraced various iterations of this work. Most of these current methods are termed **scorecards** or **dashboards**. Scorecards are similar to the original Balanced Scorecard concept that organizational managers can use to monitor progress towards all strategic goals. Dashboards are more granular, showing daily operations' data points such as current patient census, financial data, and quality indications. Useful dashboards should be able to drill down into specific patient care cases to improve operational quality, safety, and efficacy.

Both scorecards and dashboards are helpful for successful operations management. Ideally, all team members should have daily access to updated dashboards with KPIs that their work impacts. Organizational leaders should also share and discuss scorecard results at least monthly. Scorecard discussions should include interpretations of each goal's meaning and how each team member contributes to the goal's success. Celebrating successful progress towards KPIs can help to engage teams.

Activity 5.9 Dashboards in Action

As the outpatient clinic manager, you regularly review the clinical team dashboard, which displays each therapist's patient satisfaction average, average outcome measurement improvements, and percentage of time spent with direct patient care. Below is your team's most recent dashboard (see table 5.4).

Table 5.4 Sample Team Dashboard

Therapist	*Patient Satisfaction*	*Outcome Measurement % MCID* Improved*	*Percentage of Therapist Time in Patient Care*
A	60%	90%	88%
B	95%	91%	55%
C	92%	61%	85%
D	91%	92%	84%

Note: * Minimum clinically important difference

Based on this dashboard, how would you follow up with each individual and with the team as a whole?

____

____

____

____

Pragmatic Operations Management

When organizations and departments are underperforming on their KPIs, it is time to determine the breakdown forensically. Lean management tactics can provide valuable tools. Conducting an RCA of the deficit is commonly employed. During an RCA, each interprofessional team will have a representative review the case or the trend to identify errors or shortfalls. The manager must note that RCAs are retrospective studies and must be combined with proactive improvement techniques.[38] Langley et al. recommend asking three fundamental questions for improvement:[39]

1. What are we trying to accomplish?
2. How will we know that a change is an improvement?
3. What changes can we make that will result in improvement?

This philosophy evolved into the **Plan, Do, Study, Act** (PDSA) improvement cycle (see figure 5.6). Organizational managers should conduct RCAs with subsequent PDSAs with the first principle or purpose in mind. Without purpose at the center of quality improvement, "quick fix" mentalities and tactics may prevail, needlessly adding complexity while not addressing the underlying deficit. Once the interprofessional team has determined the underlying deficit and addressed the problem, the solution and correct process must be communicated to all work levels.

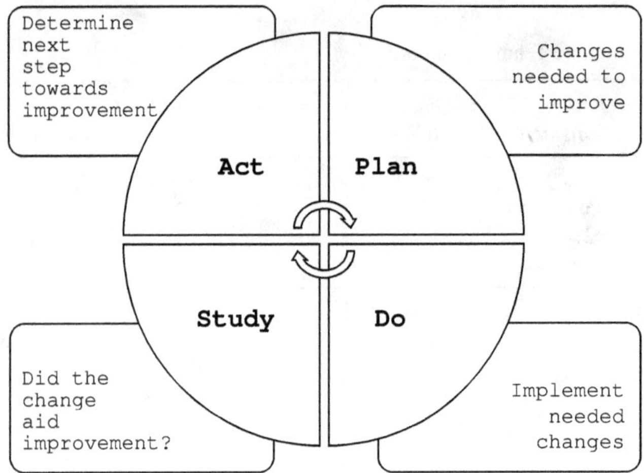

Figure 5.6 Plan, Do, Study, Act

Activity 5.10 Learning From Failure

You are the manager of an acute care hospital therapy department that has identified excessive and unwarranted bedrest as a contributor to hospital-acquired injury. You are tasked with leading the interprofessional team to address this need. What will your PDSA cycle look like?

____

____

____

____

Aha!

"Failure is success in progress."

Albert Einstein, German-born theoretical physicist best known for developing the theory of relativity

Untying the Knot to Correct the Fundamentals

If an organization finds more fundamental errors in their operations management philosophies and processes beyond individual errors that RCA and PDSAs can dissect and improve, deeper investigations are required. First, senior managers must go back to the organization's mission, vision, values, and underlying first principle. The team must refocus on the first principle building blocks of "what are we trying to accomplish, and for whom?" To do so, managers must abolish all management assumptions and start with a clean slate. Next, they should employ what Sakichi Toyoda called "The Five Whys." Managers should continue to dissect the issues by successively asking "why" until the problem or deficit is reduced to its fundamentals.[40] The dysfunctional knot is untied at that point, and a plan to rebuild properly can ensue.

Leading Human Progress

While translating the first principle into purposeful operations management process design and execution, the manager must focus on each team member and their adoption of best practices and correct processes. Communication of the first principle focused MOTM statement should be posted throughout work areas and with committee charters. Updated dashboards and scorecards should be posted and communicated each month.

Decision-Making

When decisions are needed, managers should consider and let the team know what type of input is needed and how the final decision will be made. As discussed in chapter 1, one finds that the terms *leadership* and *management* are sometimes interchanged; however, both have their nuances. For the decision-making discussion, we use the term *leadership style*. Will the decision be delegated to others to make or decided by the leader? How the final decision should be made is based on two things:

1. Which leadership style(s) a manager uses:[41]
    a. charismatic
    b. transformational
    c. transactional
    d. autocratic
    e. bureaucratic
    f. democratic

2. The parameters of choices available based on available resources, compliance requirements, ethical boundaries, and strategic direction.

Al Khajeh found that transformational, autocratic, and democratic "leadership" styles positively affect organizational performance. Within these more beneficial styles, the manager should choose whether each decision can be made democratically with the whole delegation of authority; alternatively, at the other end of the continuum, autocratic decision-making occurs when the manager remains responsible for all decision-making. A successful manager with an engaged team should rely more on democratic decision-making within the set of organizational parameters. Autocratic decision-making may be needed in emergency decision-making or other overwhelming organizational catastrophes when quick, decisive action is needed; however, it should be limited. For example, in the first few weeks of the COVID-19 pandemic in March and April 2020, the Baylor University Medical Center therapy department needed to utilize decisive action and decision-making to create and implement a temporary telehealth model to continue patient care for patients in infectious disease isolation while there was a worldwide short supply of personal protective equipment. Department management needed to utilize authority to rapidly put together a team of experts with strict directives to create and implement the novel program within two days to minimize missed patient needs. Within those strict parameters there existed a democratic interprofessional model creating a program based on the evolving evidence base.[42]

Team Communication

Communication is the chain that connects strategic direction and operations management with meaningful, safe, and effective action. In health care, communication breakdowns can lead to inefficient operations at best and catastrophic events at worst. Organizations should choose a consistent communication strategy that is employed continually.[43] One such evidence-based communication strategy is SBAR (situation, background, assessment, recommendation):[44]

1. **S**ituation (a concise statement of the problem)
2. **B**ackground (pertinent and brief information related to the situation)
3. **A**ssessment (analysis and considerations of options – what you found/think)
4. **R**ecommendation (action requested/recommended – what you want)

Organizations with standardized communication strategies such as SBAR can translate operational directions effectively, tackle communication challenges competently, and solve problems as they happen.

Working Through Conflict

Recall in chapter 2 discussions about the need to develop conflict management skills. Even the highest functioning teams will encounter conflict at times. Interprofessional teams bring together professionals with different backgrounds and perspectives through which to interpret and analyze situations and challenges. These different perspectives and professional passions to advance the organization and its patient care will invariably lead to conflict. The successful manager will utilize conflicting perspectives to dive into the situation using the power of diverse perspectives to progress.

Fisher et al. recommend looking for a shared purpose and "separate people from problems" when working through conflict and focusing on "interests instead of positions."[45] While separating people from problems, and before examining **shared interests** instead, the manager must help their conflicting team to identify any subjective interpretations or stories that may add unneeded stress and emotion. In emotional and stressful situations, we are all guilty at times of creating stories behind "why" people or situations upset us. These stories may or may not have validity, but they will limit our ability to address negotiations objectively. The manager needs to help those working through conflict to take control of their stories so that the stories do not take control and prevent collaborative communication. Helping those around us to work past their stories separates the people from the problems so that we can examine the merits of the challenge. The manager can then help the conflicted group to proceed to the next step in finding shared interests. Fisher et al. advise us to focus on interests, not each party's position. At the core lies the question, "what is important to them and to me?" The manager can then mediate to help each side to understand all the interests, including shared interests.[44]

Successful managers should continually watch for potential conflict, confusion, or ambivalence about the organizational first principle, purpose, and direction. The operative goal should be a shared purpose and applying the evidence, interprofessional strengths, and different approaches to meet that purpose.

Activity 5.11 Working Towards Shared Purpose

In your capacity as therapy department manager, two therapists come to you arguing about the best patient care treatment approach. Both clinicians are thoughtful and skilled but disagree significantly about this case.

How will you help to facilitate this disagreement beyond a simple resolution with the goal of improving overall teamwork and collaboration?

____

____

____

____

Bottom Line!

Successful operations management must be approached systematically and holistically. The manager must ensure that the team accurately understands the first principle and purpose. Each team member should relate to principled goals that fulfill that purpose and the MOTM statement. The clinic or department should construct and utilize EIP systems and structures focusing on creating value and should have quality improvement strategies and dashboards to monitor and improve quality, safety, and efficiency. Finally, the operations manager must adapt management styles that best manage the team under the circumstances, help the team members to work through conflict, and continue building team collaboration and communication.

Activity 5.12 Physical Therapy in the Emergency Department

As the therapy manager of a rural hospital and outpatient department therapy clinic, you have heard hospital concerns about increasing emergency department (ED) volumes. You are fortunate to have a small but talented group of inpatient and outpatient therapists who love pushing themselves and working at the top of their licenses. The team is interested in helping the ED, and the hospital management is interested in stationing a full-time therapist in the ED on weekdays. Now you and your team need to make this happen.

Step 1: Complete your new ED PT program MOTM statement.

____

____

Step 2: Explain how you might use a Pareto chart to determine the type of patients you will focus on.

____

____

Step 3: Explain how you will use the Six Sigma DMAIC methodology to design and implement your new program.

____

____

Suggested Readings

NEJM Catalyst. What is lean healthcare? April 27, 2018. https://catalyst.nejm.org/doi/full/10.1056/CAT.18.0193

Porter ME, Lee TH. What 21st century health care should learn from 20th century business. NEJM Catalyst. September 5, 2018. catalyst.nejm.org/doi/full/10.1056/CAT.18.0098

Rosenthal E. *An American Sickness: How Healthcare Became Big Business and How You Can Take It Back*. Penguin; 2017.

Shrank WH, Rogstad TL, Parekh N. Waste in the US Health Care System: Estimated Costs and Potential for Savings. *JAMA*. 2019; 322(15): 1501–1509. doi.org/10.1001/jama.2019.13978

References

1. Harari, O. *The Leadership Secrets of Colin Powell*. McGraw Hill; 2003; p. 164.
2. Taylor FW. *Shop Management*. Harper & Brothers; 1911.
3. Morgan G. *Images of Organization*. Updated edition. SAGE Publications, Inc.; 2006.
4. Parker LD, Ritson P. Fads, stereotypes and management gurus: Fayol and Follett today. *Manage Decis*. 2005; 43(10): 1335–1357. doi.org/10.1108/00251740510634903
5. NEJM Catalyst. What is lean healthcare? April 27, 2018. https://catalyst.nejm.org/doi/full/10.1056/CAT.18.0193
6. Rotter T, Plishka C, Lawal A, et al. What is lean management in health care? Development of an operational definition for a Cochrane systematic review. *Eval Health Prof.* 2019; 42(3): 366–390. doi.org/10.1177/0163278718756992
7. Itchhaporia D. The evolution of the quintuple aim. *J Am Coll Cardiol*. 2021; 78(22): 2262–2264. doi.org/10.1016/j.jacc.2021.10.018
8. Karbowski J. *Aristotle's Method in Ethics: Philosophy in Practice*. Cambridge University Press; 2019.
9. Martín-Velasco MJ. Popular knowledge and its rhetorical use in Aristotle. In: Muñoz Morcillo J, Robertson-von Trotha CY, eds. *Genealogy of Popular Science: From Ancient Ecphrasis to Virtual Reality*. Transcript Verlag; 2020: 131–150.
10. Baer D. Elon Musk uses this ancient critical-thinking strategy to outsmart everybody else. *Business Insider*. January 5, 2015. https://www.businessinsider.com/elon-musk-first-principles-2015-1
11. Hansen MT. The "man on the moon" standard. *Harvard Business Review*. May 25, 2011. https://hbr.org/2011/05/the-man-on-the-moon-standard
12. Bonebright CA, Clay DL, Ankenmann RD. The relationship of workaholism with work–life conflict, life satisfaction, and purpose in life. *J Couns Psychol*. 2000; 47(4): 469–477. https://doi.org/10.1037/0022-0167.47.4.469
13. Ryff CD, Singer BH. Know thyself and become what you are: A eudaimonic approach to psychological well-being. *J Happiness Stud.* 2008; 9: 13–39. doi.org/10.1007/s10902-006-9019-0
14. Rosenthal E. *An American Sickness: How Healthcare Became Big Business and How You Can Take It Back*. Penguin; 2017.
15. Kantabutra S, Avery GC. The power of vision: Statements that resonate. *J Bus Strategy.* 2010; 31(1): 37–45. doi.org/10.1108/02756661011012769
16. Porter ME. What is value in health care? *N Engl J Med*. 2010; 363(26): 2477–2481. doi.org/10.1056/NEJMp1011024

17. Porter ME, Lee TH. What 21st century health care should learn from 20th century business. NEJM Catalyst. September 5, 2018. catalyst.nejm.org/doi/full/10.1056/CAT.18.0098
18. Hull BL, Thut MC. Improving operational efficiency, effectiveness, and value in acute care physical therapy using the therapy value quotient. *J Acute Care Phys Ther.* 2019; 10(3): 107–116, p. 2. doi.org/10.1097/JAT.0000000000000101
19. Hull BL, Thut MC. A simple tool using AM-PAC "6-clicks" to measure value added in acute care physical therapy: The therapy value quotient. *J Acute Care Phys Ther*. 2018; 9(4): 155–162. doi.org/10.1097/JAT.0000000000000082
20. Morris ZS, Wooding S, Grant J. The answer is 17 years, what is the question: Understanding time lags in translational research. *J Roy Soc Med.* 2011; 104(12): 510–520. doi.org/10.1258/jrsm.2011.110180
21. Hull BL, Thut MC, Cheng SJ, Kaufhold DM, Brown SR. Changing the culture of a large multihospital acute care therapy system to value-added through best practice guidelines: A quality improvement project. *J Acute Care Phys Ther*. 2016; 7(2): 47–54. doi.org/10.1097/JAT.0000000000000025
22. Studer Q. *Hardwiring Excellence: Purpose, Worthwhile Work, Making a Difference.* 1st ed. Fire Starter Publishing; 2003.
23. Studer Q, Hagins M, Cochrane BS. The power of engagement: Creating the culture that gets your staff aligned and invested. *Healthc Manage Forum*. 2014; 27(1_suppl): S79–S87. doi.org/10.1016/j.hcmf.2014.01.008
24. Saks AM. Antecedents and consequences of employee engagement. *J Manag Psychol.* 2006; 21(7): 600–619. doi.org/10.1108/02683940610690169
25. Saks AM, Gruman JA, Zhang Q. Organization engagement: A review and comparison to job engagement. *J Organ Eff-People P*. 2021; 9(1): 20–49. https://doi.org/10.1108/JOEPP-12-2020-0253
26. American Society for Quality (2022). The define measure analyze improve control (DMAIC) process. Accessed June 24, 2024. https://asq.org/quality-resources/dmaic
27. Wysocki B, Lueck S. Just-in-time inventories make U.S. vulnerable in a pandemic. *The Wall Street Journal*. January 12, 2006. https://www.wsj.com/articles/SB113703203939544469
28. Shrank WH, Rogstad TL, Parekh N. Waste in the US Health Care System: Estimated costs and potential for savings. *JAMA*. 2019; 322(15): 1501–1509. doi.org/10.1001/jama.2019.13978
29. Institute of Medicine, Committee on Quality of Health Care in America. Kohn LT, Corrigan JM, Donaldson MS, Eds. I *To Err Is Human: Building a Safer Health System*. National Academies Press; 2000. http://www.ncbi.nlm.nih.gov/books/NBK225182/
30. Tammany JE, O'Connell JK., Allen BS, Brismée J-M. Are productivity goals in rehabilitation practice associated with unethical behaviors? *Arch Rehabil Res Clin Transl.* 2019; 1(1): 100002. doi.org/10.1016/j.arrct.2019.100002
31. Gawande A. The checklist. *The New Yorker*. December 10, 2007, http://www.newyorker.com/magazine/2007/12/10/the-checklist
32. Brennan GP, Fritz JM, Hunter SJ, Thackeray A, Delitto A, Erhard, RE. Identifying subgroups of patients with acute/subacute "nonspecific" low back pain: Results of a randomized clinical trial. *Spine*. 2006; 31(6): 623–631. https://doi.org/10.1097/01.brs.0000202807.72292.a8
33. Minick K. Using Data to Revolutionize the Practice of Physical Therapy. Paper presented at: *American Physical Therapy Association Combined Sections Meeting*, 2022; San Antonio, TX.

34. Hunter S. LAMP School of Management Quality Improvement & Monitoring Module. Paper presented at: *American Physical Therapy Association Combined Section Meeting*; 2022; San Antonio, TX.
35. Minick KI, Hunter SJ, Capin JJ, et al. Improved outcomes following a care guideline implementation: Part 1 of an analysis of 12 355 patients after total knee arthroplasty. *J Orthop Sports Phys Ther*. 2023; 53(3): 143–150. doi.org/10.2519/jospt.2022.11369
36. Hoyer EH, Young DL, Klein LM, et al. Toward a common language for measuring patient mobility in the hospital: Reliability and construct validity of interprofessional mobility measures. *Phys Ther*. 2017; 98(2): 133–142. doi.org/10.1093/ptj/pzx110
37. Kaplan RS, Norton DP. The balanced scorecard: Measures that drive performance. *Harvard Business Review*. January–February, 1992. https://hbr.org/1992/01/the-balanced-scorecard-measures-that-drive-performance-2
38. Sujan MA, Embrey D, Huang H. On the application of human reliability analysis in healthcare: Opportunities and challenges. *Reliab Eng Syst Saf*. 2020; 194: 106189. doi.org/10.1016/j.ress.2018.06.017
39. Langley GL, Moen R, Nolan KM, Nolan TW, Norman CL, Provost LP. *The Improvement Guide: A Practical Approach to Enhancing Organizational Performance*. 2nd ed. Jossey-Bass; 2009.
40. Ohno T. *Toyota Production System: Beyond Large-Scale Production*. CRC Press; 1988.
41. Al Khajeh EH. Impact of leadership styles on organizational performance. *J Hum Resour Manag Res*. 2018; 1–10. doi.org/10.5171/2018.687849
42. Exum E, Hull BL, Lee CW, et al. Applying telehealth technologies and strategies to provide acute care consultation and treatment of patients with confirmed or possible COVID-19. *J Acute Care Phys Ther*. 2020; 11(3): 103–112. https://doi.org/10.1097/JAT.0000000000000143
43. Institute for Healthcare Improvement. SBAR Tool: Situation-Background-Assessment-Recommendation. Accessed June 24, 2024. https://www.ihi.org:443/resources/Pages/Tools/SBARToolkit.aspx
44. Müller M, Jürgens J, Redaèlli M, Klingberg K, Hautz WE, Stock S. Impact of the communication and patient hand-off tool SBAR on patient safety: A systematic review. *BMJ Open*. 2018; 8(8): e022202. doi.org/10.1136/bmjopen-2018–022202
45. Fisher R, Ury WL, Patton B. *Getting to Yes: Negotiating Agreement Without Giving In*. Penguin; 2011, p. 19.

6 Managing People (Human Resources Management)

Chris Chimenti and Jennifer E. Green-Wilson

Leaders must be close enough to relate to others, but far enough ahead to motivate them.

John C. Maxwell, world-renowned speaker and
New York Times bestselling author of
The 21 Irrefutable Laws of Leadership[1]

Chapter Objectives

1. Discuss the employee life cycle.
2. Define elements that impact the employee experience.
3. Examine the essential functions of human resources management and strategic human resources management.
4. Discuss recruitment and interviewing practices for human resources management.
5. Discuss elements of compensation packages.
6. Discuss how goal-setting influences performance management.
7. Review legal considerations (i.e., employment law) for managing people.
8. Discuss managing people through leadership principles.

Management Vignette

Jason Berl, PT

The amount of time and energy it takes to manage or supervise people depends on the situation. For example, *who* you are managing and *what* you're working towards with regards to your goals will make a difference. Overall managing people – *and yourself* – takes an extensive amount of energy. Currently, I estimate that only 4% of my time is allocated for managing people, yet it's about 50% of my daily work! It takes work to understand other people's perspectives, put your ego aside, and think about the way you

DOI: 10.4324/9781003524250-8

communicate – the timing of the communication, your body language, and your tone. While managing people I've learned that *how* you say something matters a lot more than *what* you say. By *how*, I mean everything – the body language, the words you choose, being respectful and professional. When you're in a management role, all eyes are on you. You're the example (i.e., the role model).

You need to work as a team to function properly in physical therapy or in any organization. How I build and manage a team depends on where we are in the team process. You need to know the goal that everyone is trying to work towards, know what resources are needed to be successful, know "the plan," and then get the right people in those roles to do "the work." My role in the agency makes me responsible and accountable for agency-wide quality initiatives and outcomes, but I don't have any authority over the people on my team (in other words they don't report directly to me). Therefore, to manage effectively and achieve our collective goals, it's about *leading people*, inspiring people, building those relationships, and figuring out how to get people to move in the right direction without dictating the direction.

I believe that many of the problems in an organization are truly management problems. It's a management problem if you have people in the wrong positions. Managers should be identifying who needs to be in the right position at the right time for the right task or goal. It's a management problem if people don't do the work because they don't have access to the right tools and resources. It's a management problem if we're all working towards different goals or misaligned goals, changing directions frequently, using broken processes, not looking at why "something" is it not working, not getting to the root cause and then not fixing it.

Interviewing has been an interesting experience. I find it helpful to be honest and transparent in a way that might not make the open position (i.e., the role) look as great as you'd like it to be. If people join your team, they're going to find out where you're falling short. I want them to realize from the beginning that we have some things we're doing well, we have things we're not doing so well, we're working on a plan, and this is what you're going to be walking into. I want people to join our team being ready to work through those things and not see them as barriers that can't be resolved.

Onboarding provides an opportunity to meet with people one-on-one and make sure they have the right tools and resources from the very beginning. This proactive human resource strategy or approach underscores the importance of setting and clarifying expectations for each role, explaining the scope of what the team is working on and why, and outlining where the team is going. By doing this, you can address things sooner if performance isn't where you expect it to be.

Managing performance includes, "You understand what's expected, where our goals are, and if you're falling short of that, let's have a conversation." When managing performance, keep your emotions out of the various conversations. Stick to the issues. Be specific and objective, share examples, and be open to what the other person is saying. If you do that, you can walk away with an action plan that gives the person who's not meeting performance expectations the chance to change their performance. Ultimately, it's their choice whether they want to rise to that level or not or for them to tell me what else they need so that I can try to help them.

The advice I would share with physical therapist students learning to manage or supervise others is to get involved with more than what you're required to do. As a physical therapist or physical therapist student, get involved with other committees, take on students or mentor other people, whenever you can. All these experiences add up. Managing others is about relationships with people. Managing is a skill that you must learn through experience. Seek out different experiences and find mentors to help you to develop and refine your skills.

Chapter Introduction

A well-organized, responsive human resources (HR) team is vital to the success of any business. Depending on the size and structure of the organization, an HR team may be responsible for a variety of functions including hiring, recruiting, performance management, compensation, benefits, conflict resolution, compliance, workplace safety, and disciplinary action. As the term implies, HR is focused on the people, or employees, who constitute the workforce. Unlike other businesses such as manufacturing or construction, health care employees interact directly and frequently with people. Strong interpersonal relationships are paramount to the vitality of the business. As a result, health care organizations tend to rely heavily on the HR team (or HR functions) to ensure a well-staffed, effective workforce.

Employee Life Cycle

The **employee life cycle** is a model that depicts the entire employee-employer relationship within an organization.[2] This life cycle describes the different stages an employee goes through from the point when they are hired to when they leave. The seven stages in an employee life cycle model are shown in figure 6.1 and described briefly in table 6.1. Understanding the employee life cycle helps individuals *and* managers to know how to engage throughout the entire cycle. As an individual, understanding this cycle helps you to self-manage and navigate throughout each stage successfully to optimize your own **employee experience**. As a manager, understanding the employee life cycle enables you to attract the right candidate(s), optimize your employees' experiences, and improve productivity and performance in your organization.

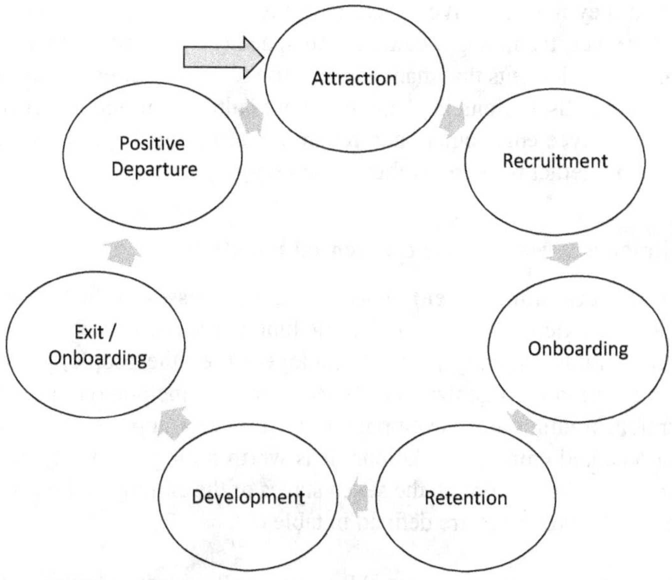

Figure 6.1 Employee Life Cycle

Table 6.1 Seven Stages of the Employee Life Cycle

Seven Stages	*Description*
1. Attraction	Eliciting potential candidates' interest towards an organization as a desirable place to work.
2. Recruitment	Process of finding, screening, and selecting qualified candidates for specific job opening(s).
3. Onboarding	Introducing new hires to the company culture, their specific roles, responsibilities, and expectations.
4. Retention	Implementing strategies to keep employees engaged and motivated to stay with the company.
5. Development	Providing opportunities for employees to gain new skills and advance their careers within the organization.
6. Exit/Offboarding	Managing the process when an individual leaves the company to ensure a smooth exit/departure.
7. Positive Departure	Creating a positive exit experience for departing employees (hopefully to retain the brand image as a "good place to work.")

Organizations can use the employee life cycle as a guide to create and implement meaningful human resources management policies and procedures that support the growth and development of their people.

Employee Experience

The **employee experience** represents how employees feel about what they encounter and observe within their companies over time. In the book, *The Employee Experience Advantage*, the author proposes that the best way to retain employees is by ensuring that they have positive experiences (i.e., are *happy*) and fulfilled in their role(s).[3] Moreover, technology, culture, and space (i.e., physical space or hybrid/remote) are three elements that managers can use to create better employee experiences. Recall the discussions in chapter 4 about culture. Culture is a critical component for employee engagement and retention because it shapes how employees feel about and interact with each other on an ongoing basis.

Human Resources Management: Essential Functions

Human resources management (HRM) is the processes performed within the organization (or external to it when the HR function is outsourced) as well as the informal (continuous) management of employees (i.e., the people) performed by all managers within an organization.[4] HRM processes include recruitment, selection, retention, training and development, performance appraisal, compensation, labor relations, and employee relations. It is worth noting that many of these essential functions align well with the seven stages of the employee life cycle model. The essential HR processes are defined in table 6.2.

Table 6.2 Essential Human Resources Management Processes: Common Terms and Definitions

HRM Process	*Definition*
Recruitment	Process of actively seeking out, finding and hiring candidates for a specific position/job. Hiring includes the process of integrating the recruit into the company (through onboarding).
Selection	Process of appraising candidates' qualities, expertise, and experience(s) to narrow the pool of applicants until the best person for the role can be identified. This process involves conducting interviews.
Retention[5]	Strategies used to reduce employee turnover, prevent attrition, increase (sustain) retention, and promote employee engagement.
Training and Development	Process of providing learning opportunities for employees to acquire specific knowledge, skills, and attitudes/abilities to improve job performance (i.e., for a particular job/task) and enable future career growth.
Performance Appraisal[6]	Appraising performance refers to the formal review (i.e., annual) of an employee's job performance (i.e., skills, achievements, and growth, or lack thereof) and overall contribution to a company (i.e. how they meet or don't meet established goals). Managers use performance appraisals to give employees feedback on their work, to confirm/support pay increases/bonuses, and to justify disciplinary action or termination decisions.
Compensation (Packages)[7]	Employers offer employees a compensation package (base salary and (fringe) benefits) in exchange for employment (doing the work); these packages vary by employer and by position(s).
Employee Relations[8]	Efforts by organizations to maintain positive relationships with employees. HRM helps to prevent and resolve problems or disputes between employees and management and assists in creating and enforcing policies that are fair and consistent with the workplace.
Labor Relations[9]	Labor relations, a sub-function of the human resources function, is focused on preventing and resolving employee-related problems, usually involving employees covered by a collective bargaining agreement or union contract.

Strategic Human Resources Management

Strategic human resources management (SHRM) is the comprehensive set of managerial activities and tasks related to developing and maintaining a qualified workforce.[4] SHRM is the process of formulating and executing HR policies and practices that produce the employee competencies and behaviors required for the organization to achieve its strategic objectives.[4] To produce the required staff competencies and behaviors, health care organizations need to implement the right mix of recruitment, selection, compensation, performance appraisal, employee development, and other HR strategies, policies, and practices. To implement these methods and practices strategically, organizations must:

- determine the requirements for positions in advance of recruiting/hiring (i.e., job analysis, job design, job descriptions);
- recruit and select qualified people;
- train and develop employees to meet future organizational needs (allow organization to grow); and
- provide adequate rewards and recognition to attract and retain top performers.

Bottom Line!

Managing human resources effectively can increase revenue and profitability, productivity and performance, market value, and organizational growth.[4]

Building the Team: Recruiting

Recruiting, interviewing, hiring, training, and retaining future team members is a labor-intensive endeavor. Depending on the specific position and job market, the manager is often confronted with one of two challenges: (1) candidates seem to be hiding away in a deep, dark cave and are nowhere to be found; or (2) resumes are piling up quickly and it simply isn't possible to interview each candidate individually. Regardless of the challenges at hand, the manager should approach each interview with one primary focus: not only to make sure that the candidate is right for both the position and the organization, but equally importantly to ensure that the position and the organization are right for the candidate. Long-term retention of your workforce brings stability, maturity, and expertise to an organization. Constructive outcomes from implementing explicit retention strategies include lower turnover, lower hiring costs, increased employee productivity, better employee experiences, stronger work relationships, less work-related stress, and less burnout.[5] Securing a team's commitment to the future also brings a promise of familiar faces, relationships, brand recognition, and, ultimately, customer loyalty.

When desperate to fill an open position due to short staffing, it can be far too tempting to hire the first candidate. Taking the time to ensure an equal fit can save considerable time, frustration, energy, and money down the road. In fact, it's estimated that the cost of turnover may be as high as two times the employee's annual salary.[10] Some candidates may interview well, but when it comes down to fitting into the culture, doing the work, and interacting with colleagues, performance may not necessarily match the interview skills that were so remarkable during the first impression. Consistently dedicating time to a thorough, objective interview process will pay dividends as the manager builds the team. **Behavioral interviewing** is a technique used to question candidates about their past experiences and is based on the premise that past performance may predict future behavior.[11] Behavioral interview questions prompt the candidate to provide concrete examples of previous actions they've taken in the workplace. Candidates' responses provide insight into how they may act (in similar situations) while immersed in your organization. An established interview evaluation form containing an objective scoring format is recommended to ensure consistency throughout the interview process. Below is an example of how an interview evaluation form may be formatted:

Describe a specific situation when you went beyond your scope of duties to help a co-worker:

____

What did you do?

____

What was the outcome?

____

Score (5 excellent, 4 good, 3 satisfactory, 2 fair, 1 poor) ________________

A practical five-step sequence or strategy for recruitment is outlined in box 6.1.

Box 6.1 Successful Recruitment Strategies

Step 1: The HR team conducts a phone interview, virtual meeting, or in some circumstances an in-person encounter to screen the candidate and establish an impression. If an organization is too small to have an HR team or the HR team isn't directly involved in various phases of the hiring process, the process would begin with step 2.

Step 2: The hiring manager contacts the candidate by phone or sets up a virtual meeting to discuss the position, probe rationale for interest in the position, and answer general questions.

Step 3: The hiring manager, along with a select group of team members, meets the candidate in person for an extensive (team) interview. Involvement of the department team members in the interview process enhances the chance of success with selecting the right candidate for the position. Also, the team is much more likely to support the final decision on candidate selection, provide assistance during the training/onboarding process, and ensure that the new employee feels welcome (included). During the interview, the team should pay particular attention to body language, level of engagement, interest in the organization, and eagerness to start. The plan for training, career development, and continuing education can be discussed to ensure long-term success is a priority. Candidates who come prepared with a list of questions and appear genuinely engaged in employment often turn out to be the ones who buy into the organization's mission, vision, and values.

Step 4: The hiring manager asks a member of the team to host a shadow experience or ride-a-long with the candidate. The team member can be asked to observe interactions with other team members, assess level of engagement, and envision the level of synergy for the team and organization.

Step 5: The hiring manager calls a brief meeting with Human Resources and the hosting team member(s) to discuss impressions and recommendations for hiring status.

You as the Hiring Manager: Interview Tips for Employers[12]

The STAR model[13] of interview design is another approach to consider when recruiting and encompasses the following:

- Situation: Ask the candidate to describe a situation where they used a key behavior or competency.
- Task: Invite the applicant to articulate the specific task(s) they had to achieve within the stated situation.
- Action: Ask the candidate to clearly convey actions they took in the face of the situation and task at hand.
- Result: Ask the individual to define the results or outcomes triggered by their actions within a broader context.

You as the Potential Employee: How to Prepare for an Interview[14]

Interviews can be highly stressful situations, especially if it's your first interview. Planning before an interview can prepare you for a successful experience. Below is a checklist of suggestions for you to consider as part of your interview planning.

☐ Research the company before the actual interview to understand the company and the role for which you are applying. Research the company's vision, mission, and values, as well as any recent news or developments that might be relevant to your interview.

- ☐ Review the job description to understand the responsibilities and qualifications required for the position.
- ☐ Practice your answers out loud (not just in your head) by role-playing a mock interview with another person. This process can help you to feel more comfortable and confident during the actual interview. Practice answering the question directly and succinctly. Use the set of common interview questions listed in the next section to start your role-play scenario.
- ☐ Dress professionally. It's better to dress too professionally, rather than too casually.
- ☐ Arrive 10–15 minutes early for your interview.
- ☐ Bring a hard copy of your resume/CV (curriculum vitae) to the interview.
- ☐ After the interview, follow up. Send a hand-written "thank you" note or email to the interviewer.

Common Interview Questions

Here are a few common interview questions that you can use to practice (role-play) for your interview:[15]

- ☐ Tell me about yourself and describe your background. (Hint: be brief.)
- ☐ How did you hear about this position?
- ☐ What type of work environment do you prefer?
- ☐ What are your strengths? What are your areas of weakness?
- ☐ Why do you want this position?
- ☐ What attracted you to our company?
- ☐ What do you know about our company?
- ☐ Why should we hire you?
- ☐ What can you do for us that other candidates can't?
- ☐ How do you deal with pressure or stressful situations?
- ☐ Do you prefer working independently or on a team?
- ☐ How do you keep yourself organized when you're balancing multiple projects?
- ☐ What did you do in the last year to improve yourself?
- ☐ What are your salary expectations? It is worth noting that it's better to discuss a salary range (rather than a specific number) during the interview to leave room for future negotiation.

Compensation Packages

Good news! Your preparation for the interview worked well and you've been offered the position. Now it's time for you to understand and assess what's included in the compensation package. Compensation packages vary by employer(s) and by the particular position that's available. Before accepting an offer, make sure you know what's included in the compensation package to help you to make a strategic decision regarding your future employment. The common components that you'll find in a compensation package are listed and described in table 6.3.

Table 6.3 Compensation: Some Common Terms and Definitions

Term	*Definition*
Salary	Base salary refers to the amount of money you make for completing your work (i.e., the money reflected in your paycheck). Bonuses or incentives (variable compensation) may be included as part of your compensation plan.
Paid Time Off (PTO or personal time off) (i.e., paid holidays, vacation days and sick days)[16]	Compensated time away from work, provided by an employer, for employees to use in different ways. Often measured in hours and classified for different types of absences (i.e., sickness or vacation time).
Health Insurance Benefits (i.e., medical, dental and vision)	Your compensation package may include a package or range of health insurance benefits.
Retirement savings plan(s)	Many employers offer retirement savings plan(s) (options) that allow you to contribute part of your pre-tax earnings to an investment account (e.g., 401(k) retirement savings plan).

In addition to these common components, some employers may include other benefits in their compensation packages to attract talent and stay competitive in their industry. For example, some employers may offer telecommuting or the option to work remotely (i.e., home office). Some employers may offer you tuition reimbursement or may subsidize/pay for training and development (i.e., continuing education).

Aha!

How to Assess a Compensation Package

It's important to consider each element of a potential compensation package (i.e., one that has been offered) and the level of importance that each component holds for you. Consider the following tips:

- Tip 1: Identify what's important to you. Consider your lifestyle, goals, what you value in life, and what aspects (in a compensation package) you value the most. Remember that the employee experience can be shaped by more than just money.
- Tip 2: Gather and understand the specific details from your potential employer, especially regarding those elements that are most important to you (i.e., health insurance plans, fringe benefits).
- Tip 3: Clarify eligibility requirements. Some benefits or "perks" may not be available to you right away (i.e., you may not receive medical coverage until you've been with the company for at least 90 days; tuition reimbursement

needs to be approved by your manager and is only available after your first year of employment).

- Tip 4: Compare your offer with current trends and other compensation benchmarks. There are several websites available that allow you to compare salary and benefits data across different companies and geographical locations (see Tool: Finding Compensation Benchmarks).

Tool

Finding Compensation Benchmarks[17]

You should have an idea about the salary range linked to the position (for which you are interviewing) before you have your first interview. Helpful websites include:

Glassdoor (https://www.glassdoor.com/Salaries/physical-therapist-salary-SRCH_KO0,18.htm)
Fishbowl (https://www.fishbowlapp.com/post/curious-on-how-much-ptptas-are-currently-making-hourly-or-salary-based-on-their-experience-level-practice-setting-and)
Vault.com (https://vault.com/professions/physical-therapists)
ZipRecruiter (https://www.ziprecruiter.com/Salaries/What-Is-the-Average-Physical-Therapist-Salary-by-State)

Activity 6.1 Researching Salaries

Take a few minutes – *right now* – to research salaries for physical therapists using at least two three different websites (from the list provided in the tool section). What did you discover?

____

____

____

Building the Team: Cultivating Talent

Once the right candidate has been selected, the manager should get to work on a plan for onboarding, training, and building relationships across the organization. New employees thrust into a new role with little preparation are destined for turnover for another position elsewhere. Ample training early on to ensure that the employee "does the job right the first time" mitigates anxiety and frustration. None of us enjoy being corrected or reprimanded for doing something wrong on the job, especially if it's a failure of the training process. Knowledge and skills are important, but teamwork, emotional intelligence/self-leadership, and self-management shouldn't be overlooked. Special attention to understanding the motivations of each individual member of the team is a key to maximizing performance. Constructive feedback, support from a peer network, and comprehensive training are a few key elements to consider. Employee recognition for a job well done creates a positive, engaging environment. Pointing out mistakes may be necessary, but it's best to catch an employee doing something right or going the extra mile and take the time to celebrate the moment. Routinely scheduled meetings with a new employee during the first 6–12 months provides the opportunity for ongoing dialogue about growth, expectations, role clarification, and performance. Goal setting and (informal) progress reviews provide the new employee with a structured understanding of how they are settling in and contributing to the organization.

Set Goals and Follow Up (Manage Performance)

During the onboarding process, every new employee should be provided with a copy of their job description (see box 6.2 for a sample job description).

Box 6.2 Job Description for a Physical Therapist18

[Intro Paragraph] Brief company introduction.

Physical Therapist Responsibilities (*examples*):

- Restores patient's function, alleviates pain, and prevents disabilities by planning and administering medically prescribed physical therapy.
- Provides quality care by assessing and interpreting evaluations and test results.
- Determines physical therapy treatment plans.
- Helps patient to accomplish treatment plan by administering and supervising the treatment plan.
- Evaluates and records patients progress, modifying treatment plans, and trying new treatments if required.
- Documents patient care services.

[Work Hours & Benefits]
Includes a description of the work hours and benefits for the position, information about flexible schedules, shift work, and travel requirements. Describes unique perks (i.e., gym discounts, continuing education, childcare reimbursements). The physical therapist salary range may be included early on to demonstrate pay transparency.

Physical Therapist's Qualifications/Skills (*examples*):

- Communication skills/interpersonal skills
- Motivation skills
- Time management skills
- Self-management skills
- Complex problem-solving skills
- Persuasion skills
- Resilience
- Basic computer skills

Education and Experience Requirements:
Clarify requirements that are preferred, rather than required. Adding things beyond the "minimum requirements" may affect the screening of other qualified candidates (*examples*):
DPT preferred
Licensed as a physical therapist (in state in which you need to practice)
Minimum of one year of physical therapy experience.

Once onboarding is complete and the employee is settled into their new role, it's time to sit down and set goals for the future. Each goal should follow the SMART format:

- **S**pecific: What you wish to accomplish should be clearly defined.
- **M**easurable: The goal is defined by a tangible metric.
- **A**ttainable: The goal should inspire motivation, is achievable, and shouldn't be too lofty.
- **R**elevant: The basis for the goal is clear and related to the overall success of the team.
- **T**ime-bound: The target date is made clear.

An example of a SMART goal may be "Consistently achieve 16 units of billable units/day for a minimum of five consecutive workdays by August 15 to establish baseline productivity needed for this position." As the employee is working towards this target date, you should be briefly checking in on progress and offering additional support as needed. By doing so, you'll show the employee that you're invested in their success. Moreover, they're much more likely to achieve the goal.

Once the employee hits their stride, it's time to step up the pace. Michelangelo once said, "a great danger (for most) is not that our aim is too high, and we miss it … but that our aim is too low and we reach it." Your team will likely strive to reach the bar that you have set, and will likely go no higher.

Legal Considerations for Managing People[19]

An important role for the HRM function (within an organization) is to ensure a safe, healthy, fair and equitable workplace for employees. HRM is responsible for strategically managing employees within an organization while remaining compliant with laws that govern employee rights and employer obligations. **HR compliance** means ensuring that company policies and actions adhere to labor laws (i.e., federal, state, or municipality). If an organization violates these complex and ever-changing regulations, it exposes itself to risk, including lawsuits, financial losses, and reputation damage.

There is a set of laws that affect HRM. It is essential for employees and managers to understand the impact of these laws affecting the workplace. Several categories of different laws are listed and described briefly in table 6.4.

Table 6.4 Categories of Laws for Human Resources Management

Category of Laws	*Description*
Workplace Discrimination Laws	Equal Employment Opportunity (EEO) laws protect against the discrimination of any individual based on age, disability, genetic information, national origin, race/color, sex, pregnancy, or religion. Examples of individual laws that safeguard **protected classes** of individuals include: • Americans with Disabilities Act (ADA) • Equal Pay Act (EPA) • Age Discrimination in Employment Act (ADEA) • Pregnancy Discrimination Act (PDA) These laws are applicable during all stages of an employee's working life cycle, from pre-hiring processes through rightful termination. A protected class, created by both federal and state laws, is a group of people with a common characteristic who are legally protected from employment discrimination based on that characteristic.
Wage and Hour Laws	These laws are regulated by the US Department of Labor and protect the wages and hours of employees. *Examples*: • The Fair Labor Standards Act (FLSA) dictates the national minimum wage, establishes the 40-hour work week, outlines requirements for overtime pay, and directs child labor regulations. • The Family and Medical Leave Act (FMLA) (1993) entitles eligible employees to 12 weeks of unpaid leave for certain family and medical reasons, with a continuance of health care coverage and job protection.

(*Continued*)

Table 6.4 (Continued)

Category of Laws	*Description*
Employee Benefits Laws	Protect employees' access to benefits. *Examples*: • The Affordable Care Act (i.e., "Obamacare") increased access to affordable health care for those living below the federal poverty level. • The Employee Retirement Income Security Act (ERISA) stipulates that any organization offering pension plans must meet certain minimum standards. • The Consolidated Omnibus Budget Reconciliation Act (COBRA) mandates that health insurance programs must provide eligible employees access to continued health insurance coverage for a period of time after leaving employment. • The Health Insurance Portability and Accountability Act (HIPAA) affords employees and their dependents protection and privacy from the release of personal medical records. It also protects employees from discrimination based on their medical condition or history.
Immigration Laws	Ensure that employers only hire candidates eligible to work in the United States, including citizens, non-citizen nationals, lawful permanent residents, and aliens authorized to work. Regulations outline the use of I-9 forms to verify compliance. *Example*: • Immigration and Nationality Act (INA)
Workplace Safety Laws	• The Occupational Safety and Health Act (OSHA) (1970) ensures that employees are provided safe working conditions. • Workers Compensation Laws outline the administration of disability programs that serve federal employees who are injured on the job. Individuals who work for private companies or state governments are protected under regulations dictated by the individual states worker compensation boards.

Important federal statutes that directly or indirectly affect the employment setting are the Fair Labor Standards Act (FLSA), the Family and Medical Leave Act (FMLA), the Americans with Disabilities Act (ADA), and the Health Insurance Portability and Accountability Act (HIPAA; 1996). Moreover, federal laws establish legal requirements for managing the workforce and include the Civil Rights Act (Title VII), the Fair Labor Standards Act, and the Americans with Disabilities Act. State and local laws also play an important role in the workplace. Examples of these employment laws are listed in table 6.5. It is worth mentioning that sometimes state and local laws extend the provisions of federal law, while in other cases, new regulations must be put in place.

Jason Berl (see the management vignette at the beginning of this chapter), Chris Chimenti (co-author of chapter 6), Brian Hull (author of chapter 5), and Jerre van den Bent (see the management vignette at the beginning of chapter 1) all emphasize that managing people successfully requires *leadership*. Recall in chapter 1 when

Table 6.5 Description of Federal and State Employment Laws[4]

Employment Law	*Description*
Equal Pay Act of 1963	Requires that men and women performing equal jobs receive equal pay.
Civil Rights Act (Title VII) of 1964	The portion of the law prohibiting discrimination in employment based on race, sex, religion, national origin, or color. Blocks discrimination in hiring, promoting, compensation, training, benefits, and other HR aspects.
Americans with Disabilities Act (ADA) of 1990	Prohibits discrimination against individuals with disabilities.
Americans with Disabilities Act Amendments Act (ADAAA) of 2008	Provides a more flexible and inclusive definition of a qualifying disability.

we discussed the differences between management and leadership. Management and leadership are complementary but require different sets of skills that can and need to be developed. Physical therapists need to develop their management and business literacy skills *as well as* leadership skills to be successful in clinical practice. The focus of this textbook is management. However, the following vignette by Chris Chimenti highlights a few key principles or "secrets of success" for *managing people effectively through real-world leadership experiences*. Moreover, that's why the quotation (discussed below) was selected for this chapter.

Management Vignette

Chris Chimenti – Managing People Through Leadership

You've assembled the "dream team." Now, how do you go about holding this team together in the long run? Can you draw out the true potential buried deep within each individual? John C. Maxwell, author of *The 21 Irrefutable Laws of Leadership*, wrote that "leaders must be close enough to relate to others, but far enough ahead to motivate them."[20] This brief quotation epitomizes several key principles inherent to managing people through successful leadership.

Five key principles that will help to guide you in managing people effectively are:

1. Build and strengthen relationships.
2. Establish the culture.
3. Make the vision crystal clear.
4. Invest in growth and development.
5. Engage in succession planning.

Principle 1: Build and Strengthen Relationships

A delicate line exists when sharing relationships with employees who report directly to you. While it's important to get to know each person, getting too close can create troublesome moral and legal conflicts, especially if the need for disciplinary action arises for issues related to performance or attendance. Be cautious when spending time with direct reports outside of work hours or sharing social media interaction. However, getting to know some things about each member of your team (i.e., hobbies, family, favorite sports team, and even their birthday) can go a long way to show you care about the person, not just the employee. After all, we're all human beings who happen to share a professional relationship. At the end of the day, the interactions we share with our direct manager are a key factor in our job satisfaction, and ultimately long-term engagement with our employer.[21] Interestingly, a recent Gallup poll indicated that "52% of voluntarily exiting employees say their manager or organization could have done something to prevent them from leaving their job."[22]

Principle 2: Establish the Culture

Culture in the workplace is critical. According to *Forbes* magazine, "A positive workplace culture improves teamwork, raises the morale, increases productivity and efficiency, and enhances retention of the workforce. Job satisfaction, collaboration, and work performance are all enhanced."[23] Based on this realization, culture is a key driver behind organizational success. Recall from chapter 4 the detailed discussions about culture. Here is a list of a few additional concepts to consider for managing people and, subsequently, culture:

- Open-door policy: Each member of the team feels comfortable (safe) raising questions and concerns.
- Recognize and celebrate: Give awards, hand-written notes, and gift cards, host luncheons and picnics, and share announcements to acknowledge a job well done.
- Follow up: Close the loop on requests and suggestions, even if the response isn't what the employee was looking for.
- Take the temperature: Every so often, ask each member of your team, "How would you rate your job satisfaction on a 0–10 scale?"
- Show support: Demonstrate compassion and flexibility when employees struggle with a personal matter.
- Communicate, communicate, communicate: Just when you think you've communicated enough with your team, communicate again.

Activity 6.2 What Matters to You?

Review the list in the management vignette. In the space provided, pick the top three things (from this list) that are important to you and reflect on why they matter.

____

____

____

____

Principle 3: Make the Vision Crystal Clear

Where do you see your team going in the next three to five years? The answer to this question is important as it reveals the common goal and direction for each member of your team. For example, in the early days of Microsoft the vision for the company was to see a computer on every desk and in every home. Fast forward to 2014 when Amazon declared, "Our vision is to be Earth's most customer-centric company, where customers can find and discover anything they might want to buy online, and endeavors to offer its customers the lowest possible prices."[24] It appears these visions have largely come to fruition and impacted our lives for years to come. It's important for your team to not only understand the vision, but to buy into it as well. An impactful and well-communicated vision has the power to harness your team's energy and make things happen.

Activity 6.3

Take a moment to reflect upon your current (or previous) employment. Answer the following questions:

Do your career goals align with the tasks of day-to-day operations?

____

Have you bought into your organization's short-term and long-term goals?

____

Is the connection clear between your individual contributions and the organization's bottom line?

Could your employer do some things differently that would optimize your performance? If so, what and why?

The answers to these questions can provide helpful insight into the "right fit" for long-term employment.

Principle 4: Invest in Growth and Development

Professionals want to feel as though they're part of something special. While formal education, board exams, and degrees are important, long-term success is largely defined through a commitment to life-long learning and ongoing skill development. As a manager, you have the power to support your team in rising to a level above the competition. This can involve financial and time-off support to obtain advanced certifications. Or it can be as simple as implementing a journal club or arranging a schedule of guest lectures by various content experts. Regardless of the path you can afford to take, make it clear to your team that you're committed to ensuring that they feel effective in and inspired by the work they are each doing.

Principle 5: Engage in Succession Planning

You've built the dream team, employee retention is at an all-time high, patients are lined up outside the door for your world-class service, and the organization is exceeding all its goals despite the fact you're not even at year end. Just when you think you've reached the summit, the bottom drops out. You need to leave town to help care for an ailing parent, your Clinical Director resigns because they are going back to school to pursue a PhD, and a married couple employed at your busiest location announce that they are relocating out of state to be closer to family. You ask yourself, "What am I going to do now?" Successful HRM practices mean that you are prepared for moments like these. Every clinical practice needs employees who are perfectly content to give 100% every day but who may have no interest in climbing the corporate ladder. At the same time, whether outspoken or not, other employees would gladly seize the opportunity to grow their skills and step on the path towards career development. To successfully weather a storm as described above, managers can prepare ahead of time by conducting a 9 Box Grid.[25] This tool is designed to place individual employees into one of nine different categories based on current performance and potential for growth in the future (see figure 6.2). The tool allows managers to identify employees who may be ripe for management development, often well in advance of the need for them to serve in a formal management position. Using this tool, some employees may be considered "High Performers, Low Potential." In contrast, your potential future managers may be considered "Moderate Performers, High Potential." By using this tool once or twice a year, managers can identify and cultivate the talent that will be ready to step up when the time is right.

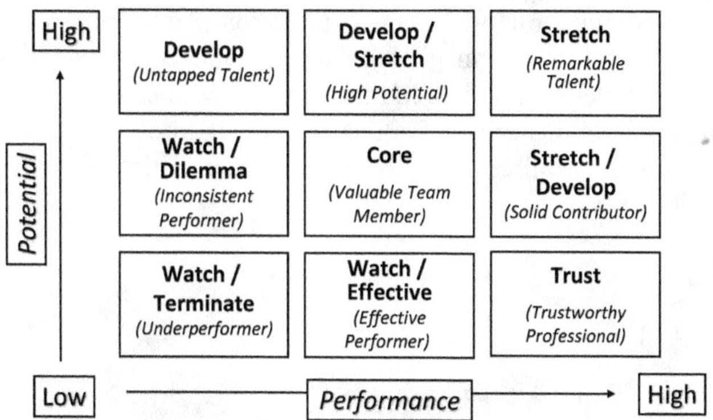

Figure 6.2 The 9 Box Grid: A Tool for Career and Succession Planning[24]

Activity 6.4 Where Do You Fit?

Review the 9 Box Grid (see figure 6.3) and identify the category in which you fit – right now – by placing an X in the appropriate box. Next, identify the category in which you aspire to fit within the next 1–2 years by placing a Y in the appropriate box.

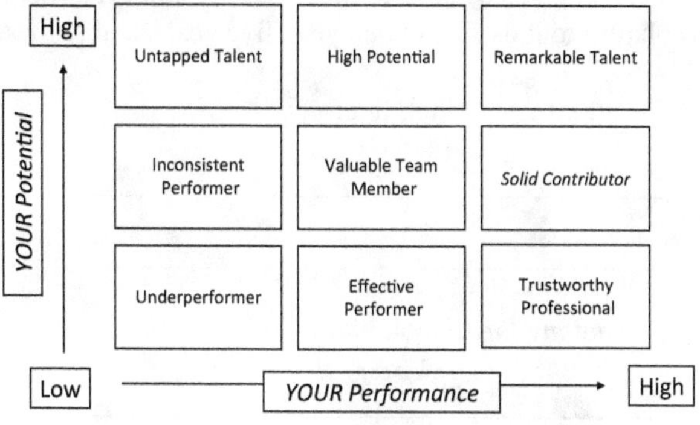

Figure 6.3 Self-Assess Your Fit

Career Management (Managing Your Career)

Career management involves purposeful planning, combined with active career development. It is the process of understanding yourself, identifying your career goals and your strategy, and implementing them with regular review and monitoring.[26] Career management[27] can help you and organizations develop strategies for ongoing professional development and succession planning. For organizations, career management supports strategic succession planning. For individuals, career management is the process of taking an active role in planning your career for the future through structured plans (i.e., action plans) and goal setting (i.e., short-term goals and long-term goals). Career management includes achieving desired positions/roles (i.e., Clinic Manager) and advancement (i.e., improved financial compensation, better benefits), or even being hired by a different organization. This process requires research, planning (i.e. action plans), networking, and goal setting.

Aha!

Your Career Plan is Up to You!

Even though you may have formal annual performance reviews (i.e., appraisals) with your manager, ultimately the responsibility for managing your career lies with you![26]

Activity 6.5 Career Planning

Answer the following questions, in the space provided, to start your process of managing *your* career.

Draft your career goals by envisioning what you want *your life* (personally and professionally) to look like in one year, five years, and ten years' time.

In one year, I want *my life* to look like:

____

____

In five years, I want *my life* to look like:

____

____

In ten years, I want *my life* to look like:

____

____

Do you want to have a prominent role in your profession?

Yes *No* *Maybe?* *Haven't considered this yet*

Are you hoping for a career with a good work/life balance? Describe how this would look for you.

____

____

Do you want to retire early by concentrating on earnings and savings (i.e., retirement planning) throughout your career?

Yes *No* *Maybe?* *Haven't considered this yet*

Career management also includes crafting a strategy or action plan by breaking down the process into multiple actionable and achievable steps aimed at achieving your specific goals. Once crafted, you can review and reflect upon the progress you are making or adjust some of your strategies as needed to keep you headed in the right direction for future success.

Bottom Line!

Invest in developing yourself! Even though many organizations invest in developing their people (especially learning organizations) by providing funding for external continuing education or internal training opportunities, it's important for you to work on the specific competencies and experiences that relate to achievement of your ultimate goals.

Suggested Readings:

Green-Wilson J, Zeigler S. *Learning to Lead in Physical Therapy*. Slack, Inc.; 2020.

Scott K. *Radical Candor: Be a Kick-Ass Boss Without Losing Your Humanity*. St. Martin's Press; 2019.

References

1. Maxwell JC. *The 21 Irrefutable Laws of Leadership*. Harper Collins Leadership; 2022.
2. Verdinden N. Employee life cycle: The ultimate guide for HR. Academy to Innovate HR. Accessed July 26, 2024. https://www.aihr.com/blog/employee-life-cycle/#:~:text=The%20employee%20life%20cycle%20consists,%2C%20offboarding%2C%20and%20happy%20leavers
3. Morgan J. *The Employee Experience Advantage*. Wiley; 2017.
4. Fried BJ, Fottler MD. *Fundamentals of Human Resources in Healthcare*. 2nd ed. Health Administration Press; 2018.
5. Retention strategy. Bamboo HR. Accessed July 26, 2024. https://www.bamboohr.com/resources/hr-glossary/retention-strategy
6. Hayes A. Performance appraisals in the workplace: Use, types, and criticisms. Investopedia. Updated June 4, 2024. https://www.investopedia.com/what-is-a-performance-appraisal-4586834
7. Indeed Editorial Team. Compensation packages: Definition and what they include. Indeed. Updated October 28, 2022. https://www.indeed.com/career-advice/career-development/compensation-packages
8. Employee relations. Bamboo HR. Accessed July 26, 2024. https://www.bamboohr.com/resources/hr-glossary/employee-relations
9. What is labor relations? Everything HR should know. HR Acuity. December 13, 2022. https://www.hracuity.com/blog/what-is-labor-relations-everything-hr-should-know/#:~:text=Labor%20relations%20is%20a%20sub,bargaining%20agreement%20or%20union%20contract
10. Mcfeely S, Wigert B. This fixable problem costs U.S. businesses $1 trillion. Workplace. March 13, 2019. https://www.gallup.com/workplace/247391/fixable-problem-costs-businesses trillion.aspx#:~:text=The%20cost%20of%20replacing%20an,to%20%242.6%20million%20per%20year
11. Elliott, J. What is behavioral interviewing? And how to use it to hire for your business. CO. July 27, 2022. https://www.uschamber.com/co/run/human-resources/behavioral-interviewing
12. Paychex Worx Blog. Essential interview tips for employers. Paychex. Accessed July 26, 2024. https://www.paychex.com/articles/human-resources/employer-best-practices-tips-for-interviews#0Topinterview
13. Birt J. How to use the STAR interview response technique. Indeed. Updated April 9, 2024. https://www.indeed.com/career-advice/interviewing/how-to-use-the-star-interview-response-technique
14. How to prepare for an interview (steps & tips). Handshake Blog. Accessed July 26, 2024. https://joinhandshake.com/blog/students/how-to-prepare-for-an-interview/
15. Oliver V. 10 Common job interview questions and how to answer them. November 11, 2021. Harvard Business Review. https://hbr.org/2021/11/10-common-job-interview-questions-and-how-to-answer-them
16. What is paid time off (PTO)? Bamboo HR. Accessed July 26, 2024. https://www.bamboohr.com/resources/hr-glossary/paid-time-off-pto
17. Occupational employment and wages, May 2023. US Bureau of Labor Statistics. Accessed July 26, 2024. https://www.bls.gov/oes/current/oes291123.htm
18. Physical therapist job description template. Monster. Accessed July 26, 2024. https://hiring.monster.com/resources/job-descriptions/healthcare/physical-therapist/
19. Legal issues affecting HR managers (know your HR law). Factorial. September 5, 2023. https://factorialhr.com/blog/legal-issues-hr-law/?variant=original-new-design

20. Maxwell JC. *The 21 Irrefutable Laws of Leadership*. Harper Collins Leadership; 2022.
21. Mann Jackson N. Manager relationships with employees can boost retention. ADP. Accessed July 26, 2024. https://www.adp.com/spark/articles/2018/11/manager-relationships-with-employees-can-boost-retention.aspx
22. Mclain D, Morgan I. Overwhelmed by employee turnover? Have stay conversations. Gallup. October 11, 2021. https://www.gallup.com/workplace/355238/overwhelmed-employee-turnover-stay-conversations.aspx
23. Agarwal P. How to create a positive workplace culture. *Forbes*. August 29, 2018. https://www.forbes.com/sites/pragyaagarwaleurope/2018/08/29/how-to-create-a-positive-work-place-culture/?sh=5c9ac3304272
24. Björklund A. Amazon's vision statement. Zooma. June 5, 2014. https://zooma.agency/en/learn/amazons-vision-statement
25. Van Vulpen E, van der Merwe M. The 9 box grid: A practitioner's guide. Academy to Innovate HR. Accessed July 26, 2024. https://www.aihr.com/blog/9-box-grid/
26. Neale P. Career management: For you and your leadership. *Forbes*. August 13, 2021. https://www.forbes.com/sites/forbescoachescouncil/2021/08/13/career-management-for-you-and-your-leadership/
27. Indeed Editorial Team. What is career management? (And how to create a plan). Indeed. Updated February 3, 2023. https://www.indeed.com/career-advice/career-development/career-managment

7 Managing the Financial Bottom Line (Financial Management)

Karen M. Hughes

Understanding the business models in the health care industry is fundamental for all clinicians, so they know how to operate when the financial marketplace continually lowers the reimbursement for services provided.

John J Petosa, Esq, JD, CPA, Syracuse University Professor of Practice Whitman School of Management

Chapter Objectives

1. Understand the importance of developing financial literacy and financial health literacy as a physical therapist.
2. Examine the financial fundamentals for financial management.
3. Examine how to analyze financial performance.
4. Examine how to implement action plans, through data-informed decision-making, to improve financial performance.
5. Discuss general aspects of the revenue cycle management process.

Management Vignette

Lori Pearlmutter, PT

Physical therapist students need to develop financial literacy for personal and professional reasons. Basically, it's important for DPT students to get through school without graduating with such high debt. Pre-physical therapy students need to understand what this decision entails – which school they should pick, the cost-benefit analysis of their choice(s), and what kinds of assistance they can access to get through school without being totally in debt for the rest of their lives. DPT students are generally younger in age and often young people don't think about the future because it's so far ahead. Adam Alter, in his book *Anatomy of a Breakthrough*,[1] talks about how young people don't think about retirement because they can't identify with their

DOI: 10.4324/9781003524250-9

70-year-old selves. Personally, thinking about the future allows us to be able to live the kind of life we want by starting to save a little bit at a time and understanding/applying financial strategies like the time value of money and compound interest or how to use money to make money. We don't think ahead to the future, which is very normal. But when we think about what we *want* to do with our lives, then, doesn't it become a discussion about money? It becomes a discussion about what our desires are, what matters to us, and how we want to live our lives. That's important. Professionally, you don't want to pick "a job" just because there's good money in it. You want to pick the opportunity that you are passionate about *and* has good money in it.

I don't think physical therapists really understand that reimbursement is going to keep changing and how little we get reimbursed. Physical therapists think that if they see six or seven patients a day and charge this amount for each patient seen, then why isn't that enough? I wish physical therapists understood that what you charge or bill insurance companies and what you actually get paid is different. Also, physical therapists don't seem to understand the costs associated with what we do (i.e., we must keep our lights and heating on, we might have equipment breaking down, and we must order supplies).

Financial literacy is like any other kind of literacy. Financial literacy means you are always learning and growing. It's not, "I understand finance" and that's it. It's being open to the fact that this is another area of my life in which I can learn; I'm going to learn more and more about finance over time. It's about not being afraid of learning and wanting to learn (i.e., by asking questions and seeking help). It's about reaching out to experts in finance and using the resources that are available. It's about understanding finance from a growth mindset and as a facet of lifelong learning. Finance is like everything else. It's not, "I took a yoga class today and that's it. I'm never taking another yoga class." You must have the same mindset about finance, but unfortunately many physical therapists often react, "No, I don't need this. This isn't important."

We are hurting ourselves, our practice, and our profession when we're not investing in understanding the financial aspect of practice because we are saying we don't value ourselves. I believe that the financial aspect of practice should be integrated into as many classes in DPT education as possible. New graduates need to understand financial management to hit the ground running. But physical therapist students, academic faculty, and physical therapist clinicians are not comfortable with financial management, and they don't like to talk about money.

Why do we tend to resist talking about our finances? Some of it might be cultural. It's not taboo to talk about money in my culture; it's just part of everything else. My parents talked to me about it all the time. But a lot of people view money as a negative thing, "It's the root of all evil." It's almost like you can't care about money to be a wholly wonderful person. But money is a part of every other aspect of your life. I've witnessed people having so much angst around fundraising, and I tell them, "Just ask them, it's only money." But if they didn't talk about it at home, they're not going to talk about it with anybody else.

I admire people who ask for more money (i.e., during the interview or employment negotiations). Women don't do that as much as men. Informally, I've asked women (we have a lot of women in physical therapy), "When you're offered a job, do you ask for more money?" Nine out of ten times women say *no*; however, men say *always*! It's interesting. It sends the message, "I'm worth more." If we start communicating that we're worth more, then others will see us as being worth more too.

Financial Literacy

Financial literacy plays a crucial role in the success of any health care professional, and physical therapists are no exception. Understanding the intricacies of finance personally, and in the health care industry can significantly impact the revenue potential for physical therapists. Financial literacy can be a key driver in unlocking revenue potential for physical therapists and prepare physical therapists for management positions in health care organizations.[2]

A financially literate physical therapist can effectively navigate the financial aspects of their practice, ensuring optimal revenue generation. This means you have an understanding and an ability to use different financial skills effectively, including managing your personal finances, budgeting, and investing.[3] Developing your financial literacy – sooner rather than later – can support many personal and professional goals, such as paying for education, saving for retirement, using debt responsibly, and, perhaps, managing your own business/practice.[4]

Activity 7.1 Assess Your Level of Financial Literacy

Answer the following questions by circling the best response.

Do you prepare/use a budget?

Always Sometimes/Occasionally Never Sporadically

Do you keep track of expenses (how often)?

Always Sometimes/Occasionally Never Sporadically

Did you pick your bank based on convenience, fees, or interest rates?

Always Sometimes/Occasionally Never Sporadically

Do you understand impacts to credit?

Always Sometimes/Occasionally Never Sporadically

Do you make timely payments on all bills?

Always Sometimes/Occasionally Never Sporadically

Do you periodically check your credit report?

Always Sometimes/Occasionally Never Sporadically

Do you know how much to save; do you save?

Always Sometimes/Occasionally Never Sporadically

Do you know how to determine favorable loan terms?

Always Sometimes/Occasionally Never Sporadically

Do you have a plan for retirement; are you investing for the future?

Always Sometimes/Occasionally Never Sporadically

Aha!

Of Course, There's an App for That!

Technology is always changing, but according to Nerdwallet,[5] some of the best budgeting apps that connect with your financial accounts, track spending, and categorize expenses so you can see where your money is going, are:

- Mint, for just about everything;
- YNAB, for hands-on zero-based budgeting;
- Goodbudget, for hands-on envelope budgeting;
- EveryDollar, for simple zero-based budgeting;
- Empower Personal Wealth, for tracking wealth and spending;
- PocketGuard, for a simplified budgeting snapshot;
- Honeydue, for budgeting with a partner; and
- Fudget, for budgeting without syncing accounts.

Activity 7.2 Millennials, Gen Z and Debt

Answer the following questions in the spaces provided.

How much debt will you have after you receive your graduate degree?

____

What percentage rate did you borrow the money at?

____

How long will it take for you to pay off your student loan?

____

What strategies will you employ to pay off your debt?

____

Low levels of financial literacy prevailing among the largest share of the American workforce mean that millennials (and Gen Z) are unprepared for possible financial crises and that they (over 44%) also carry considerable amounts of student loan and mortgage debt.[6]

Aha!

DPT Student Debt

The American Physical Therapy Association (APTA) has documented how physical therapist student debt has limited trainees' career choices, further education, and professional expansion, as well as adding stress to find additional jobs to pay back their student loan debt.[6] Students and therapists need to have a better understanding of financial literacy to understand the ratio between student debt and their expected earnings, in order to help them to calculate the net present value of their student loans over the duration of their career.[7]

Further compounding matters, a financial crisis is being created for the uninformed with the additional health care environment pressures of reducing reimbursements for therapy services, while the cost of education continues to skyrocket. This is why it is important to err on the side of being fiscally more conservative in borrowing and to research all other opportunities to help to finance education and loan repayment strategies. According to the APTA,[8] 90% of physical therapists have education-related loans.

- The average physical therapy student loan debt amounts to $116,183.
- The average total education debt for physical therapists amounts to $142,489 *including undergraduate debt.*

Tool

What Can *You* Do Before Executing Your Loan Repayment Plan?

Sara Cates, PT, DPT, FAFS, HHP,[9] has some helpful advice for you.

1. Know how much you owe, to what lender, and at what percentage rate.
2. Don't do income-based repayment if you can afford it, as the long-term hit on interest can end up doubling your loan amount.
3. Use a monthly budget to plan your expenses, but don't be too hard on yourself.
4. Decide which debts to pay off first using highest interest rate as your focus.
5. Make at least the minimum payment on time each month so that you stay out of delinquent status.
6. Build an emergency fund to fall back on.
7. Work for an employer who matches 401k or another retirement account (aka *free* money!)
8. Open a Roth IRA (pre-taxed retirement account) as soon as you start working.
9. Consider your significant other/family in the "big picture."
10. Don't take your foot off the repayment gas pedal until the debt has been paid off.
11. Review the possibility of a public service loan forgiveness program, especially if you are dedicated to working ten years in a non-profit health service department. The government will repay all outstanding federal loan amounts (see https://studentaid.gov/pslf/).
12. Watch the interest rates and consider loan consolidation. This is a great way to combine all your loans that qualify to create a lower interest rate.

Bottom Line!

Financial literacy means that you know how to make smart decisions about money. Becoming financially literate involves learning and practicing different skills related to budgeting, managing, and paying off debts, and understanding credit and investment products/strategies.[2]

Tool

The US government-sponsored Financial Literacy and Education Commission offers a range of free learning resources.[9,10]

Financial Health Literacy

Financial health literacy refers to the knowledge and understanding of financial concepts, practices, and strategies that are specific to the health care industry. It involves being familiar with health care coding, billing procedures, and the revenue cycle. Investing in financial health literacy training yields numerous benefits for physical therapists. First, it empowers you to take control of your financial future by making informed decisions about budgeting, saving, investing, and retirement planning. Second, it helps to improve the financial stability and revenue potential of your work environment, which will enhance the overall efficiency of a practice. Physical therapists who are well versed in financial management can optimize processes, reduce administrative burdens, and allocate resources effectively. This efficiency translates into cost savings and improved patient care.

Third, financial health literacy training instills confidence in physical therapists when negotiating contracts with health insurance companies or collaborating with other health care professionals. A strong financial foundation enables them to advocate for fair reimbursement rates and make informed decisions that align with their practice's financial goals.

Financial health literacy is your ability to access, understand, and utilize financial health information to achieve improved health and financial outcomes.[11] In order to increase the frequency and effectiveness of collaborative conversations related to health care finances and to assist patients to make sense of the costs associated with their health care, such as medical bills, prescription medications, or **price transparency**, the health care provider needs to have a clear understanding of health care financial literacy themselves. They should be able to discuss financial health literacy, identify common problems such as price transparency and financial responsibility, and provide recommendations on improving interprofessional shared decision-making as a central tenant to patient-centered care.[11]

At the organizational level, financial health literacy is critical to understanding the unique demands it imposes on budgets; this skill set is even more critical.[11] Understanding how resources are allocated and how to negotiate and self-advocate during financial discussions has never been more important than it is now at a time when the health care system is very stressed. The key is for health care providers to learn to speak the language of business and finance well enough to understand and influence financial experts, as well as patients. Physical therapists who are able to demonstrate strong financial literacy will be well positioned to thrive in this changing landscape, maximizing revenue potential and delivering high-quality care.

To unlock your full revenue potential and enhance your financial literacy as a physical therapist, explore the various resources and courses available from reputable organizations such as the APTA and the Healthcare Financial Management Association (HFMA). Invest in your financial future and help to take operational control of your practice's financial health. With the right knowledge and skills, you can help to maximize revenue and deliver high-quality care to your patients.

Tool

APTA Financial Solutions Center

The APTA provides resources and tools to support solid financial management decisions and to manage student debt. The APTA encourages physical therapists, physical therapist assistants, and students to be knowledgeable about their financial health in order to secure their long-term career success. Visit the APTA's Financial Solutions Center at:
https://www.apta.org/your-career/financial-solutions-center

Business Models

Health care financial models are slightly different from normal business models (see chapter 10 for examples of business models). In a typical transactional business model, you provide a product or service, provide an invoice, and the company earns revenue for every item or transaction that was billed in a relatively short period of time. To increase profits, business owners and corporations usually start reducing their costs and keeping their prices the same. This is commonly referred to as *shrinkflation*, as coined by British economist Pippa Malmgren. Your ice cream and cereal containers are a good example of this. Over the past two years the size of the container has shrunk, but the price has stayed the same. However, in health care, it is virtually impossible to deliver a lower level of service for the same price to make more money. For example, a hospital can't reduce the expense of cleaning and disinfecting the operating theater between surgeries or reduce the cost of the anesthetic medication used during procedures because this would affect the patient outcome and revenue generated from value-based purchasing models. Furthermore, hospitals and private practices are not able to set their prices according to each individual payor. Federal laws and regulations require a uniform charge structure; however, payments do not correspond to those charges and vary greatly between payors. Sometimes the payment is less than the cost of providing the service.[12]

Activity 7.3 Paying for Services

Answer the questions that apply to you in the space provided.

How do you determine how much you're going to pay for the following services:
Haircut and Color: ____________________
Boutique Fitness Class: ____________________
Manicure/Pedicure: ____________________
Overhead Light Fixture Replacement: ____________________
Auto Collision Work: ____________________
MRI of the Knee: ____________________
Physical Therapy for a Stroke: ____________________
Physical Therapy for a Knee Replacement: ____________________
Neurologic Consult for Dizziness: ____________________

Review your list and put an asterisk (*) next to the service providers that can tell you exactly how much you will be paying out-of-pocket. Why can they do this?

____

Are health care services transactional? (Circle one answer.)

Yes No Depends

Can health care services become more comparable and shoppable, too? (Circle one answer.)

Yes No Depends

Operational Definitions

The purpose of this section is to start to build your financial vocabulary by providing you with *operational definitions* to help you to understand the jargon used in financial management. You need to know these terms because it will help you to: (1) contribute to better conversations with colleagues; (2) negotiate a better compensation package; (3) make better financial decisions; and (4) provide better care for

Table 7.1 Operational Definitions

Financial Term	*Operational Definition*
Gross *charges* (revenue)	Billed to patient; total patient revenue generated = *price* x billing quantity
Contractual obligations	Number of gross charges not collected due to contractual allowances by payor (typically ranges from 30%–70% of charges)
Patient responsibility	Number of gross charges owed by patient for co-payment or co-insurance or deductible
Denied amount	Charges denied due to varied reasons, such as non-coverage, no prior authorization, services considered medically unnecessary, or liability of different payor
Uncompensated care	Charity, pro bono, and bad debt that will never be collected
Net patient revenue	Total amount of payments collected for the services provided
Operating expense	*Cost* of running a business in day-to-day transactions
Net operating income	Bottom line, i.e., total operating revenue less total operating expense

your patients. These terms will be discussed further in the Revenue Cycle Management section and in other chapters in this book.

Revenue

One of the financial mistakes made in health care finance is when organizations use charges to monitor revenue instead of actual net revenue based on payments.[13,14] There are a variety of sources of revenue in health care, but the largest source is from patient care, and smaller amounts can be derived from grants, donations, and investments. The patient care payment sources are either government payors, like Medicare and Medicaid, or private payors, including commercial payors, employee-sponsored payors, and self-pay. Each payor will have a different contracted rate for every health care service provided, regardless of the charges or costs. The distribution of the sources of these payors is referred to as the "payor mix."

Charges, Price, and Cost

According to the HFMA, charges, price, and cost are three distinctly different definitions in health care finance.

Table 7.2 Charges versus Price versus Cost

Financial Term	*Definition*
Charges	The amount in US dollars that a health care provider sets for services rendered before negotiating any discounts. The charges can be different from the amount paid.
Price	The total amount that a health care provider expects to be paid by payors and patients for health care services, usually based on contracted rates.

(*Continued*)

Table 7.2 (Continued)

Financial Term	*Definition*
Cost	The definition of cost varies according to the perspective: • To the patient, cost is the amount payable out-of-pocket for health care services. This may include deductibles, co-payments, co-insurance, amounts payable by the patients for services that are not included in the patient's benefit design and amounts balance-billed by out-of-network providers. Health insurance premiums constitute a separate category of health care costs for patients, independent of health care service use. • To the health care provider, cost is the expense (direct and indirect) incurred to deliver health care services to patients. • To the insurer, cost is the amount payable to the health care provider (or reimbursable to the patient) for services rendered. • To the employer, cost is the expense related to providing health benefits (premiums or claims paid).

Price Shopping

Patients and health care consumers are becoming more and more computer savvy and are using the internet for many of their health care questions, including costs. One-third of health care consumers use the internet to compare the quality and cost of medical services before seeking a provider (see https://www.inovalon.com/blog/the-impact-of-patient-satisfaction-on-your-revenue-cycle/). As more health care insurance responsibilities shift to patients with high-deductible plans, they are becoming more astute and careful with their bills. In addition to wanting a good outcome from the services they receive, patients also want simple, stress-free payment processes. Therefore, it is important for all providers to have smooth, accurate revenue cycle processes in place that don't cause mistakes in billing to patients or on their behalf.

Historically, payor reimbursement prices were taken from comparative charges from other organizations, or a factor of a Medicare reimbursement then increased arbitrarily by a certain percentage every year, possibly corresponding with a cost-of-living increase percentage. Consumers of health care never knew what their charges or prices were going to be for the services that they received, until they received their bill. The **Hospital Price Transparency Rule**[15] that came into effect on January 1, 2021 helps Americans to know the cost of a hospital item or service before receiving it. It requires each hospital operating in the United States to provide clear, accessible pricing information online about the items and services they provide. This information makes it easier for consumers to shop and compare prices across hospitals and to estimate their cost of care before going to hospital.

American consumers have another new protection in place when seeking medical care. As of January 1, 2022, the **No Surprises Medical Billing Act**[16] established a new set of rules to help to protect people in job-related and individual health plans from having to pay surprise bills for emergency care, non-emergency care from out-of-network providers at in-network facilities, and air ambulance services from out-of-network providers. In many cases, the out-of-network provider could bill consumers for the difference between the charges the provider billed, and the amount paid by the consumer's health plan. This is known as *balance billing*. An unexpected balance bill is called a *surprise bill*. This bill eliminates the responsibility to pay these surprise bills, while still receiving the services.

Both the Hospital Price Transparency Rule and the No Surprises Medical Billing Act aim to empower patients with information and protections that lead to more predictable and manageable health care costs. Together, they promote a more transparent, fair, and patient-friendly health care system.

Activity 7.4 Review Physical Therapy Charges

Review the charges for a physical therapy evaluation (CPT codes 97161, 97162, or 97163) for three hospitals in your vicinity. By how much do they differ and why? Do you believe that these charges will correlate to the therapists' salaries?

____

____

____

Costs

The *cost* of delivering health care services is the largest amount of the operating expenses. Costs are usually divided into *fixed costs* and *variable costs*.

Fixed costs are ones which do not change and are generally part of long-term agreements. For instance, full-time staff, rent, and malpractice premiums are common examples of fixed costs in medical practices. Other examples include capital expenditures, building maintenance, and utilities.

Variable costs would change in the same direction as patient volume changes. As the workload increases, so does the variable cost. Examples of variable costs are hourly staffing expenses, medications administered, or procedural supplies.

A fundamental concept in business management is understanding whether you are making money and how many patients you need to see in order to break even and pay all the fixed costs at minimum. To do this analysis, you need to know your *net profit*, which is the difference between your *total revenue* and *total expenses*. Then a breakeven analysis can be completed. The formula to calculate the *breakeven point* is (number of patients) = total fixed costs/contribution margin per patient (which is equal to revenue per patient – variable cost per patient).

This tells you the number of patients that you need to see in order to pay all your bills (your fixed costs), excluding the additional increment additional costs associated with more volume identified in the variable costs.

Table 7.3 Breakeven Calculation Example

Estimate for Clinic with 5,000 Patient Visits with an Average Revenue of $100 per Visit	*Total*	*Per Patient (PP) Calculation*
Revenue	$500,000	$100
Variable costs	–$250,000	$15
Fixed costs (overheads, full-time salaries, benefits)	–$350,000	
Net profit	$125,000	
Breakeven point	= $350,000/(100–15)	4,118 patients
= (Fixed Costs / (Rev PP-Variable Cost PP))	= $350,000/85	

Bottom Line!

In a health care organization, total costs are very difficult to calculate without technologies with advanced data analytics and with the integration of multiple software. Pricing does not always reflect the actual cost of the care that was provided due to this historic inability to define these costs. Most department managers in hospital organizations seldom get to see the actual costs or revenue associated with their departments. It takes very sophisticated and integrated software to provide that decision-making information to department managers.

Activity 7.5 Identifying Your Expenses (Costs)

In a physical therapy clinic, what are examples of three fixed costs and three variable costs?

____

____

____

Cost Shifting

To maintain a sustainable financial status, hospitals negotiate payment rates from private insurance groups. The margins on these payments subsidize hospital losses from public payor underpayment, bad debts, and charity care. This is known as

cost shifting and can result in higher premiums for privately insured individuals. However, hospitals have no ability to negotiate payments from the public payors – Medicare and Medicaid – that pay for most of the clinical services provided. This poses a tremendous financial challenge for hospitals because these payments do not cover actual costs. To overcome these shortfalls, hospitals negotiate higher rates from private insurance groups. For this reason, continuing cuts to Medicare and Medicaid payments create an unsustainable business environment and put undue financial pressure on private payor contract negotiations. Hospitals and health systems are working to solve this problem. Payment methodology changes and improved delivery system alignment may provide some relief over the next few years.[13]

Activity 7.6 Payor Mix

Why is it important to understand the payor mix? What would you do with this information?

____

____

Compare the reimbursement for three different payors paying for neuromuscular re-education (CPT code 97112).

____

____

____

Bottom Line!

Delivering health care is expensive, labor intensive, and has narrow operating margins. Unlike luxury items, higher prices do not equate to higher quality. In fact, the National Bureau of Economic Research found that higher-priced hospitals will not necessarily lead to better health outcomes.[17]

Revenue Cycle Overview and Management

Revenue cycle management is the process used by health care systems in the United States and all over the world to track the revenue from patients, from their initial appointment or encounter with the health care system to their final payment of balance.[12] It is a normal part of health care management/administration and the

Table 7.4 Revenue Cycle Management Operational Definitions

Term	*Definition*
Beneficiary	Person entitled to health insurance benefits.
Benefits	Specific services that members or the policyholder are entitled to use in their health plan.
Charge Capture	Process of ensuring that all services provided to a patient are accurately documented so that providers can bill appropriately.
Claim	Information submitted by a provider or covered person to establish that medical services were provided to a covered person from which processing for payment to the provider or covered person is made.
Episode of Care	All treatments rendered in a specific time frame for a specific disease or condition.
Guarantor	Person who is financially responsible for an account.
Out-of-Pocket Costs	Portion of payments for health services required to be paid by the enrollee, including copayments, coinsurance, and deductibles. This is sometimes referred to as patient responsibility or liability.
Patient- Focused Billing	Techniques used by health care organizations to make the billing process clearer for patients by making bills easier to read and understand, thus minimizing patient confusion and increasing patient satisfaction and timely payment.

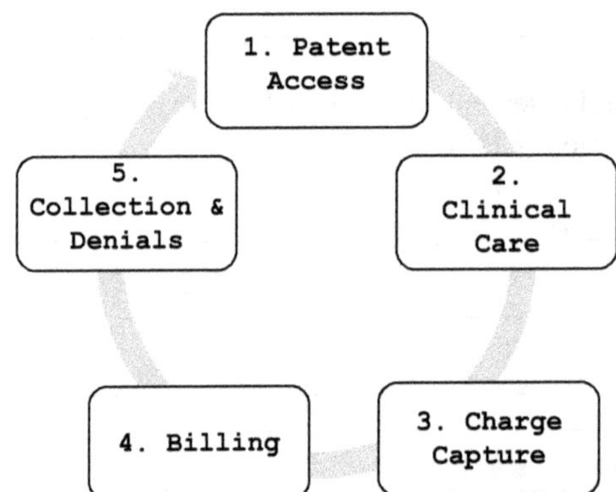

Figure 7.1 Revenue Cycle Schematic

goal of revenue cycle management is to ensure that processes and technologies are in place to help organizations to receive payment in full for services, as quickly as possible, from the point when you begin scheduling an appointment until there is no further balance owed on the account. Refer to table 7.4 for revenue cycle management operational definitions.

Overview of a Simple Revenue Cycle[18]

In this section, each main step of the revenue cycle process will be introduced and discussed (see figure 7.1). The key steps are outlined in table 7.5.

Table 7.5 Key Steps in the Revenue Cycle Process

Step 1: Patient Access	Patient Scheduling
	Pre-registration/Registration/Demographic Verification
	Authorization/Pre-certification
	Point of Service Collection
	Financial Counseling
	Insurance Verification
Step 2: Clinical Care	Documentation
Step 3: Charge Capture	Coding
	i. Diagnosis
	ii. Procedural
Step 4: Billing	Adding Modifiers/NCCI Edits
Step 5: Collection and Denials	

Revenue cycle management is a critical component of the health care system that ensures financial stability, regulatory compliance, and operational efficiency for providers. For patients, it translates to reduced financial stress, improved access to care, and a better overall health care experience. By optimizing the revenue cycle, health care providers can focus more on delivering high-quality care, and patients can have greater confidence in their health care journey. Yet there are many opportunities for errors to take place throughout the revenue cycle where data can be missing or inaccurate and result in delayed payment or non-payment for services. However, if organizations minimize these errors, they can collect the appropriate revenue and ensure that they are paid for the services and supplies that were provided in a more timely manner. As they say, "No money, no mission."

Aha!

Wrong Bill!

Have you ever received a bill for the wrong amount of money? What did you do? Did you dispute the bill? Did you trust the person who gave you the bill? Would it make you scrutinize everything that this company sent you in the future? Would you tell your friends?

What if you did not have a completely delightful experience either? Can you see how something as simple as getting a bill wrong could not only impact the patient's experience but also the company's future word-of-mouth advertising in the community?

Activity 7.7 Your Role in the Revenue Cycle Management Process

As you review each step in the section that follows, consider your role and responsibilities as a physical therapist in contributing to a positive (or negative) outcome to the organization in which you are employed, and ultimately to your patient.

Step 1: Patient Access

The activities associated with the registration process include scheduling, pre-registration/registration, authorization/pre-authorization, point of service collections as well as financial counseling. The information gathered during the registration process is crucial to the revenue cycle process. If any of this information is inaccurate it will cause errors throughout the patient's period of care in this instant and it also may follow the patient into future periods of care. This information also drives an organization's ability to collect and receive reimbursement. Some 20% of denials are caused by errors related to patient access.

a. *Scheduling*: Often the first point of contact made between the patient and the organization. The scheduler sets the patient's appointment, gathers basic demographic and payor information for registration, and advises the patient about the financial and clinical process that will follow.
b. *Pre-registration/Registration*: Usually the trigger that activates the patient in the electronic system. The registrar is responsible for collecting all the accurate patient financial and demographic data points to be used during patient treatment and all the billing phases of the revenue cycle. Best practice organizations pre-register at least 95% of their scheduled patients and verify insurance policies for at least 85% of those patients.
c. *Authorization/Pre-certification*: When a patient's insurance company requires authorization or pre-certification for services received. An authorization number is secured from the insurance provider either by phone or electronically. Best practice organizations secure pre-authorization prior to services for at least 95% of those for whom it is required.
d. *Point of Service Collection*: Refers to the process of identifying and requesting the amount of patient responsibility prior to the patient leaving the facility. As mentioned earlier the amount the patient owes is sometimes referred to as liability responsibility balance or out-of-pocket expense. Even for patients with a high deductible health plan, providers typically ask for some out-of-pocket payments towards the entire bill. Prior to the outbreak of the COVID-19 pandemic, point of service collections at top-performing organizations was at least 1.1% of net revenue; however, since the pandemic these percentages have fallen significantly.

e. *Financial Counseling*: Usually available at the point of patient access to help uninsured and underinsured patients to resolve potential payment issues by providing opportunities to investigate other options. Financial counselors work proactively to help patients to understand their payment options and explore non-traditional methods of payment like private funding resources or lesser-known state funding programs.

To reduce or eliminate delayed payment or non-payment for services due to missing or inaccurate data, access service personnel should adhere to and be mindful of the following points:

f. *Insurance Verification*

   i. *Verify insurance*: Insurance verification, pre-certification, and pre-authorization processes must be completed prior to the patient's scheduled visit. An incorrect estimate or incorrect application of the combination of health plan contract rules and patient benefit rules may later result in debits or credits on the patient's account, after the insurance company has processed the claim.
   ii. *Verify identification*: Key personal information should be verified by means of a photographic ID and an insurance card.
   iii. *Verify historic visits*: Information obtained during a previous visit should be reviewed and re-verified during admission/registration. This will also reduce costs associated with and denials for duplicate testing.
   iv. *Verify patient responsibility*: To improve cash flow and reduce delays in payment, any co-payments, co-insurance amounts, deductibles or other self-pay balances should be collected on site as part of the access process. Co-payments are usually straightforward; however, co-insurance balances often require charge estimation. On-site, self-pay collection is improved by the ability to accept payments not only as cash or checks but also as debit or credit cards.
   v. *Assist* with any alternate funding required.

A successful encounter has occurred if the information necessary to bill and collect the patient's account is completed in a friendly, courteous, and timely manner. The importance of creating positive patient experiences will be discussed further in chapter 8.

Step 2: Clinical Care and Documentation

Documentation of the clinical care delivered is required to record pertinent facts, findings, and observations about an individual's examinations, tests, treatments, and outcomes of each therapy session billed. Documentation supports the medical necessity and appropriateness of the therapeutic services provided and ensures that those services have been accurately reported. Since payors have a contractual obligation to their enrollees, the required documentation is used to support the insurance coverage being provided.

To mitigate risks during this phase:

1. Therapists need to understand the contractual coverage of the patient's payor during the episode of care. Patients could be billed for non-covered services, if the therapist is unaware of contractual coverage by the patient's specific insurer or doesn't understand how many units are allowed by Medicare for a date of service or has exceeded the number of authorized visits.
2. Documentation needs to support medical necessity *every visit*! The intervention and skills of a therapist need to be documented in every note, every day, with evidence of functional improvement and progress.
3. Documentation needs to support the diagnosis and billing codes charged on the bills.

Step 3: Coding and Charge Capture

Providers or professional coders usually assign codes in the electronic health record. These codes translate the narrative documentation into concise terms that payors and other data analysts use to understand the services provided.

The **International Classification of Diseases (ICD-10-CM) codes** are required as part of the Health Insurance Portability and Accountability Act. They are the United States' clinical modification of the World Health Organization's ICD-10. They are used to describe the clinical picture of the patient and are more precise than those needed for statistical grouping and trend analysis purposes. Every year, on October 1, the Centers for Medicare and Medicaid Services (CMS) and the National Center for Health Statistics release an updated ICD-10-CM Official Guidelines as well as any changes to the code set.

The *healthcare common procedure coding system* (HCPCS) is divided into two principal subsystems referred to as level one and level two of the HCPCS. Level one of the HCPCS comprises *current procedural terminology* (CPT) a numeric coding system maintained by the American Medical Association (AMA) which is used to describe the services rendered to a patient by a health care provider. These codes will most commonly be used by therapists to report the services and procedures performed. Most physical therapy codes will fall under the physical medicine and rehabilitation section of the CPT code book 97000–97799. When a Medicare or Medicaid patient is being billed for CPT codes they are referred to as HCPCS codes. Depending on payor contracts the organization may utilize some level 3 HCPCS codes required for local insurers. See table 7.6 which offers clarification of the HCPCS and CPT coding systems.

Due to annual updates of ICD-10-CM and CPT codes, this phase of the revenue cycle is at great risk of causing delays in the revenue cycle or denials of payments. Most organizations do not have professional coders to assist in determining codes for therapy departments and need to rely on the therapist to carry out this task.

Table 7.6 HCPCS Codes versus CPT Codes

Basic Terms	*HCPCS (CMS 1983)*	*CPT (AMA 1966)*
Maintenance	Updated quarterly by the CMS.	Updated annually by the American Medical Association.
Divisions	Operate under three levels: Level 1: CPT Category 1 Level 2: Codes A–E, including dental, Outpatient Prospective Payment System (OPPS) and Durable Medical Equipment (DME) Level 3: Local Codes	Operate under three categories: Category 1: Five numeric digits with their own set of guidelines (00100–99499). Category 2: Supplemental tracking codes ending with an F (0001F-90007F). Category 3: Temporary codes for emerging technology or services (four digits ending with a T (0042T-0737T).

Therefore, to ensure good management practice, the following recommendations need to be considered to mitigate risk:

1. Update ICD-10-CM codes whenever there is an opportunity for them to be picked, e.g., the Electronic Health Record, intake records, registration, or chargemaster, on an annual basis.
2. Ensure that the ICD-10-CM code supports medical necessity for the intervention being delivered for the diagnosis, condition, problem, or other reason for encounter/visit shown in the medical record to be chiefly responsible for the services provided. List additional codes that describe any coexisting conditions.
3. ICD-10-CM codes for symptoms, signs, and ill-defined conditions (from chapter 18 of the ICD-10-CM book) are not to be used as principal diagnosis when a related definitive diagnosis has been established.
4. ICD-10-CM codes that describe symptoms and signs, as opposed to diagnoses, are acceptable for reporting purposes when a diagnosis has not been established (confirmed) by the provider. Include all codes that are going to affect the prognosis and outcome of the care being delivered.
5. Make sure that the CPT codes accurately reflect the services delivered to the patient and are supported by the relevant documentation. Was the service coded 97110 (therapeutic exercise) or was the service coded 97112 (neuromuscular re-education)? Do you and your staff understand the difference? Can you clearly document the differences?
6. For Medicare patients, ensure that the "8 Minute Rule" is followed and that all codes have times documented in the medical record, including the total time that the patient was in your care.
7. Make sure that there is a charge capture reconciliation process in place that guarantees that there are charges associated for all services delivered daily. If charges are not submitted in a timely manner, payors have limitations and can deny outright for untimely filing.

As therapists, we need to ensure that we are always providing services at the "top of our license." This means that if another provider can provide the service, such as a physical therapy assistant or a personal trainer in a gym, then they should. The idea behind this is that the value of physical therapy provided by a therapist will cost more money and therefore the outcome should be greater. So, as therapists are delivering care, it is imperative to ensure that their documentation supports the complicated patients that are being treated by describing all of the co-morbidities with the multiple diagnosis codes, as well as the applying all of the most appropriate CPT codes, not just the "easiest or most common codes," but what you actually did with the patient and described in your documentation. Many therapists' documentation shows that the therapist has either copied and pasted the same treatment intervention from one day to the next, without any critical analysis or documented need for physical therapy intervention. Others might miss billing for a more complex CPT with a heavier weighted relative value unit (and usually a higher reimbursed) code. There is never a time that you should bill for services based on greater reimbursement only, but always bill for services provided. Often, therapists underbill for their services, with an expressed concern for the patient's personal responsibility for the services. The value of physical therapy is being determined by claims data being generated in these diagnosis and procedural codes. These days insurance companies, researchers, and bots are scouring our data and making assumptions about the value, outcomes, and possible future of physical therapy services.

Aha!

Coding Onboarding Process

How were you onboarded during your clinical rotations to the documentation, coding, and billing process for the department? Who educated you on how to determine the correct diagnosis and procedure codes to choose?

Step 4: Billing

During the billing and collections phase, the patient's account is finalized and reimbursement is collected after the bill has been sent to the insurance company or patient. **Billing** includes the preparation and submission of claims to an insurance provider or patient to obtain payment for the services rendered. It also includes the generation and resolution of all bill edits. Most claims are now submitted electronically, although some insurance companies are still required to submit paper claims in outpatient therapy departments.

Applying Modifiers/NCCI Edits

As part of the Omnibus Budget Reconciliation Act of 1989, the CMS developed the National Correct Coding Initiative (NCCI). The goal was to promote national correct coding methodologies and to control improper coding leading to inappropriate payment, fraud, and abuse of Part B claims. These are pre-payment edits and are updated on a quarterly basis. The program includes three different types of edits:

1. *Procedure to Procedure Edit* (PTP): These are services that should not be reported together or are not typically performed together based on research and best practice. As the example below from the CMS website indicates, 97112 (neuromuscular re-education should not typically be reported with 97022 (whirlpool therapy). However, it is indicated by the "1" in Column E that an NCCI PTP-associated modifier can be used for this combination to show that a clinical circumstance justifies the modifier. *Modifier 59* signifies to Medicare that you performed a service or procedure separately and distinctly from another non-evaluation and management service provided on the same day. It's a way to tell Medicare that payment for both services complies with the NCCI. You can also use this modifier when you perform a procedure on a separate and distinct body part, or at a different time. Documentation to support modifier 59 is critical. There are also other valid modifiers, e.g., XE (separate encounter), XS (separate structure), XP (separate practitioner), and XU (unusual non-overlapping service), that provide even greater reporting specificity than modifier 59. These modifiers need to be used when multiple rehabilitation professionals are using PTP edits, as the CMS does not differentiate therapy-specific modifiers (GN, GO, GP) with NCCI edits.[19]

Review the following case examples in box 7.1.

Box 7.1 Case Examples in Therapy

1. You are treating a patient with an ankle sprain, and you are billing 15 minutes of manual therapy (CPT code 97140) and 15 minutes of therapeutic activity (CPT code 97530) on the same date of service. Add the 59 modifier to code 97530, and it allows you to receive payment for both of these timed codes (provided you performed them during separate 15-minute increments).
2. You are providing therapeutic exercise services to a patient, but you note she is not making progress and opt to perform a re-evaluation during the same visit to update the plan of care. The 59 modifier allows you to bill for both the re-evaluation and the therapeutic exercise.

2. *Medically Unlikely Edits* (MUE): These are the maximum number of units of service that are reportable under most circumstances by the same provider for the same beneficiary on the same data service. This prevents payment for an inappropriately high quantity of units of the same service on the same date. Table 7.7 shows some examples from the Medicare website.[19]

Table 7.7 Medically Unlikely Edits

CPT Code	*MUE Value*	*MUE Rationale*
97010 (hot/cold packs)	0	CMS Policy
97012 (mechanical traction)	1	Clinical: Data
97014 (unattended stim)	0	CMS Policy
97018 (paraffin)	1	Clinical: Data
97139 (unlisted)	1	Clinical: CMS Workgroup

3. *Add On Code Edits* (AOC): These consist of a list of HCPCS and CPT add-on codes that cannot be performed without their respective primary code. An add-on code is eligible for payment when its primary code is also eligible for payment.

If edits are not applied properly, charges will either be rejected in a hospital charge scrubber system or denied by a payor and result in staff having to rework that account in order to get paid.

Step 5: Collection and Denials

1. *Following up on collections* includes all activities associated with obtaining full payment from the health insurance carrier – the primary insurance carrier – sending the balance to a secondary or tertiary insurance carrier or to the patient when there is an outstanding balance on the account.
2. *Payment posting* is an activity that is required to ensure that all the payments and adjustments that are received back from the insurance company are accurately recorded and applied against the patient's financial record.
3. *Payment variance resolution* is the set of activities that supports the identification and resolution of payment discrepancies either in an underpayment/overpayment situation or a denial.
4. *Customer service* is the link between patients and the health care organization, and this role is extremely important in continuing to provide patient satisfaction in answering questions and concerns correcting demographic and financial information and communicating with insurance carriers on behalf of the patient.

Once the total payments received from the health plan and patient equal the amount specified in the contract with the health plan, the health care provider or physician office can close the account.

Bottom Line!

The importance of customer service carried out by the revenue integrity team is critical in creating a positive patient experience. Sometimes this is the patient's last memory of the services that you provided, so it needs to be positive.

Aha!

Management Practice Tip

Opportunities to reduce risks to an organization during this phase include:

Tip 1: Many organizations leave the addition of modifiers up to the rehabilitation (rehab) department. Since the NCCI edits are updated quarterly, it is imperative that someone from the rehab department is designated as the billing compliance person tasked with monitoring and updating the staff about these changes. Billing is monitored and invoices are sent out in a timely manner after all the edits have been applied and scrubbed.

Tip 2: Secondary and tertiary billing is handled electronically.

Tip 3: Payment variances are identified and resolved quickly with corrections of any upstream problems which many have created the payment variance.

Tip 4: A solid third-party denial management team is prepared to appeal all denials.

Tip 5: A collection agency is used to assist with old collections, and its performance is also monitored.

Activity 7.8 Data Tells the Picture

The old adage used to be that your documentation should tell the story of your patient. However, the truth is that real-world data needs to tell the story of your patient and all the services that you provide including their outcomes.

How confident are you that a complete picture of your patient, the physical therapy intervention, and the outcome achieved was provided in the codes that you submitted?

____

____

What will you do to improve it?

____

____

Tool

The Top Five Tips for Improving Your Revenue Cycle

- Tip 1: Understand the payor rules:
  - How many visits do they allow?
  - Do you need pre-authorization or re-authorization?
  - What are the diagnosis to procedural code crosswalks? (i.e., can you bill Canalith repositioning (CPT code 95992) for a diagnosis of dizziness and giddiness?).
- Tip 2: Have *stellar* documentation:
  - Complete all documentation daily (including evaluations);
  - Always demonstrate skilled therapy services;
  - Write progress notes regularly with documented signs of objective improvement towards the patient's long-term goals.
- Tip 3: Understand diagnosis coding and apply it appropriately.
- Tip 4: Understand procedural coding and the application of modifiers.
- Tip 5: Always provide the care the patient needs to improve, not what you think they can afford. There is always a way to assist with financial arrangements to pay for services.

Analyzing Financial Performance

Financial performance is an outcome measure of how well an organization, practice, or department has used its assets to generate revenue over a given period.[20] Financial performance can use multiple measures to determine the outcome of all of the work that was implemented, beginning from the strategic plan (see chapter 11) through the operationalization of the budget during the same time period.[18]

Below is an example of a Financial Performance Review (see table 7.8) including a revenue analysis, expense analysis, profitability analysis, cash flow analysis, and key performance indicators.

Table 7.8 Summer Off Physical Therapy Practice Financial Performance Review for the Years Ending December 31, 2023, and December 31, 2024

Revenue Analysis

Metric	*2023*	*2023*	*% Change*
Total Revenue	$1,200,000	$1,320,000	+10%
Number of Patients	3,000	3,150	+5%
Average Revenue per Patient	$400	$419	+4.75%

Analysis

Total Revenue: The practice saw a 10% increase in total revenue, driven by a 5% increase in the number of patients and a 4.75% increase in average revenue per patient.

Number of Patients: The increase in patient volume indicates successful patient retention and acquisition strategies.

Expense Analysis

Expense Category	*2023*	*2024*	*% Change*
Salaries and Wages	$600,000	$650,000	+8.3%
Rent and Utilities	$120,000	$130,000	+8.3%
Medical Supplies	$90,000	$95,000	+5.6%
Administrative Expenses	$50,000	$55,000	+10%
Marketing Expenses	$30,000	$35,000	+16.7%
Total Expenses	$890,000	$965,000	+8.4%

Analysis

Salaries and Wages: An 8.3% increase due to additional staffing to accommodate the increased patient volume and ensure quality care.

Marketing Expenses: A significant increase of 16.7%, reflecting enhanced efforts in patient acquisition and brand visibility.

Profitability Analysis

Metric	*2023*	*2024*	*% Change*
Gross Profit	$310,000	$355,000	+14.5%
Gross Profit Margin (%)	25.8%	26.9%	+1.1%
Net Profit	$210,000	$245,000	+16.7%
Net Profit Margin (%)	17.5%	18.6%	+1.1%

Analysis

Gross Profit and Margin: The practice saw an improvement in both gross profit and gross profit margin, indicating effective cost management and revenue growth.

Net Profit and Margin: Net profit increased by 16.7%, demonstrating strong overall financial health and efficient operations.

Cash Flow Analysis

Metric	*2023*	*2024*	*% Change*
Operating Cash Flow	$220,000	$260,000	+18.2%
Investing Cash Flow	($40,000)	($30,000)	–25%
Financing Cash Flow	($20,000)	($15,000)	–25%
Net Cash Flow	$160,000	$215,000	+34.4%

Analysis

Operating Cash Flow: Increased by 18.2%, reflecting improved profitability and efficient cash management.

Investing and Financing Cash Flow: Decreased outflows in both categories indicate reduced capital expenditures and debt repayments, contributing to better net cash flow.

Key Performance Indicators

KPI	*2023*	*2024*	*Target*
Patient Retention Rate	85%	88%	90%
New Patient Growth Rate	10%	12%	15%
Days in Accounts Receivable	45	40	30
Staff Utilization Rate	75%	80%	85%

Analysis

Patient Retention Rate: Increased to 88%, indicating improved patient satisfaction and loyalty.

New Patient Growth Rate: Growth in new patients is positive but still below the target, suggesting room for improvement in marketing and outreach strategies.

Days in Accounts Receivable: Improvement to 40 days, showing better collections efficiency, though still above the target.

Staff Utilization Rate: Increased to 80%, reflecting more effective use of clinical staff, but still short of the optimal target.

Conclusion: The physical therapy practice demonstrated strong financial performance and growth over the past two years. Revenue and profit margins improved, driven by increased patient volume and effective cost management. Cash flow also saw significant improvement, ensuring financial stability. While there are areas for further enhancement, such as patient growth and collections efficiency, the overall outlook is positive with a solid foundation for continued success.

Key Performance Indicators

Since most of these financial statements are provided annually, managers need some indication of how well they are doing during the year. Therefore, **key performance indicators** (KPIs) are monitored on a weekly or monthly basis, so there are no surprises at year end. Some of the critical KPIs that therapy managers should monitor for financial performance[18] are (see also chapters 5 and 11):

Revenue: Reviewing incoming cash to ensure that it is sufficient to cover expenses and comparing it to what was budgeted is critical. Managers should monitor revenue per therapist, revenue per visit, or revenue per payor contract. Revenue includes payments received from insurance companies as well as patients' responsibilities.

Patient volume: Since the primary source of revenue is from patient visits, the number of patients attending therapy is critical. Furthermore, since reimbursement depends directly on the amount of RVUs that were billed for the patient, many managers track billing units or RVUs instead of just the number of patients to understand the number of charges that were billed for the month better, and to assist in managing staffing levels.

Total expense: Monitoring total cost per month, in comparison to budget and income, is essential. This includes fixed and variable costs (discussed earlier).

Payor mix: Understanding the types of health insurance (private versus public) your patients have and how that impacts your financial bottom line helps you to understand how their reimbursement will affect your financial performance.

Decision-Making and Implementing Action Plans

When financial margins are at risk, in a typical transactional business, most managers' initial actions are to raise prices or reduce operating costs. However, as mentioned earlier, health care differs from other businesses in that prices are set by the payor contracts, so managers need to evaluate the volume of patients and clinician productivity levels. This is not a easy fix; if you simply increase the patient-to-therapist ratio the clinical outcome may be impacted negatively, which is not desirable. However, there are many productivity metrics that managers monitor to ensure that work is equally distributed among the team. Productivity can be measured in many ways; some managers use billable units per day or billable minutes per hour.

Activity 7.9 Revenue Variance

The first quarter budget variance report shows that your department is well below *reimbursed revenue*, as compared to budget.

Which metric would you look at first to determine the cause of the variance and why? Circle the one that applies.

a. Payor mix
b. Point of service collection rate
c. Patient volume
d. Therapist productivity rate
e. Variable costs
f. Fixed costs

Expense Variance

The second quarter budget variance report shows that your department has exceeded its *expenses*, as compared to budget.

Which metric would you look at first to determine the cause of the variance and why? Circle the one that applies.

a. Payor mix
b. Point of service collection rate
c. Patient volume
d. Therapist productivity rate

e. Variable costs
f. Fixed costs

Net Profit Variance

The third quarter budget variance report shows that your department has exceeded its *net profit*, as compared to budget.

Which metric would you look at first to determine the cause of the variance and why? Circle the one that applies.
a. Payor mix
b. Point of service collection rate
c. Patient volume
d. Therapist productivity rate
e. Variable costs
f. Fixed costs

Growth Evaluation

What information do you need/want in order to make the decision to hire another physical therapist? What would the data tell you?

____

____

As the health care industry continues to evolve (and it will), financial literacy will become even more important for physical therapists. Advances in technology, changes in reimbursement models, and shifting regulatory landscapes will require physical therapists to stay agile and adapt to new financial challenges. Furthermore, the increasing emphasis on value-based care and the transition from fee-for-service reimbursement models to alternative payment models necessitates a deep understanding of financial management. Physical therapists who possess strong financial literacy skills will be well positioned to thrive in this changing landscape, maximizing revenue potential and delivering high-quality care.

Suggested Readings

Gapenski L. *Healthcare Finance: An Introduction to Accounting and Financial Management.* 6th ed. AUPHA/HAP; 2013.

Hayhurst C. The economic value of physical therapy in the United States. American Physical Therapy Association. Published December 1, 2023. Accessed May 21, 2024. https://www.apta.org/apta-magazine/2023/12/01/economic-value-physical-therapy-united-states

Hoffmann T, Bakhit M, Michaleff Z. Shared decision making and physical therapy: What, when, how, and why? *Braz J Phys Ther*. 2022; 26(1): 100382. doi:10.1016/j.bjpt.2021.100382

James BD, Boyle PA, Bennett JS, Bennett DA. The impact of health and financial literacy on decision making in community-based older adults. *Gerontol*. 2012; 58: 531–539. doi:10.1159/000339094

References

1. Alter A. *Anatomy of a Breakthrough: How to Get Unstuck When It Matters Most*. Simon & Schuster; 2023.
2. Igoe KJ. It's more important than ever for physician leaders to develop financial literacy – here's how to start. Harvard T.H. Chan School of Public Health. Published December 14, 2021. Accessed May 21, 2024. https://www.hsph.harvard.edu/ecpe/its-more-important-than-ever-for-physician-leaders-to-develop-financial-literacy-heres-how-to-start/
3. Fernando J. Financial literacy. Investopedia. Updated June 29, 2024. Accessed May 21, 2024. https://www.investopedia.com/terms/f/financial-literacy.asp
4. What is financial literacy? Financial Literacy 101. Accessed May 21, 2024. https://www.financialliteracy101.org/financial-literacy/index.cfm
5. Ayoola E. The best budget apps for 2024. Nerdwallet. Updated February 20, 2024. Accessed May 21, 2024. https://www.nerdwallet.com/article/finance/best-budget-apps
6. Bolognesi A, Hasler A, Lusardi A. Millennials and money: Financial preparedness and money management practices before COVID-19. TIAA Institute, Global Financial Literacy Excellence Center. Published August 2020. Accessed May 21, 2024. https://gflec.org/wp-content/uploads/2020/08/Millennials-and-Money-Technical-Report-August2020.pdf
7. Shields RK, Dudley-Javoroski S. Physiotherapy education is a good financial investment, up to a certain level of student debt: An inter-professional economic analysis. *J Physiother*. 2018 Jul;64(3):183–191. doi:10.1016/j.jphys.2018.05.009
8. American Physical Therapy Association. Impact of student debt on the physical therapy profession. Published June 1, 2020. Accessed May 21, 2024. https://www.apta.org/apta-and-you/news-publications/reports/2020/impact-of-student-debt-on-the-physical-therapy-profession
9. Cates, S. PT school put me in debt – now what? Core Medical Group. Accessed May 21, 2024. https://www.coremedicalgroup.com/blog/pt-school-debt
10. Financial literacy and education commission. US Department of the Treasury. Accessed May 21, 2024. https://home.treasury.gov/policy-issues/consumer-policy/financial-literacy-and-education-commission
11. O'Mara CS, Young JP, Winkelmann ZK. Financial health literacy and the shared decision-making process in healthcare. *Int J Environ Res Public Health*. 2022; 19(11): 6510. doi:10.3390/ijerph19116510 https://www.ncbi.nlm.nih.gov/pmc/articles/PMC9180139/
12. Fact sheet: Hospital billing explained. American Hospital Association. Published September 2017. Accessed May 21, 2024. https://www.aha.org/system/files/2018-01/factsheet-hospital-billing-explained-9-2017.pdf
13. Florida Hospital Government & Public Affairs. Hospital finance basics part 1: Revenue. Texas Health Huguley Hospital. Published 2013. Accessed May 21, 2024. https://www.texashealthhuguley.org/sites/default/files/assets/hospital-finance-basics-part-1-revenue-2013.pdf

14. Goehle JJ. 10 key financial metrics to measure in a surgery center. Becker's ASC Review. Published December 19, 2011. Accessed May 21, 2024. https://www.beckersasc.com/asc-news/10-key-financial-metrics-to-measure-in-a-surgery-center.html
15. Centers for Medicare & Medicaid Services. Hospital price transparency. CMS.gov. Updated November 2, 2023. Accessed May 21, 2024. https://www.cms.gov/priorities/key-initiatives/hospital-price-transparency
16. Centers for Medicare & Medicaid Services. Ending surprise medical bills. CMS.gov. Updated April 9, 2024. Accessed May 21, 2024. https://www.cms.gov/nosurprises
17. Cooper Z, Doyle JJ, Graves JA, Gruber J. Do higher-priced hospitals deliver higher-quality care? National Bureau of Economic Research. Working Paper w29809. Published February 2022. Updated January 2023. Accessed May 21, 2024. https://www.nber.org/system/files/working_papers/w29809/w29809.pdf
18. 6 Essential Performance Metrics to Start Tracking Right Now. BetterPT. Accessed May 21, 2024. https://www.betterpt.com/post/6-essential-performance-metrics-to-start-tracking-right-now
19. Centers for Medicare & Medicaid Services. National correct coding initiative (NCCI) coding edits. CMS.gov. Updated June 3, 2024. Accessed July 8, 2024. https://www.cms.gov/Medicare/Coding/NationalCorrectCodInitEd/NCCI-Coding-Edits.html
20. Healthcare Financial Management Association. Cost analysis and management: Part 6 – variance analysis. Accessed May 21, 2024. https://learn.hfma.org/learn/course/cost-analysis-and-management/cost-analysis-and-management-1/part-6-variance-analysis?page=2

8 Marketing a Physical Therapy Practice (Marketing Management)

Brandonne Ouillette Rankin

We talk about *marketing* in physical therapy, instead of *selling*, because we resist the notion of sales (or selling) as something that we need to do in clinical practice. Yet selling is a process of building authentic relationships and as physical therapists we build relationships every day in clinical practice. We need to get more comfortable with marketing *and* selling our value, by leveraging our inherent ability to build genuine relationships.

Dr. Jennifer E. Green-Wilson

Chapter Objectives

1. Describe the future health care landscape and its impact on patient care and outcomes.
2. Outline various demographic behaviors of health care consumers, their decision-making influences, and desires.
3. Identify your practice's business focus.
4. Develop mission, vision, values, goals, and brand identity for your physical therapy practice.
5. Using the three Ps of physical therapy practice marketing (Practice, Principles, and People), and the four Ps of traditional marketing, create a comprehensive marketing strategy for a physical therapy practitioner and practice.

Management Vignette

Dr. Tracy Sher, PT, DPT

Pelvic health is my passion. I'm dedicated to destigmatizing the topic and to improving both the quality of and access to information for patients and practitioners alike. I started out with my free blog, *The Pelvic Guru*, using stock images to provide depth to my content. I wasn't fully satisfied with

DOI: 10.4324/9781003524250-10

them, though, because many images were either anatomically incorrect or they lacked crucial details. So, I hired an illustrator to create the specific images I needed, and over time these have evolved into a library of around 200 copyrighted illustrations. When we started getting image use requests from organizations like universities and medical centers, that was an impetus for me. I thought, "There's an opportunity here."

I built my clinical practice, Sher Pelvic Health and Healing, LLC, around the mission of providing exceptional, inclusive pelvic health care. To me, exceptional care starts with expert practitioners. I've been fortunate to collaborate with and learn from some of the best in the world, and I thought, "What if we brought these experts together in a multidisciplinary, supported global network to share and teach what they know?" So my team and I created the Global Pelvic Health Alliance Membership (https://www.academy.pelvicglobal.com/gpham-select) through which we offer access to clinical and business webinars, podcasts, and our copyrighted images, as well as licensing opportunities for our learning materials. We also offer continuing education courses through our Pelvic Global Academy (https://www.academy.pelvicglobal.com/home). We emphasize a strong, communicative practitioner–patient relationship to help to reduce embarrassment and normalize conversations about pelvic health to help patients to achieve their physical and emotional health goals.

On the patient side of our services, we created social media groups and the world's largest free directory of pelvic health providers so that people can find what they're looking for, whether that's information, professional help, or peer support. It works because we're satisfying innate patient curiosity and desire for better care. Good leaders and innovators know how to transform consumer needs and preferences into a relevant products or services.

Chapter Introduction

So, you're a qualified physical therapist and you've decided to open your own physical therapy practice. At this point, you may even have chosen your business name and thought about where you'll set up shop. Congratulations! But before you send out those grand opening invitations, take some time now to ensure the future success and longevity of your practice. According to the Bureau of Labor Statistics, while 45% of the fastest growing US industries are in health care, nearly 19% of those businesses fail within one year of opening. At the three-year mark, the failure rate increased to 35.5%; after five years, it was 45.2%.[1]

Why do some businesses fail? The main reasons are low new customer/patient attraction rates and cash flow issues. It's just as important to know, however, that business owners who plan for future technological growth and diversified revenue streams are more likely to succeed. What this means is that physical therapists who want to go into business for themselves need to know four things: first, how the health care landscape will change and evolve over the next five to ten years; second, how to structure your business; third, who your target patients are and what they want; and finally, how to build the right marketing strategy for you as a physical therapist and for your practice. These four components can vary from practitioner to practitioner and from practice to practice, but together they help to inform the direction you should take so that, over time, you can effectively market and grow your professional brand, and grow your physical therapy practice with your team, target audiences, prospective patients, and brand partners.

The Future Health Care Landscape: What Does It Look Like?

No matter how hard we try to suppress or avoid them, we are continuously inundated with marketing messages urging us to try a new diet, supplement, or pain management regimen, to ask our doctor if a specific medication is "right" for us, or even to join a class action lawsuit against a faulty medication or medical device. These messages are far more sophisticated and targeted than the newspaper ads, highway billboards, and television commercials of traditional marketing campaigns. They appear in our social media feeds and text messages, on uniforms and equipment at sporting events, and are subtly placed in the dialogue and sets of our favorite TV shows and films. In other words, marketing teams have found newer, more subtle, and effective ways to reach their target consumers.

The future health care landscape is taking shape now, and it's heavily influenced by evolving technology and social trends, including the following:

- *Telehealth*, used by health care providers to connect with patients via smart devices, videoconferencing, telephone, wireless, satellite, and similar technologies to deliver clinical health care, information, records, and resources. Providers often refer to this service as a "virtual visit." Telehealth is especially helpful to patients who have health, mobility, or travel issues, and those who live in remote areas.[2]
- *Personalized medicine*, an approach providers use to tailor treatments and interventions to the individual patient using a combination of genetic data and medical history for more effective and efficient health outcomes. The patient collaborates with the practitioner in this approach, providing information on their lifestyle, emotional wellbeing, and self-care habits to paint a more detailed picture of their current and desired states of health.
- *Artificial intelligence (AI) and machine learning*, which help health care practitioners to find the root cause of patient issues using diagnostic tools such as imaging scans, wearable devices, and electronic medical records to anticipate potential issues, develop personalized treatment plans, monitor patient progress remotely, and predict outcomes. Machine learning algorithms, including classification, regression, clustering, and time series analysis, can help physical therapists to analyze data that can be used to help them to identify specific conditions or injuries in their patients.[3] At the beginning of this chapter, we discussed the high rate of small business failures, so it's worth noting that 60% of those that

did succeed used digital tools such as AI and social media to improve their reach, services, and practice efficiency.[4]

- *Preventive care*, which helps health care practitioners to identify and mitigate specific risk factors in their patients and, to the extent that it is possible, to avoid the expenses and complications of chronic diseases. Examples of preventive care vary depending according to a patient's age, current health, and care team, but it typically includes vaccinations (e.g., influenza, COVID-19, pneumonia, shingles, meningitis), cancer screenings (mammograms, colonoscopies, dermatology visits), tests (blood pressure, cholesterol, diabetes), and counseling (nutrition, exercise, weight management, mental health, substance use).[5]

The future health care landscape and its associated technologies will not only improve patient outcomes, they will also help physical therapists to find their target audiences and build trusting relationships based on personalized care. It's already happening: between 1997 and 2016, medical marketing spending, particularly direct to consumer marketing, increased by $12.2 billion, contributing to greater consumer awareness of certain diseases and associated treatments, as well as more frequent medical visits.[6] So, how can practitioners and practices promote the value of physical therapy in an already crowded health care information marketplace? Ultimately, we need to align ourselves with the right partners, strategies, and channels to reach our target consumers, but first we need to understand the health care landscape.

Successful physical therapy practitioners and practice managers know what their patients want (we'll discuss that topic later in this chapter). They also understand how health care evolves and changes. The health care landscape is shaped by a myriad of factors, including policy, regulation, epidemiology, geography, population, patient preferences, cost, medical, and technological innovations.[7,8] Over the past 50 years, there has been a shift towards more patient-centered care, which prioritizes individual health needs, desired outcomes, and decisions shared between practitioner and patient.[9] More recently, advances in telehealth video conferencing, telephone encounters, and mobile notifications have afforded practitioners greater patient reach and scheduling flexibility than ever before.[10] What do these and other changes mean for the future of the health care landscape, as well as for physical therapy practices and practitioners?

Trends and trajectories across the health care landscape may change over time, but the overarching goal remains firm – to provide fast, accurate, and cost-effective diagnoses and treatment, as well as preventive health screenings and vaccinations. This virtual care delivery is increasingly guided by analytical and statistical data gathered from tech resources and software that offer virtual care solutions, engagement rate boosting, practice growth opportunities, electronic health record options, and more. Most software is configurable or customizable for individual practice needs and goals in alignment with regulatory compliance. Many software programs pair well with the current preferences of over 60% of health care consumers, who want options such as online scheduling and changing of health care appointments, medical record and test result review, and prescription renewal. Patients who have online and mobile communication and scheduling options report higher satisfaction rates, are less likely to change health care providers, and are more likely to use related services from the same provider, so while the software can be costly initially, it can be a worthwhile expense.[11]

Success in the competitive health care marketplace is largely dependent upon practices and practitioners operating with a growth mindset; that is, through continuous learning and improvement of skills, services, and operations that blend seamlessly with field advances and patient desires.

Activity 8.1 Explore Tech-Driven Practice Solutions

The patient experience influences individual health outcomes, satisfaction scores, and trust in practitioners. Think about the health care you've received over the course of your life. From routine visits to your primary care physician or dentist, to specialty visits for vision or allergies, to trips to urgent care or your local emergency department for broken bones or cuts, what did those patient experiences have in common? How did they differ? Were you consulted about your treatment? Were you informed about your choices? Were your questions answered and concerns addressed? How did you feel about your overall care? What factors most impacted your experience? Using table 8.1 below, compare a few of your different visits and record how you can apply those experiences and lessons learned from them to your own physical therapy patients and practice.

Table 8.1 Evaluate Your Patient Experience

Visit Type	*I Felt ...*	*Because ...*	*My Practice Takeaways*	*Solutions I Can Offer*
Example: Primary care	Satisfied	My doctor listened to my neck pain concerns and referred me to a specific physical therapist for treatment.	Be solution oriented. Connect patients to next steps.	Offer telehealth visits. Provide exercises and instructions in patient portal.

Incorporating Total Mind and Body Wellness

The future health care landscape isn't solely focused on digital transformation. In recent years, individual health care consumers have begun to view their health in terms of a physical and emotional balance. Loosely defined as total mind and body wellness, this trend addresses spiritual, emotional, social, intellectual, occupational, and physical dimensions, incorporated with stress reduction and management techniques, sleep routines, socialization, healthy eating, supplements, and physical activity.[12] People are also living longer and want the quality of life that comes with longevity. Individuals are increasingly turning to health care professionals, including primary care physicians, nutritionists, and, yes, physical therapists, to achieve and maintain lifelong mind and body wellness.

Activity 8.2 Tying Physical Therapy to Total Mind and Body Wellness

Previously in this chapter, we discussed the health care landscape as well as emerging and future trends in the field. Now let's explore physical therapy's relationship to mind and body wellness and consider the ways that it can be incorporated into everyday practice using table 8.2 below.

Table 8.2 Connect Physical Therapy and Mind-Body Wellness

Mind-Body Wellness Issue	*My Physical Therapy Solution for My Patient*	*Physical/Emotional Benefits for My Patient*
Example: Sleeplessness	Guided stretching techniques	Mind and body relaxation, flexibility maintenance
Stress		
Tech neck		
Back pain		
Social anxiety		

Bottom Line!

While the overarching goals of health care will always be to provide the fastest, most accurate, and most cost-effective treatments to patients, the future health care landscape's advancing technologies, patient involvement and preferences (such as personalized care and preventive focus) will dictate how that care is delivered by practitioners. Anticipation of, and adaptation to these changes is essential for a thriving physical therapy practice.

What Influences Consumer Behavior?

A poll found that 57% of consumer health care respondents want quality service and engagement from their health care providers, similar to that of other important purchasing experiences, such as buying a car.[10] Both the COVID-19 pandemic and the ever-increasing retail presence of giants such as Amazon, Walmart, and CVS in the health care space have helped to create a patient experience economy, in which individual encounters with health care providers significantly impact their continuation of and loyalty to specific practices, providers, and services.[13] So, what are consumers' expectations for this enhanced experience? Across all demographics, information accessibility and credibility are key components, as are personalized care where and when the patient wants it. As we discussed earlier in this chapter, health care practices and providers, as well as consumers, are increasingly using the internet to share and review health records, schedule and conduct medical appointments, and gather basic information. In fact, 7% of Google's daily searches – more than one billion each day – are health care related.[14]

Online services may allow greater flexibility and points of connection for both provider and patient, but it's also important to know which patient groups do and don't regularly use online resources, and when services such as telehealth appointments are appropriate and preferred. Most initial patient physical therapy assessments, for example, need the physical practitioner–patient contact of an in-person visit, whereas established patients may benefit from or even prefer telehealth appointments. Advances in medicine and associated technologies may be key drivers of the future health care landscape, but to reach and connect with your target audiences, you need to meet them where they are. Before you find out *where* your target audiences are, however, you need to know *who* they are. Broadly, health care consumers include patients, caregivers, insurance brokers, employers, and government purchasers. The needs and wants of these groups tend to vary by generation. For our purpose, we'll focus on the defining characteristics, health care preferences, concerns, and decisioning influences of baby boomers, Generation X, millennials, and Generation Z in the following two infographics.

Generation	Defining Characteristics	What They Want	What Influences Decisions
BABY BOOMERS (1946–1964)	• Follow MD advice more than other generations • Account for 26% of annual MD visits	• Reputable MDs & care • Quality care & service coverage • Attention to health conditions	• Word of mouth recommendations • Practice reputation • Trusted MD recommendations
GENERATION X (1965–1980)	• Grew up at start of internet use • Visit MDs often for themselves, their children & their parents	• High-quality service • Flexible appointment options • Convenience	• Comparison of various sources to determine best options • Ease of finding sources
MILLENNIALS (1981–1996)	• Grew up with mass internet use • Lowest # of annual MD visits • 51% don't visit MD annually	• Price transparency • Online MD chats • Digital comparison tools	• Peer recommendations & patient testimonials • Cost
GENERATION Z (1997–2012)	• Least likely to see MD because of cost, inconvenience & lack of time • 45% don't have PCP	• Telehealth • Wearable devices • Access to health care data	• Parental advice • Convenience • Digital offerings

Figure 8.1 Defining Health Care Consumer Characteristics by Generation[15,16]

INTERNET SEARCH TOPIC	% OF SEARCHERS BY AGE GROUP			
	18–29 yrs.	30–49 yrs.	50–64 yrs.	65+ yrs.
Specific disease or medical problem	60%	70%	69%	62%
Specific treatment or procedure	48%	60%	59%	55%
Chronic pain management	14%	16%	12%	14%
Doctors & other health practitioners	37%	53%	41%	30%
Services covered by health insurance	32%	36%	32%	30%

Figure 8.2 Internet Health Care Search Topics by Age Group[17]

With this basic understanding of generational health care consumer behaviors, we can learn even more about key target audiences through other demographics, such as education, income, and geographic location. When put together, different data points tell the story of who target audiences are, as well as how to reach and retain them as patients. For example, rural areas tend to have less consistent broadband and high-speed internet access than suburban and metropolitan areas, so rural physical therapy practices may not wish to rely heavily on telehealth and digital marketing to grow patient volume. It's also helpful to know that 88% of caregivers, 78% of adults with physical disabilities, and more women than men use the internet to search for health-related information. Similarly, people with college degrees and higher household incomes are more likely to research injuries, medical conditions, treatments, and specific practitioners online. They use more health services, too, so internet outreach and communication will likely be a more effective marketing tactic with these groups.[18]

Activity 8.3 Identify Your Target Audiences

Armed with your knowledge of how to identify and reach various health care consumer groups, use table 8.3 (which follows) to build a high-level profile of your own target audiences, their preferences, and examples of physical therapy services and settings you can offer to attract and retain patients to your practice.

Table 8.3 Create a Demographic Profile of Your Target Audiences

Target Audience	*Patient Needs and Concerns I Will Focus On*	*Services I Can Offer*
Example: Baby boomers	• Chronic condition management • Rehabilitation from injury	Teach classes and see patients at 55+ facilities and community centers

Bottom Line!

Patients across generations want superior outcomes delivered in a timely manner, as well as a simple, convenient care experience at an affordable cost. The type of care and experience sought by patients differs by age, socioeconomic status, education, health status, and geographic location. Understanding these differences will help practitioners and practice managers to connect meaningfully with each target audience and meet individual patient needs. Multi-channel marketing, communication, and care options are therefore crucial to meeting your target audiences where they live, delivering care the way they want it, and growing your practice. We'll examine these options in closer detail in the next section of this chapter.

Building the Right Marketing Strategy for Practitioners and Practices

At the beginning of this chapter, we discussed the changing health care landscape. We learned how to identify and reach target audiences for your physical therapy practice. Now it's time to turn our focus to marketing, both for yourself as a physical therapist, and for your practice.

We will start by examining the differences that occur between selling and marketing. Although each team's work impacts the other, their purposes are distinctly separate. Put simply, selling is a short-term process of persuading customers to buy a product or service and delivering volumes at a profit to gain market share and meet revenue goals.

Marketing, on the other hand, is a long-term process focused on anticipating, identifying, and satisfying customer needs and desires with products and services. This is done in two ways: first, by marketing the principal physical therapist(s) of your practice as thought leaders, and second, by marketing the practice itself.

Thought leadership positioning takes reflection and strategy that is worth the investment of time it requires. A thought leader is a well-known, trusted source of information who shares their original ideas, research, and experience to grow their practice and to build relationships with colleagues and potential patients. Dr. Tracy Sher, who is profiled in this chapter's management vignette and who is widely known as the *Pelvic Guru*, is a prime example of a thought leader. First, she identified pelvic health as her physical therapy passion and studied it extensively. As she developed her expertise, Dr. Sher started a blog to share her findings and best practices with other physical therapists, using illustrations to help to explain specific issues and therapeutic techniques. She found her differentiator when she realized that the existing portfolio of pelvic health illustrations was insufficient for her needs, so she commissioned a set of her own, branded and shared them on her website, and began to grow her practice and reputation.

Activity 8.4 Positioning You as a Physical Therapy "Thought Leader": What's Your Potential Brand?

To begin positioning yourself as a physical therapy thought leader, answer the following questions in the spaces provided.

What are your areas of interest and strength?

____

____

What makes your practice (*you* as "the practice") different from your peers? (i.e., how are you different/unique?)

____

____

What information and tools are underdeveloped or lacking in your specialized area?

____

____

How can you as a practitioner develop and deliver what is lacking?

____

How will you share your unique knowledge with colleagues and potential patients?

____

____

Having answered those questions, you can focus on tactics to begin positioning yourself as a thought leader. Here are a few examples:

- *Newsjacking*: Follow reputable news outlets and set alerts for coverage in your specialized area. When a relevant story appears, blog about it, sharing your unique insights and practices, and link back to the original story. If you have media connections (or a public relations firm who can make them for you), reach out and offer your expertise on the subject to amplify media coverage and social media engagement.
- *Socialization*: Establish a consistent communication cadence across multiple platforms (mobile operating systems, your practice website, social media) and channels (email, push notifications, SMS).[19] Get into the habit of posting succinct, relevant content throughout each week. It's an effective way to attract and grow your target audiences, and you can make the process easier by creating an editorial calendar to organize content topics, promotions, channels, assets, and posting dates.
- *Public speaking*: Conferences, trade shows, and exhibitions are solid opportunities to grow your professional network and establish your reputation. Events typically post calls for speaker submissions at least six months ahead of the event. Review previous event themes and itineraries to familiarize yourself with the types of content each organization offers and develop one or two high-level proposal submissions that can be adapted to fit the specifications of each event. Each proposal should include a thought-provoking title, brief session description and estimated length, objectives, keywords, any conflict of interest, target audience skill level, and a short professional biography. Similarly, physical therapy journals and health care periodicals publish original research, studies, clinical trials, reviews, and other relevant articles. Research each publication's submission guidelines to determine where you can offer your expertise.

Practice marketing is mainly done using the **four traditional Ps of marketing**: Product, Placement, Price, and Promotion. We'll discuss the four traditional Ps later in this chapter, but before you can develop products and services, you must

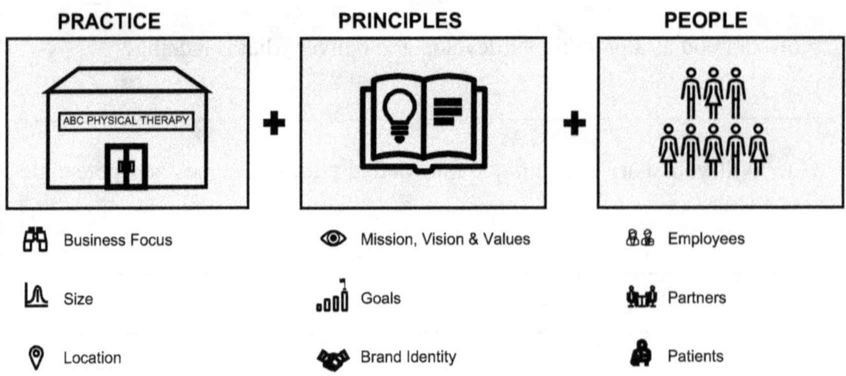

Figure 8.3 The Three Ps of Physical Therapy Practice Marketing

first build the foundations of your practice. To do that, we'll examine a different but equally important set of Ps: the **three Ps of physical therapy practice marketing**. The three Ps are Practice, Principles, and People, and together they form the DNA of your business. The three Ps are established first because they guide and impact most of your future practice decisions. The infographic above offers an overview of the three Ps of physical therapy practice marketing.

Now, let's dive into the three Ps of physical therapy practice marketing. The first category is Practice, which includes Business Focus, or the area of physical therapy you plan to practice in your new business. You may decide to open a general practice, which would enable you to offer a variety of services in one place to a broader spectrum of potential patients, or you may choose to have a specific care focus, such as neurological, pediatric, orthopedic, geriatric, sports, pelvic health, or other specialized type of physical therapy.

Keep your Business Focus in mind as we turn to the second Practice P, which is Size. Begin with your staff. Will you open a small, solo practice, or will you employ other physical therapists, receptionists, accountants, human resources personnel, or cleaners? Will you have salaried, hourly, or per diem employees? Will you have business partners? Answering these questions will help you to determine the amount of continuous cash you'll need to have to hand. Next, you'll need to consider how much actual space you need for your practice type, employees, and patients. Most importantly, you'll need to know how much you can afford to pay for any necessary space renovations, as well as monthly rent, utilities, insurance, and payroll. Size can change, of course, as your practice grows and evolves over time.

The third Practice P, Location, is a set of choices that determine how potential patients initially find and perceive your business in both the physical and online communities. Researching where your target audiences/potential patients regularly shop, dine, socialize, exercise, and even where they receive other medical care is a good place to start. This area is the ideal spot for your practice location if appropriate space is available and the price is right. If the "ideal spot" is out of your price range, another option is finding an affordable spot that can be easily found with simple directions. The other important factor is your website. Hiring a website designer who incorporates attractive design with search engine optimization (SEO) can be a sound investment in your practice's success. SEO not only improves search engine rankings, it builds trust with your target audiences, many of whom perceive websites at the top of their search as more credible. It also improves organic site traffic and can enhance user experience by making your site easily navigable and accessible. SEO can be integrated into site design, in on-page material such as keyword search, meta tags, and headers, as well as off-page sections like backlinks and social media sharing buttons.

The second P in the three Ps of physical therapy practice marketing is Principles. This is a category of evergreen or unchanging elements that are unique to your practice, including your mission, vision, values, goals, and brand identity. They describe who you are, what you stand for, what you offer, and what drives you as both a physical therapist and as a business owner.

Principles include your practice mission, which is a concise "right now" statement that explains why and how you do what you do, and what you strive to achieve for your patients. Let's assume we're starting a business called ABC PT, with a general physical therapy business focus. First, we'll need a purpose, which explains why your practice exists (beyond producing revenue). ABC PT's purpose might be "to improve our patients' overall health outcomes."

Along with purpose, your practice's overarching goals support the mission. Goals are described in generalized yet aspirational terms such as "providing individualized plans for each patient" or "innovating in the patient service model." And finally, the mission provides guidance to ensure future strategies and decisions stay true to it.

If we combine our purpose and goals to form ABC PT's mission, it might look like this: "To improve patients' overall health outcomes through service model innovation and individualized patient plans."

A vision statement complements the practice's mission, but with subtle differences. While the mission concentrates on what the practice is currently doing, the vision focuses on its future aspirations. It is an inspiring summary of what the company wants to achieve. Pulling in our knowledge of the future health care landscape, ABC PT's vision could aim "to be the region's leading provider of preventive and therapeutic patient wellness solutions."

Values are a statement of practice and practitioner beliefs that guide how a business operates, both internally and externally. Building upon the previous examples of ABC PT's mission and vision, its values could include:

- *Authentic connection*: Within the practice, to the health care field, and with our patients so we can understand, develop, and deliver the right physical therapy solutions at the right time.
- *Innovation*: We are curious, continuous learners who seek new information, insight, techniques, and technology to advance the field of physical therapy and patient health outcomes.
- *Flexibility*: We meet patients where they're most comfortable, whether that's in our clinic, via video appointment, or out in the community.

The final Principle category is **brand identity**, which is a group of assets that shape how your practice is perceived by current and potential patients and partners. Brand identity components include your practice logo, text fonts, customized colors used for internal and external branding materials, and brand voice, which is the tone and feeling evoked by the language you use about your practice. It also includes a brief tagline that captures the spirit of the practice. Famous tagline examples such as Nike's "Just Do It," Walmart's "Save Money, Live Better," and Subway's "Eat Fresh" succinctly sum up their mission, vision, and values with a simple, action-oriented statement.

Activity 8.5 Define Your Mission, Vision, Values, and Brand Identity

Using your knowledge of your target audiences, Principles, and table 8.4 below, develop a high-level version of your new practice's unique mission, vision, values, brand identity, and tagline.

Table 8.4 Define Your Business

Define Your Mission	
Find your purpose: why does your practice exist?	
What are the overarching goals of your practice?	
Summarizing your answers to the two questions above, what is your mission?	
Describe Your Vision	
What do you want your practice to achieve, and be known for, in the future?	
Detail Your Values	
As a physical therapist and as a business owner, what practices and behaviors do you believe in?	
Develop Your Brand Identity	
What colors will you use to convey the essence of your practice?	
What imaging elements and text font types will you use in your logo to represent your practice?	
What consistent tone/language will you use in your internal and external marketing materials?	
Incorporating the mission, vision, values, and brand identity components listed above, what is your tagline?	

Methodically and meticulously mapping out who you are, what you value, what you offer, who your target audiences are, and how you'll operate as a practice and as a practitioner can help you to avoid making some of the common mistakes that cause many small businesses to fail. You'll also find that performing the exercise in Table 8.4 can help you to efficiently build upon and expand your ideas in an organized and consistently branded way.

The third P of physical therapy practice marketing is People. These are the individuals and groups who you will work with to maintain, grow, and expand your practice. The People category includes any business partners you may have, as well as your employees, physicians, and patients who refer potential patient clients to you, topical influencers who act as brand and/or product evangelists to their own target audiences, fitness clubs, senior centers, and other groups whose target audiences overlap with yours. Creative, outside-the-box thinking is encouraged when considering potential partners for your practice.

With the three Ps of physical therapy practice marketing in place, we can now bring the four traditional marketing Ps (Product, Placement, Price, and Promotion), into the mix. When fully developed, the four traditional Ps form the basis of your strategy.

The first traditional P is the Product or service you'll develop for your practice. Product is a detailed process that begins with market research to help you to identify trends, marketplace need gaps, and target audiences. It then delves into what differentiates your product or service from others already on the market and what would make target audiences more likely to choose it, such as clever packaging, value, and usability.

Product also includes multiple personas, which are characters that you and your team create to represent the types of people likely to use your developing product

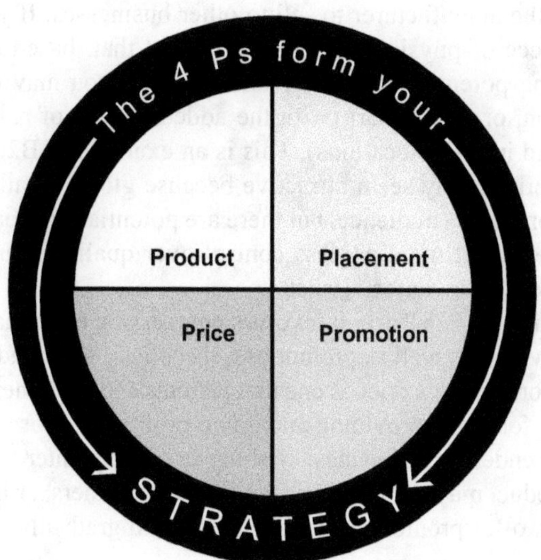

Figure 8.4 The Four Traditional Ps

or service, as well as their health goals and pain points. Let's assume that ABC PT has identified a gap in the current market for a physical therapy app. The app will remind the patient which exercise(s) to do, when to do them, offers a quick video refresher on how to do each one correctly, and provides a daily rep tracker that can be shared with their physical therapist. Here's a description of one possible persona for the new app: "38-year-old finance executive, wife, and mother of two active middle school kids. She injured her shoulder while windsurfing on her family's annual tropical vacation but has difficulty finding time to schedule rehabilitative treatments and keep up with the exercises recommended for her." Personas are used in the product development, design, and testing phases to ensure the product meets the target audiences' expectations for function, design, features, and usability. In later phases, the same personas will be used to help to position the product in the marketplace. The Product will also go through design, testing, and adaptation phases before it's considered ready to go to market.

Although the purpose and function of the second P, Placement, may seem obvious (it is where and how you'll sell your product or service), it also includes how much product to manufacture and distribute. Placement is a highly detailed, crucial component of the overall marketing strategy, encompassing the process of selecting where the product will be available for purchase, as well as the direct or indirect distribution channels you'll use. Direct distribution channels are those that sell from business to consumer (B2C). They include your business's website and physical locations. Direct distribution channels offer a few key advantages: greater branding, marketing, pricing, profit margin, and customer experience control, as well as brand loyalty influence.

Indirect distribution channels are primarily business to business (B2B) markets. They include partner retailers selected for their traffic, easily accessible location and desirability, and distributors that can help products to go from the manufacturing facility to retailers or wholesalers, who buy the product in large quantities from the manufacturer to sell to other businesses. If your practice develops a new piece of physical therapy equipment that, based upon market research, has strong potential for mass market appeal, you may choose to sell it online at Amazon, or at Walmart (with the added benefit of reaching their customers online and in retail locations). This is an example of B2C indirect distribution. These options may seem attractive because global retail giants can help to expand your practice's audience, but there are potential drawbacks to consider, including smaller profit margins, less control over quality, brand identity, customer experience, and inventory issues.

The third traditional P is Price. It involves comparison of similar or comparable products and services, as well as promotions, discounts, and bundled pricing. Ideally, the product or service's price is one that patients and customers can afford and be willing to pay for while providing maximum profitability for the practice. Pricing is a strategic endeavor: a business wishing to quickly enter a market and gain share with its product may set a low price to attract customers, or it can set a higher initial price, then offer promotions and discounts and gradually lower the market price to maximize profit gained from as many different target audiences as possible. There are different tiers of market position pricing, ranging from premium, which is the most expensive, to mid-range, to budget, and the tier selected should reflect the practice's brand identity. The quality and availability of materials, labor, and manufacturing facilities factor heavily into price, and they can also be affected by unforeseen circumstances such as natural disasters, or even by other health care factors, such as the outbreak of the COVID-19 pandemic in 2020.

The fourth and final traditional marketing P is Promotion, which combines strategy and tactics that capture its target audiences' attention and creates desire to try it. The process begins with product or service awareness, continues by piquing interest in and desire for it by touting its benefits, and then encourages target audiences to purchase or try it. This can be accomplished through paid promotion, which includes online, television, radio, and print media advertisements, social media, affiliate, and influencer marketing, direct mail campaigns, trade show exhibitions, event sponsoring, discounts, and limited time offers.

Take the time to pursue earned media coverage. Earned media is content created and published about your product or service, but without your creative ownership or control. It is the most difficult content to obtain because it cannot be bought, but that is precisely what makes it the most trusted form of marketing among consumers.[20] Examples include digital, video, or print news stories, organic social media mentions, independent product and service reviews, and other user generated content, such as forum discussions or threads, and blog comments. Engaging a public relations team can help to build media connections and objective product coverage, but if your budget doesn't allow for that, content marketing, such as blogs, podcasts, and short videos on the practice's website can be a less costly way to reach target audiences and create opportunities to build patient and customer relations.

The three Ps of physical therapy practice marketing help to guide the marketing strategy and plan by developing the four traditional Ps of marketing (Product, Placement, Price, and Promotion). The strategy includes Product details and conceptual elements of Placement, Price, and Promotion. The plan is the tactical arm of the strategy, detailing the actions to be taken, the collateral and budget required to support the product or service launch, as well as a timeline and team members responsible for execution. The difference between marketing and strategy is a common question, and a broad overview of each appears in figure 8.5 below.

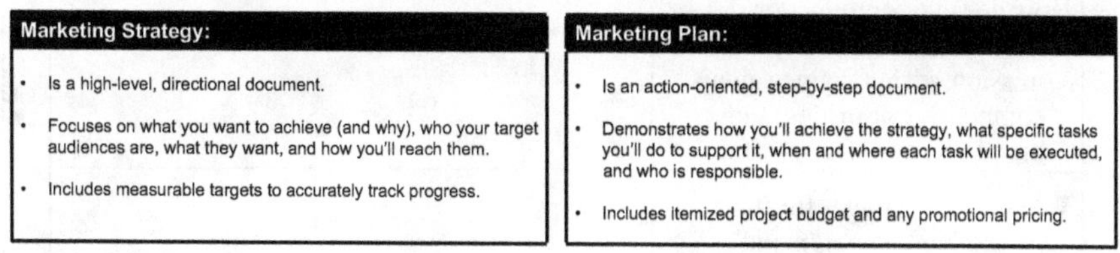

Marketing Strategy:
• Is a high-level, directional document.
• Focuses on what you want to achieve (and why), who your target audiences are, what they want, and how you'll reach them.
• Includes measurable targets to accurately track progress.
Marketing Plan:
• Is an action-oriented, step-by-step document.
• Demonstrates how you'll achieve the strategy, what specific tasks you'll do to support it, when and where each task will be executed, and who is responsible.
• Includes itemized project budget and any promotional pricing.

Figure 8.5 Marketing Strategy and Plan: What's the Difference?

Activity 8.6 Outline Your Marketing Strategy and Plan

Using your knowledge of the health care marketplace, your target audiences, the three Ps of physical therapy practice marketing and the four traditional marketing Ps, and guided by table 8.5 below, create a high-level plan for a fictional product or service that your practice intends to launch. The column on the left will prompt you to enter your responses in the column on the right.

Table 8.5 Develop Your Marketing Strategy and Plan

Market and Target Audience Research	
What customer needs or marketplace gaps did you find during the research phase?	
Do competitors currently offer a similar product or service? Describe in detail.	
What product or service will you develop in response to your research?	
Who are your target audiences?	
Product	
What is the working name of your product or service?	
Detail the design and quality features of your product or service. What differentiates it from competitor products?	
Using the target audiences listed above, what persona(s) have you created?	
What do you aim to achieve through the sale of your product or service, and why?	
How does your product or service advance your practice's mission, vision, values, goals, competitive priorities, and brand identity? Be specific.	
What is your budget for your marketing campaign and product launch? How will you divide and allocate funds for it?	

Placement	
What quantities of your product or service will you initially make available, and why?	
What direct distribution channels will your product or service be available on? Include physical retail and online locations and why you chose them.	
Will you use indirect distribution channels to sell your product or service? Why or why not? Which channels will you use?	
Price	
What price range (premium, mid-range, or budget) will you choose to market your product or service? Explain why, including how your price range supports your practice's mission, vision, values, goals and brand identity.	
What is your pricing objective? (Examples: to achieve quick marketing entry and share, to maximize profit and target audience appeal, etc.)	
What will the initial price of your product or service be?	
Will you offer discounts, promotions, sales, or bundling options? Explain when and for how long special pricing will be in effect.	
Promotion	
How will you create awareness of your new product or service? How will you create interest in your product or service? How will you create desire for your product or service with your target audiences?	

How will you use social media to market your product or service? Is there room in your budget for social media ads? Which channels will you use, and why? Have you allocated part of your budget for social media analytics? If so, what software will you use? (Examples: HootSuite, Sprout Social). If you don't have a budget for software tracking, how will you do this manually? Will you use email marketing? If so, list specifics (examples: newsletters, email campaigns).	
Will you use paid search marketing? If so, where, when, and how often?	
Will you use networking and community outreach to generate new patient referrals? Give a detailed description of each.	
Will you use local advertising options? List specific outlets and companies (examples: television, community newspapers, radio spots, billboards).	
Will you list your practice and products in online physical therapy indexes? (examples: Psychology Today, Good Therapy)	
Will you engage a public relations agency to help position your product for the public?	
How will you ensure that all of your marketing channels have consistent product messaging?	

KPIs and Measurement	
What KPIs will you use to evaluate the progress of your campaign? At what intervals will you assess and adjust them if necessary?	
Tactics and Timing	
Create a timeline and schedule that details when and where each marketing activity happens, what materials you need to develop or have to hand, and who is responsible for them.	

Bottom Line!

Once you've completed your marketing plan, don't just place it on a shelf. It's important that the plan and those executing its tactics stay flexible and adapt its components as needed to reach the practice and plan's goals and objectives. Consider the plan to be a living document that needs cyclic assessment and refinement to ensure that it still aligns with your practice goals, planned KPIs, and resonates with your target audiences. Assessment frequency will depend upon various factors, such as industry trends, product or service sales, and target audience behaviors. Here are a few guidelines on marketing plan assessment frequency:

- Quarterly: It's good practice to review and adjust at the start and end of each fiscal quarter to analyze your performance data and make any necessary adjustments to the plan to keep it on track with your KPIs and sales goals.
- Monthly: If you have a more dynamic practice scope or are in a highly competitive market, it may be necessary to assess your plan more frequently so that you can stay agile and adapt quickly to market changes and target audience behavior.
- Weekly: Even a quick review of current and upcoming tactics can allow you to spot trends and identify areas for improvement in real time.

Positioning both the physical therapist and physical therapy practice for success drastically reduces its chances of failure. In the health care field, it's critically important to familiarize yourself with key consumer demographics, as well as the present and projected future health care landscapes.

As a physical therapist, take inventory of your strengths, interests, and differentiators to help to determine how to brand and market yourself as a practitioner and thought leader. Within your physical therapy practice, taking the time to thoroughly define the three Ps of physical therapy practice marketing (Practice, Principles, and People), which form the core of your practice's DNA, helps to determine your business focus, size, location, and cash needs, as well as who you'll work and partner with. When defined properly, the three Ps tell the evergreen story of your practice's purpose, aspirations, and treatment philosophy.

When your practice is ready to begin offering your own products and services, the four traditional marketing Ps (Product, Placement, Price, and Promotion) will build upon the foundations created by the unchanging three Ps of physical therapy practice marketing to develop the marketing strategy and plan for each new offering. The strategic and tactical details built into the four traditional Ps will vary by annual plans, campaigns, and product or service launches, but their formulaic nature ensures effective time management, branding, and messaging consistency. As your marketing skills, practice, and health care marketplace knowledge increase, the process will become easier, and yet more detailed, as well. That's because repetition of these exercises positions you as a highly skilled thought leader who expertly and consistently promotes the value and growth of physical therapy through expert marketing.

Suggested Readings

How we can expect the healthcare industry to change in the future. The George Washington University School of Business. March 5, 2019. Accessed September 27, 2022. https://healthcaremba.gwu.edu/blog/technology-is-leading-a-healthcare-revolution/

Hsieh T. *Delivering Happiness: A Path to Profits, Passion and Purpose*. Grand Central Publishing; 2010.

What is patient-centered care? NEJM Catalyst. January 1, 2017. Accessed September 6, 2022. https://catalyst.nejm.org/doi/full/10.1056/CAT.17.0559

References

1. Parker E. What percentage of businesses fail? Clarify Capital. Accessed June 14, 2024. https://clarifycapital.com/blog/what-percentage-of-businesses-fail
2. Gali C. History of telemedicine. Curogram. February 8, 2022. Accessed January 17, 2023. https://blog.curogram.com/history-of-telemedicine
3. Gong D. Top 6 machine learning algorithms for classification. Towards Data Science. February 22, 2022. Accessed January 17, 2023. https://towardsdatascience.com/top-machine-learning-algorithms-for-classification-2197870ff501

4. Office of Advocacy. Frequently asked questions about small business 2023. US Small Business Administration. March 7, 2023. Accessed June 16, 2024. https://advocacy.sba.gov/2023/03/07/frequently-asked-questions-about-small-business-2023/
5. Preventive care. US Department of Health and Human Services. Accessed June 16, 2024. https://www.hhs.gov/healthcare/about-the-aca/preventive-care/index.html
6. Schwartz LM, Woloshin S. Medical marketing in the United States, 1997–2016. *JAMA*. 2019; 321(1): 80–96. doi:10.1001/jama.2018.19320
7. Technology is leading a healthcare revolution. The George Washington University School of Business. March 5, 2019. Accessed September 27, 2022.https://healthcaremba.gwu.edu/blog/technology-is-leading-a-healthcare-revolution/
8. Gulis G, Fujino Y. Epidemiology, population health, and health impact assessment. *J Epidemiol*. 2015; 25(3): 179–180. doi:10.2188/jea.JE20140212
9. What is patient-centered care? NEJM Catalyst. January 1, 2017. Accessed September 6, 2022. https://catalyst.nejm.org/doi/full/10.1056/CAT.17.0559
10. Preston B, Kaye M, Joseph J, et al. Future-proofing the business: Building a superior experience for health plan consumers through digital transformation. Deloitte Insights. May 20, 2021. Accessed October 22, 2022. https://www2.deloitte.com/us/en/insights/industry/health-care/transforming-the-health-plan-experience-with-technology.html
11. Roop L. What are your patients finding when they search for PT help? Practice Promotions. Updated February 22, 2024. https://practicepromotions.net/seo-keywords-physical-therapy-websites/?inf_contact_key=ac941c3b3cc6978f0e19a2fc5f39f922680f8914173f9191b1c0223e68310bb1
12. 6 tips to improve mind-body well-being. University Hospitals. July 10, 2022. Accessed January 5, 2023. https://www.uhhospitals.org/blog/articles/2022/07/6-tips-to-improve-mind-body-well-being
13. Healthcare 3.0: Building an intelligent omnichannel healthcare strategy. TTEC Digital, January 13, 2023, Accessed August 1, 2024. https://ttecdigital.com/articles/healthcare-3-0-building-an-intelligent-omnichannel-healthcare-strategy
14. Drees J. Google receives more than 1 billion health questions every day. Becker's Health IT. March 11, 2019. Accessed January 17, 2023. https://www.beckershospitalreview.com/healthcare-information-technology/google-receives-more-than-1-billion-health-questions-every-day.html
15. The generational influence on patient preferences. TTEC Digital, June 9, 2021. Accessed January 17, 2023. https://avtex.com/articles/the-generational-influence-on-patient-preferences
16. Dimock M. Defining generations: Where millennials end and generation Z begins. Pew Research Center. January 17, 2019. Accessed January 17, 2023. https://www.pewresearch.org/fact-tank/2019/01/17/where-millennials-end-and-generation-z-begins/
17. Fox S. Health topics. Pew Research Center. February 1, 2011. Accessed September 6, 2022. https://www.pewresearch.org/internet/2011/02/01/summary-charts/
18. Fox S. Profiles of health information seekers. Pew Research Center. February 1, 2011. Accessed January 17, 2023. https://www.pewresearch.org/internet/2011/02/01/profiles-of-health-information-seekers/

19. Team Braze. Platforms vs. channels: What's the difference? Braze. March 4, 2022. Accessed July 9, 2024. https://www.braze.com/resources/articles/platforms-vs-channels-whats-the-difference
20. BMV's 2019 digital brand: Awareness, engagement, and action index. Beantown Media Ventures. Accessed September 6, 2022. https://beantownmv.com/wp-content/uploads/dlm_uploads/2019/08/BMVs-2019-Digital-Brand-Index-1.pdf

Unit 3
Introduction

In unit 3, we pull together many of the pieces of the "management puzzle" presented so far in units 1 and 2, so that you can start to apply these fundamental practices, strategies, and tools intentionally in developing your management "style" (i.e., approach, philosophy) and crafting your ideal practice model for the future. Overall this plan might mean that you:

- ✓ practice uniquely and confidently, using your management skills (i.e., self-management) and business literacy, as an individual contributor to demonstrate value within an established system, or
- ✓ seek out opportunities to move into a formal management role, or
- ✓ start the planning process to open your own practice at some point in your career, or
- ✓ seek out ways to innovate and drive change within an existing system (i.e., health care organization or community) to improve outcomes (through intrapreneurship or social entrepreneurship).

In this unit, we continue to share stories, especially in chapter 10 (i.e., business model case studies), of real-world experiences because we firmly believe that we can learn from one another. Moreover, we hope that these authentic narratives will help to inspire and guide you when you hit the ground running in professional practice.

The three chapters comprising Unit 3 are:

- Chapter 9: "Entrepreneurship, Innovation, and Change"
- Chapter 10: "Business Modeling: Identifying Successful Practices and Avoiding Unsuccessful Ones"
- Chapter 11: "Getting Started: Planning for the Future"

We urge you to tap into your newly discovered knowledge, skills and practices to be the change agent – wherever you are – as a physical therapist. Our potential as a profession is enormously exciting and it will take *each* of us and *all* of us to collaborate and innovate to craft our future. Change is inevitable – especially in health care and physical therapy. Managing change requires planning, envisioning, and action. Change takes courage.

DOI: 10.4324/9781003524250-11

9 Entrepreneurship, Innovation, and Change

Chris Petrosino and Kristin Schweizer

The entrepreneur always searches for change, responds to it, and exploits it as an opportunity.

Peter Drucker, Austrian-American consultant, educator and author[1]

Chapter Objectives

1. Explain the differences between entrepreneurship, intrapreneurship, and innovation.
2. Describe the characteristics of an entrepreneur.
3. Discuss strategies for developing, implementing, maintaining, and assessing an entrepreneurial endeavor.
4. Explore your personal characteristics, ideas, and opportunities to become an entrepreneur.

Management Vignette

Chris Petrosino, PT, PhD

I am blessed to have had a fulfilling career in the amazing profession of physical therapy. My entrepreneurial experience, particularly my intrapreneurial experience, stems from the early 1990s when I began to develop occupational health programs in health care and industrial settings as a new clinician. While working in a hospital system, a request for on-site health care came from a steel foundry and finishing corporation. Recognizing the lucrative opportunity, a physician and I developed a proposal. The physician developed the emergency care and dispensary services while I developed the preventative and rehabilitative services. I gathered resources and expanded the original request beyond rehabilitation services to work reconditioning, work hardening, post-offer employment testing, preventative educational

DOI: 10.4324/9781003524250-12

programs, ergonomic interventions, and functional job analysis, as well as writing functional job descriptions in adherence with the Americans with Disabilities Act, and providing workers with resources for performance improvement. After earning the direct-to-employer contract and the successful implementation thereof, the demand for our services grew exponentially. Through word-of-mouth publicity other industries began requesting our services to the point that we were unable to accommodate their requests. Driven by passion, a sense of focused purpose, and a strong work ethic, my career hit the ground running and it could not have been less challenging or gratifying.

Imbued with a love of learning and teaching, I transitioned to academia as a Director of Clinical Education (termed Academic Coordinator of Clinical Education at that time). In my new academic role, I developed my own clinical student placement tracking spreadsheet at the same time as other entrepreneurs were developing software to assist in managing student records, affiliation agreements, and clinical placements. Like the occupational health venture, the spreadsheet was another small step in the development of an entrepreneurial spirit. Years later, as a Program Director teaching business concepts, the connection between detailed billing software and clinical education needs that were not being met by current software led me to reach out to a private practice physical therapist entrepreneur and billing software owner. Together with our university clinical education team and a software engineer we initiated the development of a successful clinical education software program. This entrepreneurial endeavor necessitated the building of relationships with a range of people, all of whom had different talents to mine, in order to bring this successful venture to fruition. In addition, seeing the opportunity to leverage insights from other disciplines and successfully adapting those insights to meet the needs of our own project was very advantageous. Synthesizing ideas, products, and processes from other industries and disciplines often leads to innovative endeavors. For instance, the clinical education and classroom scheduling software used by universities may prompt an entrepreneur to integrate the functionality of restaurant reservation systems into their software products. Likewise, developing clinic-based software that integrates clinical education needs and employer recruitment efforts within university-based software systems may be very beneficial in meeting the multiple needs of health care educators and service providers. The successful entrepreneur recognizes that resources are finite, yet ideas are limitless, and can discern and agilely adjust the path to desired outcomes.

I cannot emphasize strongly enough the need to surround yourself with the right people. Although we may recognize and act upon an opportunity or lead an initiative, we are hardly ever the most knowledgeable person on all aspects of what is needed in most successful entrepreneurial endeavors. You also never know when your experience as a physical therapist and the contacts you've made will stretch beyond our profession. For instance, as a

Dean of Graduate Studies at a faith-based university, I used my experience as a spiritual person, learning from physical therapy practice decision-making and curriculum development, and application of an entrepreneurial spirit to transform a theology degree into concentrations that created greater market demand. After hiring and working with an amazing theologian and priest, we were able to develop a robust core curriculum in the Department of Theology and pastoral ministry concentration within the traditional academic master's degree program. Recognizing the needs of priests in the administration of their parishes and religious educators' need for teaching skills, I engaged the right people in the business and education departments to develop concentrations in parish administration and religious education. The master's degree program expanded to four specific concentrations. Two of the concentrations required expertise from other disciplines which proved successful in increasing enrollment and providing fulfilling opportunities for students and religious organizations alike.

The skills I gained while working as a physical therapist in data gathering, examination, evaluation, and intervention, with a focus on desired outcomes in an energizing workplace, served me well as a Dean, Department Chair, and Program Director. Being ever vigilant in recognizing and acting upon opportunities and intrapreneurial initiatives, and assisting others in their own entrepreneurial adventures, have contributed to my fulfilling career in service to others. Many initiatives were very successful, while others fell short of expectations, yet all of them required calculated risk, courage, resilience, and hard work. All my entrepreneurial endeavors proved to be amazing learning experiences. The lessons learned from these experiences continue to be essential to my daily work and consulting services. The skills we develop in our profession can translate into entrepreneurial ventures in our lives if we recognize and act upon opportunities as they arise.

Entrepreneurs Thrive on Change

Peter Drucker, often referred to as "the founder of modern management,"[2] argues that the **entrepreneur** is constantly searching for change and responding to change in innovative ways. In other words, the entrepreneur "exploits [change] as an opportunity." You may have heard the quote attributed to the Greek philosopher Heraclitus that "change is the only constant in life." Do you embrace change with passion and seek the opportunities that change brings? Entrepreneurs do embrace change and are vigilant in observing the impact or potential impact of change with a focus on seizing opportunities. Through serious and thoughtful consideration, the entrepreneur transitions an idea into a plausible initiative followed by a feasible plan to implement and sustain the vision. This formation process may be instantaneous or it may take time. Regardless, there are usually risks in embarking on potentially lucrative ventures which involve time, energy, money, and specific skill sets. Alongside risk can come great rewards or failures from those efforts. Successful entrepreneurs learn from their failures and the resulting discouragement is fleeting. You may have heard a version of John C. Maxwell's quote, "fail early, fail often, but always fail forward."[3]

Activity 9.1 How Do You Manage Failure?

Think about and reflect deeply upon a time when you failed at managing change. Answer the following reflective/discussion questions.

Describe the setting (place, persons involved, atmosphere, etc.).

____

____

____

Describe the situation.

____

____

____

What did you have control over; what was under the control of others, and what was outside your control?

____

____

____

What action(s) did you take initially?

____

____

____

What action(s) did you take in attempt to succeed once failure was probable?

____

____

____

In retrospect, what actions would you take now if you could do it over again?

____

____

____

In the spaces below provide your interpretation of the situation, event(s), actions.

____

____

____

How did you feel at the time and how do you currently feel about your failure?

____

____

____

What did you learn from this failure?

____

____

____

Failure can be part of learning and growth if you engage what you have learned and strategize future approaches to similar situations. Allow your failures to enhance your passion, resilience, and desire to thrive. Furthermore, the mindset of "thriving on change" helps to build your character if you are willing to take calculated risks, and work hard with a sustained effort to achieve desired outcomes.

Activity 9.2 How Do You Manage Change?

Think back to a time of major change in your career path and answer the following questions in the spaces below.

How did you react?

____

____

____

How did your action(s) make you feel?

____

____

____

List the opportunities that you identified during that time of change.

____

____

____

Did you recognize that change was coming before it arrived? If so, what were the signs and how did you act before it arrived?

____

____

____

What Is an Intrapreneur?

When an entrepreneurial effort is sanctioned and resourced by an employer the term used is *intrapreneurship.* In other words, **intrapreneurs** are individuals who engage in entrepreneurial activities for their employer. The intrapreneur who championed the idea or innovation has limited liability in taking on a risky endeavor while the employer takes most of the risk, reward, and effect of failures. As a physical therapist, being an intrapreneur has less risk when employed in a productive business or department, unless your job description is based upon developing new and successful service lines or products.

Case Study 9.1

Developing an Intrapreneurial Endeavor

A partner in a private practice recognized that their pelvic health patients could benefit from prenatal and postpartum massage. Her successful physical therapy interventions which demonstrated effective outcomes and high patient satisfaction developed into a strong referral base for pelvic health patients. Being an astute clinician, she found ample evidence in the literature to support the benefits of prenatal perineal massage on postpartum complications.[4] Many patients began requesting her specifically as their physical therapist. Recognizing the opportunity to provide an additional benefit to her patients and an added revenue source, the practice partner began her research into the feasibility of providing perineal massage for patients experiencing stress, pain, hormone regulation issues, and sleep concerns.

Having a good understanding of her clientele and the community in which they reside, she began her investigation into developing this intervention as a revenue source. She started a needs assessment to better understand the magnitude of the health concerns and the perspective of those seeking pelvic health services.

Activity 9.3 Case Analysis

Be creative and list in the spaces provided the resources that may be available to the practice partner to gather information about the health needs of her patients.

____

____

____

What does she need to know about her patients and her community?

____

____

____

What are the secondary sources, such as the American Physical Therapy Association (APTA) Academy of Pelvic Health, that would inform her needs analysis?

____

____

____

What would you do to engage the primary sources in providing feedback? Consider the advantages and disadvantages of the information gathering methods you would choose.

____

____

____

Would this be a good time for the practice partner to develop a business plan, or conduct a SWOT analysis? (See chapter 11.) Why or why not?

____

____

____

What are the calculated risks that the practice partner needs to consider? (Consider risk/benefit, return-on-investment, access, etc.)

____

____

____

Intrapreneurs must recognize the need to understand the environment in which their employer functions to identify which services they should develop. Successful intrapreneurs consider the geographical area that is reasonable to draw clients or patients, the number of patients or clients within that area who would benefit from the service, who will help to recruit or refer those clients and patients to your employer, and what other health care facilities have captured a share of the market by offering the same or similar services. The analysis of the market is used to determine what percentage of the market share the proposed service intends to capture. Capturing market share depends upon meeting unmet needs, providing a better quality of service, increasing access to those in need, and providing the service at a reasonable or competitive cost. After undertaking the market analysis the intrapreneur can determine how to target the intended audience and market the services to potential patients or clients (see chapter 8). From all the preparatory work, a business or program plan can be created which identifies the human and material resources needed and the projected patient volume required for the venture to be successful.

Embracing Change through Innovation

Business owners and business leaders may engage in entrepreneurial endeavors that focus on products, processes for improved efficiency or effectiveness, or marketing to enhance gains in market share. **Market share** is typically represented by the percentage of the total sales that a company makes over a fiscal period. When not driven by a passionate individual, the impetus to innovate and change is typically forced by competition and market forces. An innovation may involve creating something new, expanding or improving something that already exists, or combining something to form a new product, service, or application. For instance, physical therapist private practice owners develop specialty areas or niche practices or programs that expand current services to gain market share, which is considered **product or service innovation**. Some employers have invested in employee development and training in examination and intervention approaches such as point of service diagnostic ultrasound, pelvic health, direct-to-employer occupational health services, dry needling, and low load blood flow restriction exercise. Product innovation also includes the creation or development of new equipment, software, and other resources used in the provision of physical therapy. Innovations that are focused on improving the efficiency and effectiveness of processes within the practice enabling better service are intended to decrease employee workload and provide faster turnaround on profit. This could involve patient scheduling, documentation systems, workflow, or other work practices. This type of innovation is termed **process innovation**. Health professionals must stay on top of developing and using evidence-based examination and intervention techniques to maintain appropriate contemporary practice but also develop a better reputation than competitors. Through **marketing innovation**, the entrepreneur intends to capture a larger clientele than competitors through innovative marketing strategies such as design and packaging of marketing materials, events for referral sources and consumers, giveaway items, or other enticements for clients and patients to seek their services or products over others. When considering marketing innovations, entrepreneurs should keep in mind legal and ethical issues, especially enticements that could be considered referral for profit. At times the leaders of a business may make significant changes in organizational structure, reporting lines, decision-making ability of personnel, or other business practices which are intended to improve the profitability of the business. These changes are **organizational innovations**. In general, successful innovations and changes in physical therapy are based on effective and efficient practice, adaptability, and migration of capabilities to current and future demands of patients/clients.

Creativity, drive, and energy are characteristics that are valued in entrepreneurial people. Whether individual characteristics can be developed or if some individuals are born with these traits is occasionally questioned. Regardless of a genetic predisposition, physical therapists and physical therapist assistants must nurture the traits and skills required for developing and sustaining an entrepreneurial spirit to optimize and/or overcome barriers. Some individuals are very perceptive in recognizing opportunities, while others seem to have an innate passion and drive to innovate, develop, build, explore, or bring a project to fruition. Others find or happen upon their passion which creates the spirit and energy to pursue an entrepreneurial endeavor. Knowing yourself is a big step in overcoming barriers to success and recognizing opportunities. Having a strong sense of purpose drives passion and builds energy that can bring success.

Activity 9.4 Entrepreneurial Spirit

Consider the personal characteristics of someone you believe is innovative or a successful entrepreneur.

Was that person born with a gift or did they develop the necessary skills over time? If the latter, how?

____

____

____

List that person's characteristics that you believe are from nature/innate and list those that are nurtured through skill development.

____

____

____

Compare and contrast the lists.

____

____

____

Of these characteristics, which ones do you possess? Which characteristics are ones you can improve upon?

____

____

____

Respond to the following questions.
Consider a time when you had a new idea. Briefly describe the situation.

____

____

____

Did you have the initiative to be a change agent or a catalyst for change? Circle one response.

Yes *No*

Did you develop steps to implement the change? Circle one response.

Yes *No*

Did you make a change? Circle one response.

Yes *No*

If you took the initiative to act, what was the outcome?

____

____

____

What would you have done differently knowing what you know now?

____

____

____

If you did not take the initiative to act, why?

____

____

____

SWOT Your Entrepreneurial Prowess

In chapter 11 you will learn more about the SWOT (strengths, weaknesses, opportunities, and threats) analysis. In the same way that you can assess the internal strengths and weaknesses of a business and the external environment that provides opportunities and threats, so can you self-assess your entrepreneurism. Gaining a greater insight into your own strengths and weaknesses will optimize your potential to succeed in an entrepreneurial endeavor. You have talents that can be used to earn small and large successes along the way to your entrepreneurial objectives. You will also discover weaknesses that provide insight into the need for refinement, learning, and/or development of skills that can optimize your potential for success. A SWOT analysis of yourself is very beneficial when developing a personal strategic plan to become an entrepreneur. Likewise, implementing a SWOT analysis once you identify an entrepreneurial endeavor will help you to decide on the need for partners, a team, or others with different skill sets to bring your business vision to fruition. Returning to the current opportunities and threats that can help or hinder you to become an entrepreneur, scanning external environmental factors to determine the advantages and disadvantages to your personal and professional development can be brought to awareness. An analysis of the opportunities and threats should identify the available resources and need for resources, knowledge of contemporary physical therapy practice, areas outside of physical therapy that may be integrated into future endeavors, your ability to gain market share and create consumer demand, and projections of future demand and ability to produce the sustaining work needed to succeed. Identifying opportunities and threats often brings to light issues of your competing obligations, time available, financial wherewithal, available mentors, potential stakeholders, supporters, or contributors that could be optimized to achieve your entrepreneurial vision.

Activity 9.5 SWOT Yourself

Complete table 9.1 below by following these steps:

1. Brainstorm the strengths and weaknesses you possess that would help you to become an entrepreneur. List as many as you can in the space of one minute in the space given below.
2. Brainstorm external opportunities and threats you are currently aware of that would help or hinder your ability to become an entrepreneur. List all that you can within one minute in the space below.
3. Next, reflect upon your lists in the left column. Read each question in the second column to the right and respond with an answer in the space below.

Table 9.1 A Personal SWOT Analysis

Strengths (list all)	What are your three most promising entrepreneurial strengths and how will they benefit you in an entrepreneurial endeavor?
Weaknesses (list all)	What are your three most challenging entrepreneurial weaknesses and how can you turn them into strengths?
Opportunities (list all)	What are the three most promising external resources, beyond your talents, that could help you to be successful as an entrepreneur? How can these resources be used?
Threats (list all)	What are three of the biggest external threats, beyond your own weaknesses, that you need to overcome as an entrepreneur? Which three steps might you take to overcome these challenges?

How to Recognize an Entrepreneurial Opportunity and Decide to Act

Physical therapists and physical therapist assistants become competent experts through learning from many sources (i.e., knowledge and understanding) and effectively applying their learning in practice (i.e., clinical reasoning and problem solving). Over 20 years ago, Dr. Gail Jensen and colleagues identified four dimensions of expert physical therapist practice: knowledge, clinical reasoning, movement, and virtues.[5] Largely unbeknown to the expert therapist, their expertise is recognized in the application of all dimensions in the moment of patient care through being unconsciously competent in identifying the primary problem and applying the correct technique to facilitate healing. Like the expert therapist, the entrepreneur can assimilate information through reflection-in-action to apply and adjust their understanding and perception of context for a desired outcome. Part of this skill is identifying barriers or constraints that hinder the desired outcome in the moment.

Analogous to an entrepreneur having an "aha!" moment sparking a great endeavor and acting upon it, Keith Davids and colleagues postulated that "movement emerges from the self-organizing resolution of specific constraints to achieve the successful performance of an activity."[6] The integration of perception, cognition, motivation, and contextual factors produces a goal-driving action in functional movement which translates to the entrepreneur's taking goal-driven action once an opportunity is recognized. For "expert" entrepreneurs, recognizing opportunity is seemingly an innate ability, yet this ability has been honed through practice, knowledge, and skill. Successful entrepreneurs quickly orient for action then appropriately adapt to the constraint for the desired outcome.

Learning from other professions, we can draw insights from a decision-making strategy developed for fighter pilots. Col. John Boyd of the US Airforce developed the concept of the OODA (Observe, Orient, Decide, and Act) loop to highlight the decision-making strategy used in combat operations (figure 9.1). Fighter pilots must quickly observe a situation, filter the available information to orient to the environmental context, make an appropriate decision, and act in an instant. Physical therapists and physical therapist assistants who hone their observation skills and identify opportunities in the moment seem to act through a reflexive behavior not unlike fighter pilots. Some entrepreneurs may keep a notebook handy to document insights whether at a conference, in the middle of the night, or while working with a patient. The term used by fighter pilots is "implicit guidance and control," which means that the person is trained and experienced to act without the need to bring observations to full consciousness. The physical therapist or physical therapist assistant can learn strategies to identify opportunities and act upon innovations or entrepreneurial endeavors.

Physical therapists and physical therapist assistants use clinical decision-making models similar to the OODA loop that are central to providing an effective service. In figure 9.1, we see that our decision-making does not differ much from the agile decision-making required of a fighter pilot or, indeed, an entrepreneur. In any setting physical therapists and physical therapist assistants are prepared to act in the best interests of those under their care. They bring evidence and outside

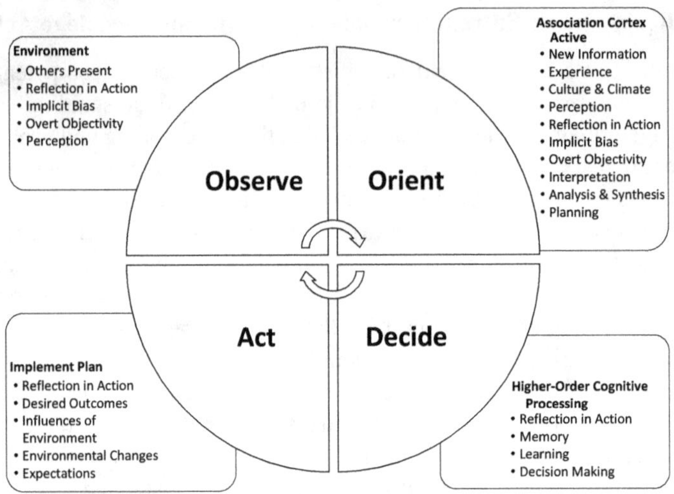

Figure 9.1 John Boyd's OODA Loop

Source: Permission is granted to copy, distribute and/or modify this document under the terms of the GNU Free Documentation License, Version 1.2 or any later version published by the Free Software Foundation; with no Invariant Sections, no Front-Cover Texts, and no Back-Cover Texts. A copy of the license is included in the section entitled GNU Free Documentation License. Found at: https://commons.wikimedia.org/wiki/File:OODA.Boyd.svg

information, such as patients' past medical history, to an unfolding circumstance in patient care, along with consideration of the environment. Physical therapists and physical therapist assistants become highly skilled at observation. They quickly orient to the patient's presentation of injury or illness, work or home environment, and social determinants of health to decide on a plan of care. They act in implementing the plan and constantly attend to unfolding information about the patient's response to the intervention so that we can adjust as needed. With clinical experience physical therapists and physical therapist assistants develop a "clinical edge" to recognize safety concerns or patient needs. They often execute an action without bringing an observation to consciousness. This implicit guidance and control in clinical practice is efficiently and effectively honed to the point whereby clinical decisions are seamlessly transitioned into action through their observations (i.e., the OODA loop). Physical therapists and physical therapist assistants who have been practicing for a few years almost instantaneously move to execute an action, just as a fighter pilot might too. This skill can develop in entrepreneurial skill given sufficient experience and vigilant observation to recognize opportunity.

Entrepreneurs are prepared to vigilantly attend to change, and they are prepared to act when an opportunity arises. Once an opportunity is recognized they seek the information needed to act, including evidence and outside information relevant to the unfolding circumstance, with consideration of the environment. Entrepreneurs are highly skilled at observation. They quickly orient themselves to the opportunity, considering many aspects of the situation. They continuously refine their approach and implement strategies based upon new information and learning. Entrepreneurs develop and refine their "entrepreneurial spirit" through experience by acting upon their insights.

Activity 9.6 Innovative Practices: Interview with an Entrepreneur

Answer the following reflective/discussion questions regarding an entrepreneur. If an entrepreneur is available first answer the questions yourself then conduct an interview using the following questions (revise as needed).

1. Do you know of an innovative physical therapy practice or physical therapist you believe is innovative? What makes the practice or physical therapist innovative?

____

____

____

2. How did the entrepreneur recognize an opportunity and act (Observe, Orient, Decide, and Act)?

____

____

____

3. How does the business gain market share and how does the physical therapist gain supporters?

____

____

____

4. What are the behaviors and decisions that the innovator made or is making?

____

____

____

Entrepreneurs innovate with expectations of financial gain, yet not all innovators are entrepreneurs. Innovators are passionate people who are energized by creating something new or better than what is currently used. The best innovators have a thirst for learning and can integrate new information and feedback from others into their ideas. Innovators are characterized by their honed skills in literature search, critical thinking and decision-making, problem solving, interpersonal skills, and communication. Many of the characteristics and behaviors of "leaders," as described in the textbook *Learning to Lead in Physical Therapy*,[7] mirror those of successful entrepreneurs and innovators. Innovators keep an open mind when others contribute valid ideas, while guarding against making all the decisions or veering from the desired vision. Innovators realize that information and feedback may take an idea or initiative to a new and better level. Skilled innovators empower others to contribute without losing control of the vision or focus. For instance, a physical therapist may propagate a conceptual model, intervention technique, or product at a conference and implement refinements from insights of those that attended the conference. Physical therapists readily share insights and ask questions following engaging presentations of innovative ideas at conferences.

Entrepreneurs manage conflicting ideas and challenge people with appropriate application of conflict management strategies. Interaction with people regarding new innovations often creates conflicting opinions and an innovator knowing when to compete, compromise, collaborate, accommodate, or avoid a conflict to produce a better product or outcome could be essential to the development, support, and sustainability of an initiative.

Activity 9.7 How Would You Handle This Conflict?

Recall from chapter 2 the discussions highlighting the need to develop conflict management skills. Now review the following case scenario:

> An expert clinician and manual therapist was at a continuing education course for treatment of temporomandibular dysfunction (TMD). In a lab session the participants were practicing a technique that was demonstrated by the presenter. While the presenter observed the expert therapist, the expert inquired, "Why not stabilize the cervical spine in this way." Their impromptu technique, based upon experience and skill, optimized the ability to mobilize the temporomandibular joint while producing the desired effect. The presenter reflected briefly and praised the expert for her revision of the technique. The expert therapist transitioned their manual therapy skill and clinical competence in treating TMD into a new intervention that combined the two skill sets. The presenter, on returning to the large group after the lab activity, proceeded to demonstrate the new adaptation to the presented intervention

and stated, "I may have discovered a new technique." Unfortunately, the presenter did not credit the expert physical therapist when it was clearly their insight to the intervention.

1. With a partner role-play the scenario demonstrating conflict management strategies. Decide who will be the "expert physical therapist" or the "presenter" and choose to compete, compromise, collaborate, accommodate, or avoid a conflict without disclosure to your partner.
2. Role-play for approximately five minutes. Once completed, identify the strategy used by each participant.
3. Discuss whether the interaction produced a positive or negative outcome for each participant.
4. Discuss how the conflict could have been better managed.

Developing a Team: The RACI Model

In consideration of your role-play scenario, the expert therapist was able to initiate the OODA loop to create a better technique. If the expert were to market and present this technique for financial gain, they would be an entrepreneur. In addition, they would need to claim the technique as intellectual property in some way to protect their innovative intervention. If the innovation required further development and the entrepreneur wanted assistance in the development a priori expectations should be established. The entrepreneur must explicitly state the parameters of the authority of those they entrust with assisting in the development of the innovation. A balance is needed between empowering decision-makers and delegating responsibility for executing and maintaining the progress of an initiative within the vision of the entrepreneur. One tool to assist in this process is the development of a RACI matrix.[8] RACI is an acronym for:

- **R**esponsible: One or more persons assigned to the task.
- **A**ccountable: Sign off when complete; it's important that only one person is accountable so that the buck stops there, and that person should be …
- **C**onsulted: Seek input during development, as a final check prior to going to full implementation, or consulted for adaptations during a soft start; furthermore, that person should be …
- **I**nformed: Typically people who are charged with a task in the developed process or desired outcome.

If the expert therapist wanted to become an entrepreneur and market their technique through educational programs, they could develop a RACI matrix to move the process along (see table 9.2). The RACI matrix is a table developed to assist in the completion of a project with appropriate lines of communication, authority, and responsibility. Projects typically require several steps to reach completion.

Table 9.2 RACI Matrix: TMD

Steps	*Project Initiation Tasks*	*Entre-preneurial Leader*	*Consultant 1: TMD*	*Consultant 2: Manual Therapy*	*Consultant 3: Research Co-investigator(s)*	*Consultant 4: Education/ Marketing Associate*
Step 1	Check face validity of technique with mentors	A/R	C	C	I	I
Step 2	Perfect technique	A/R	C	C	I	I
Step 3	Validity and reliability	A	I	I	R	I
Step 4	Publish article	A	C	C	R	I
Step 5	Book speaking engagements	A	I	I	I	R

The first column in the matrix shows the number of steps. The second breaks down the tasks that should be completed in sequence to complete the project. The following columns define responsibility and accountability for effective and efficient completion of the project.

Improvement without Innovation

Physical therapists typically start a private practice for financial gain (i.e., to earn a living), for the opportunity to provide higher quality services on their own terms (i.e., practice autonomy), or to focus on a niche practice that they believe is in demand in the health care market. All new private practices, or partnerships, are entrepreneurial endeavors which incur risk and rewards, yet most are not substantively innovative. The objective is to gradually grow a customer base from the quality of services provided. Private practice owners need to be aware of the best available evidence for quality services and possess the business acumen to grow their practice. The business owner must also be vigilantly aware of changes to contemporary practice and react in an agile and appropriate manner to maintain and grow market share. A business can be seen as an organic entity that needs to be appropriately nurtured to grow or sustain viability. Businesses tend to gain market share through continuous and incremental growth that is based on conventional ways of developing practices. The majority of physical therapists break into private practice without an abrupt, new innovative way of capturing a share of the market.

Physical therapists who have watched others venture into private practice may come to realize that they have all the capabilities to start a practice of their own. The time, energy, talents, and financial resources needed to start a physical therapy private practice may dissuade an individual from committing to business ownership. Larger private practices have been successful in providing "innovative" ways to entice physical therapists to manage and/or become part-owners of an established business. These relationships limit the risk to an individual physical therapist inclined to start a business, while optimizing the resources of the group of practices that make up the company.

Activity 9.8 Are *All* Business Owners Entrepreneurs and Are *All* Entrepreneurs Innovative?

All entrepreneurs realize opportunities, take risks, and have the tenacity to bring ideas to fruition, but are these ideas innovative or are they acting on customary practices? Physical therapy practice owners are entrepreneurial but are they innovative? Answer the following reflective/discussion questions in the spaces provided.

Can entrepreneurs succeed without being innovative?

____

____

Describe a situation where an entrepreneur is successful without being innovative (i.e., they have not introduced a new, original, or distinctly creative idea).

____

____

Can individuals be business owners without being entrepreneurial? If so, provide an example.

____

____

Describe a situation where an entrepreneur is successful without being innovative (i.e., they have not introduced a new, original, or distinctly creative idea).

____

____

Disruptive Innovation versus Sustaining Innovation

Large corporations and private companies dominate a health care field in a region by utilizing their resources to capture a majority market share of the patient population requiring their services. These companies tend to set the level of performance expected by customers. Retaining their market share can be accomplished by providing greater access, less cost, or a higher quality of services. These companies, working at the higher end of the market that is most lucrative, may offer a lower level of care than smaller competitors by becoming "in-network" at less cost to insurance companies, which in turn increases their access to patients. How do the smaller private practices break this cycle? How many patients can go to a clinic of their choice without worrying that their insurance company will not cover the cost? Are there smaller private practices working at the lower end of the market in innovative ways to gain a foothold in delivering more desirable services? When does or can this foothold become a critical mass of patients/consumers to become mainstream and potentially disrupt companies that "own" the higher end of the market? Are private practices targeting the overlooked services of the larger companies to deliver what patients and employers want in order to improve their health?

Several basic tenets of **disruptive innovation** must be met to be a truly innovative strategy to break the competition in a way that changes the demand in a market. The term disruptive innovation should not be used to describe any imposed situation that challenges the prior successful practices of an industry. Take, for example, the vice president who, under the guise of disruptive innovation, used the power of his position to flatten the organizational structure and have mid-level directors report to him directly in order to make himself appear indispensable to the CEO. While this initiative did prolong his tenure in that he appeared to resolve the chaos he created under the guise of disruptive innovation it also led to the departure of valued employees and set back the company from years of successful growth in sustaining innovation. The administrative change shifted the focus of employees from external competition to internal restructuring. The initiative was never intended to gain a foothold in a market by delivering a product or service with better functionality at a lower cost. As a leader, employees at all levels should challenge those in power who value self-interest at the expense of those that the organization is serving. In contrast, disruptive innovation must have the following tenets to meet the needs of the desired change:

1. The businesses that dominate the market are overreaching with a blind focus on innovation in products or services that consumers don't understand or need in attempt to improve their product or service and gain market share.
2. While dominant businesses are distracted with their overreach, innovative businesses begin to meet consumers' needs with simple, more focused, products or services.
3. The simple and more focused products and services continue to be refined and improved to the point of gaining a critical mass of consumers.
4. The increased demand for the services that best meet the needs of the consumer reaches a point where the once-dominant businesses are seen as failing to meet the needs of the customer.

In sum, while businesses that dominate the market are focused on advanced products and services that are targeted at the more sophisticated purchasers who are willing to pay more for them, at the higher end of the market price a less dominant business can slip in at the lower end of the market, create substantial demand and gain a substantial share of the market by meeting customers' needs or wants. How often do we over-buy things that we need for a computer, vehicle, or even entertainment cable services? How often do we change our cable services to a package that allows us to view more of the kind of shows we enjoy? In the field of health care, how often do patients go to providers that order unnecessary tests or provide unwarranted treatment interventions?

While disruptive innovation may be successful in a market where the external climate is primed for an innovative business to gain market share, sustaining innovation requires an entrepreneurial culture inside the business. Recall from chapter 4 the importance of organizational culture in creating a successful business. An organization that has an **entrepreneurial culture** can also be characterized as a learning organization that embraces change, encourages appropriate risk-taking for innovation, develops relationships that promotes the sharing of ideas, and continuously assesses the outcomes of initiatives to agilely adapt to change when needed. Developing an entrepreneurial culture that produces sustaining innovation is grounded in change management. One of the best change management approaches has been established by John Kotter in his Eight Step Change Model[9] that consists of the following steps to transforming an organization:

1. Establishing a sense of urgency;
2. Forming a powerful coalition;
3. Creating a vision;
4. Communicating the vision;
5. Empowering others to act to remove obstacles;
6. Planning and creating short-term wins;
7. Consolidating gains; and
8. Institutionalizing change in the corporate culture.

Case Study 9.2

Occupational Health Services as Disruptive and Sustained Innovations

The time could be right for disruptive and sustained innovation in occupational health services. Providing customers with direct access to physical therapists can lower the health care costs for patients who are able to receive the appropriate care in a timely manner. Shifting from individual to more effective and efficient organizational access to physical therapy and occupational health services through directly contracting with employers can have an even greater impact on lowering health care costs and increasing the quality of care and the quality of life for employees (see also Dr. Barb Tschoepe's mini-vignette in chapter 10). Strategies to improve access and provide physical therapy as the primary entry point of care are becoming more prevalent while providing evidence of reduced costs for individuals and employers. Continuing to work and to return earlier to work after injury or illness as a result of receiving physical therapy is a measure of quality of care. In addition, health care services that apply a **Total Worker Health®** approach have strong potential for improving the health and wellness of employees. Total Worker Health® is defined as policies, programs, and practices that integrate protection from work-related safety and health hazards with the promotion of injury and illness-prevention efforts to advance worker wellbeing.[10] Employers who adopt and employ a Total Worker Health® perspective with sustaining innovation to match the contemporary needs of their employees will create a strong and productive workforce. Through improved health of employees there is a decreased risk of injury and illness which can enable employers to have greater negotiating power over purchasing insurance benefit packages.

The time may be right for disruptive innovation in providing occupational health services to gain ground in breaking the hold of insurance companies having undue authority to dictate patient care through denying needed services. The dominant third-party payors are focused on improving their profit margins. These payors develop insurance policies and service packages that meet the needs of the profitable high-end customers. For instance, insurance companies are known to heavily market to older adults to purchase Medicare Advantage plans in which they can control patient care through requiring pre-authorization of services, limiting visits, or denials of services. These third-party payors may even become third-party administrators of injury claims for employers further controlling their influence on the health care of employees. There are signs that the "improved products" of third-party payors are overshooting the needs of most individuals and employers, while making large profits in the health care market. This makes a market ripe for providers to introduce cheaper, simpler, more convenient products or services aimed at the lower end of the market (disruptive innovation). Providers can offer services that increase access, decrease costs, and increase the quality of care for employers through negotiating direct contracts with employers. As mentioned earlier, there is growing evidence that demonstrates that seeking physical therapy first can result in the desired outcome of improved worker health and productivity. In 2022, the APTA House of Delegates passed two motions, one to support direct-to-employer services[11] and the other for the APTA Board of Directors to develop collaborations across the national, component, and grassroots levels of the association to produce sustaining work in pursuit of direct-to-employer physical therapy services by providers (HOD RC12–22 Charge). While building upon the strong foundation of resources the APTA developed on direct-to-employer services, the APTA is mobilizing members at all levels of the organization to create an impact on demand for physical therapy services by employers. The 2022 APTA House of Delegates established the urgency of mitigating payors from inappropriately controlling patient care for profit. The APTA started forming a powerful coalition of APTA components with a shared vision of improving access, decreasing costs, and improving quality. The APTA is working on breaking down silos between components to focus on short-term wins and consolidating gains for propagating physical therapy direct-to-employer services. The intent is to create a critical mass of providers engaged in direct-to-employer services, thereby increasing the market demand for these services and transforming society by creating a healthier population. The desired outcome is a healthier workforce with less risk of injury. A healthier workforce should enable employers to purchase insurance policies that best serve their needs without undue influence of the third-party payor. The hope is that over time direct-to-employer services will meet the needs of most of the market. For this to be accomplished, the APTA needs to develop a culture of sustaining innovation around improving access, decreasing costs, improving quality, and assisting in the establishment of direct-to-employer services.

Once the APTA realizes the groundswell of practice participating in direct-to-employer services, other means to ensure leadership development and sustaining changes that have been institutionalized within the association will emerge. With sustained success and new innovations there is potential for developing board certification in Occupational Health, greater access to provide initiatives within companies for Total Worker Health® and realizing the vision of the APTA in "transforming society by optimizing movement to improve the human experience."[12]

Where disruptive innovation is a way to break into a market dominated by sophisticated businesses overreaching on the needs of the consumers, successful businesses at all levels of a market remain active and lucrative businesses through sustaining innovation. The occupational health case study demonstrates how innovation, change, and entrepreneurship need to happen concurrently, continuously, and organically to keep up with the ever-changing environment and demands of consumers. Entrepreneurs must be vigilant and agile to respond to opportunities, embrace change, and capitalize on insightful innovations.

Champion Your Innovation

How do you get the word out about your innovation? How do you get people to "buy in" both literally and figuratively? In 1962, Everett Rogers published his first book on the diffusion of innovations theory, now in its fifth edition."[13] The theory provides insight into how an idea gets passed along to individuals and how people begin using the innovation. The two elements of the theory are "diffusion," the process through which the innovation is communicated to others via various channels over time, and "adoption" which is the process through which individuals accept and utilize the innovation over time. Adoption of the innovation relies upon successful diffusion. For example, imagine that you are a new Doctor of Physical Therapy (DPT) graduate seeking an employment opportunity. You believe you are unique and innovative, and you would like to be hired; you are the innovation to be adopted. How do you get the word out? Writing a concise and convincing letter of inquiry about your qualifications and unique abilities to see if a job is open at your preferred facility is one channel. In addition, after scouring the market for the most promising jobs and doing research on each, you write letters of application to your top three facilities. The letters are written to address the presumed specific needs of the respective facilities of interest. You also ask your professors what they know about the facilities. You decide to send the letters of inquiry first and wait a month then send the letters of application. Along with the letters you write a strong resume, once again geared towards the individual facilities. This example of "diffusion" has the elements of the following:

- **What** is communicated: qualities of the new graduate;
- **How** communication will move through formal and informal channels: letter to the facilities and speaking with professors respectively;
- **When** the letters will be sent: planned timing of the mailings; and
- **Who** will be the focus of the diffusion strategy: employers. Note that the decision to hire may be:
    - Optional: the employer may choose to hire you or not dependent upon need;
    - Collective: a group of employees may decide on who to hire; or
    - Authority: the decision to hire is made by one person in authority.

The "champion" of the innovation has most control over a diffusion strategy that may optimize adoption of the idea, product, or service. In the case above the graduate has determined how to address the elements of diffusion.

However, there are many more variables influencing the rate of adoption of an innovation. Many of the variables considered in adoption are not under the direct control of the champion of the innovation. For the person considering adoption, positive and negative perceived attributes of the innovation may help or hinder the decision to buy into the innovation. Positive perceived attributes contribute to adoption, such as:

1. having a positive perception that the innovation is better than other options or the current situation (relative advantage);
2. if there is a strong belief that the innovation fits with the values, attitudes, and needs of the individual considering adoption (compatibility);
3. if the innovation is easy to understand and use (complexity);
4. if there is a trial period (trialability); and
5. positive testimonials from others (observability).

Returning to our example of a DPT graduate looking for a job, if the cover letter and resume positively distinguished the individual from other applicants, a "relative advantage" has been gained and an interview would be imminent. If candidate interview question responses resonate with the interviewer and the desired values and potential skill set are apparent in the candidate, the potential for hire is promising. The interview provides some assurance that the attribute of compatibility has been demonstrated. After hire, if the newly licensed physical therapist meets all the supervisor's performance expectations including competent demonstration of skills, creating good rapport with patients and colleagues, and appropriately responding to constructive feedback a successful trial period would be completed. If the trial period is positive the attribute of trialability would be met. In addition, if the new employee was easy to manage without close supervision the attribute of complexity would be met. If colleagues praise the performance of the new hire the attribute of observability may secure the new physical therapist's employment.

The champion has less direct control over perceived attributes influencing adoption, which contributes to nearly 50% of the variation in adoption rate. However, the champion may optimize adoption through a thorough understanding of interconnectedness of social system that is intended to propagate the innovation, an appropriate use of strategy and timing in utilizing communication channels, and sustaining work on changing the likelihood of adoption of those who are skeptical of the innovation.

Taking a closer look at those we hope will adopt the innovation, the diffusion of innovations theory established five "adopter categories" based upon the time during which an individual adopts an innovation, with innovators being the first adopters and laggards being the last:

1. Innovators (2.5%);
2. Early adopters (13.5%);
3. Early majority (34%);
4. Late majority (34%); and
5. Laggards (16%).

Innovators are willing to be the first to try the innovation and welcome risks associated with taking on the new idea, product, or venture. The early adopters embrace change and are typically those who may be developed into leaders of the initiative. The early majority follow those who lead and are willing to adopt the innovation based upon positive evidence that the outcomes of the innovation are beneficial. The late majority typically wait until the innovation is tried by the majority to appease their skepticism, and the laggards are very skeptical and the most difficult to influence towards adopting the innovation.

To persuade the late majority and laggards to adopt an innovation, let us return to the case study example of the direct-to-employer initiative in the APTA presented earlier in this chapter. As discussed previously, the APTA is working on mobilizing members at all levels of the organization to create an impact on demand for direct-to-employer physical therapy services. The innovators championing the efforts are coming from the Academy of Orthopedics (AOPT) Occupational Health Special Interest Group and a group of members from the Private Practice Section (PPS). Many of the early adopters are from these components and are aware of the benefits and demand for these services. These members may be seeking more information on how to best implement strategies to get employer buy-in. Some are taking specific continuing education courses through the AOPT and the PPS to facilitate their practice in occupational health. Individuals in the early majority learning aspects of Total Worker Health® started to implement direct-to-employer services that are particularly beneficial to their practice. The early majority still need support for developing contracts with employers, mentoring in other service lines that benefit employers, and are seeking evidence to venture into all services offered in a Total Worker Health® initiative. The late majority are still skeptical and need active engagement and encouragement from those who have experienced the success of providing occupational health services. The laggards are the most reluctant to change and the most difficult to move towards adopting direct-to-employer services. For instance, a laggard may express concern that providing preventative health services are below the practice expectations of a DPT. Innovators are tasked with providing more research on the outcomes of direct-to-employer services and persuading others of the lucrative practice of offering these services to employers. The laggards will only move towards adoption through pressure from leaders who have experienced the benefit of providing direct-to-employer services and/or the fear of even greater control by third-party payors in dictating patient care through policies, barriers to access, and administrative bloat to deter payment for appropriate care. In sum, the diffusion of innovations theory, also known as the diffusion adoption theory, can be used to accelerate the adoption of many important innovations and initiatives in physical therapy. The theory has been successfully implemented in many fields.

Bottom Line!

Innovators are creative people who are energized by change and who are vigilantly observant of opportunities. Innovators not only act on opportunities, they create them. An innovator becomes an entrepreneur when they develop the business acumen to capture market share.

Suggested Readings

Harvard Business Review. *HBR's 10 Must Reads*. Harvard Business School Press; 2017.
Kotter JP. *Leading Change*. Harvard Business Review; 2012.
Maxwell JC. *Failing Forward: Turning Mistakes into Stepping Stones for Success*. HarperCollins Leadership; 2007.

References

1. Drucker P. *Innovation and Entrepreneurship.* Routledge; 2014.
2. Denning S. The Best of Peter Drucker. *Forbes*. July 29, 2014. Updated December 10, 2021.https://www.forbes.com/sites/stevedenning/2014/07/29/the-best-of-peter-drucker/
3. Maxwell J. *Failing Forward: Turning Mistakes into Steppingstones for Success.* HarperCollins Leadership; 2007.
4. Chen Q, Qiu X, Fu A, Han Y. Effect of prenatal perineal massage on postpartum perineal injury and postpartum complications: A meta-analysis. *Comput Math Methods Med.* 2022; 2022: 3315638. doi:10.1155/2022/3315638
5. Jensen G, Gwyer J, Shepard K, Hack L, Expert practice in physical therapy. *Phys Ther*. 2000; 80(1): 28–43. doi.org/10.1093/ptj/80.1.28
6. Davids K, Glazier P, Araújo D, et al. Movement systems as dynamical systems. *Sports Med.* 2003; 33: 245–260. doi.org/10.2165/00007256–200333040-00001
7. Green-Wilson J, Zeigler S. *Learning to Lead in Physical Therapy.* Slack Incorporated; 2020.

8. Kantor B, CIO Staff. The RACI matrix: Your blueprint for project success. CIO. June 7, 2024. Accessed June 23, 2024. https://www.cio.com/article/287088/project-management-how-to-design-a-successful-raci-project-plan.html
9. Kotter, J. Leading Change: Why transformation efforts fail, In: *HBR's Ten Must Reads on Change Management*. Harvard Business School Publishing Corporation; 2011: 1–16.
10. National Institute for Occupational Safety and Health. Total Worker Health® program. US Centers for Disease Control and Prevention. Accessed May 30, 2024. https://www.cdc.gov/niosh/twh/programs/index.html
11. American Physical Therapy Association. Direct-to-employer physical therapy services. Updated October 26, 2022. Accessed May 30, 2024. https://www.apta.org/apta-and-you/leadership-and-governance/policies/direct-employer-services#
12. American Physical Therapy Association. Vision, mission, and strategic plan. Accessed June 23, 2024. https://www.apta.org/apta-and-you/leadership-and-governance/vision-mission-and-strategic-plan
13. Rogers E. *The Diffusion of Innovations*. 5th ed. The Free Press; 2003.

10 Business Modeling

Identifying Successful Practices and Avoiding Unsuccessful Ones

Jennifer E. Green-Wilson

A principled purpose inspires sacrifice, stimulates innovation, and encourages perseverance.

Gary P. Hamel, American management consultant and founder of an international management consulting firm

Chapter Objectives

1. Define business models.
2. Discuss strategies for building value into business models.
3. Examine real-world business models and business modeling practices in physical therapy.
4. Examine successful and unsuccessful business practices in physical therapy.
5. Discuss ideas for starting your own practice in physical therapy.

Management Vignette

Karen M. Hughes, PT

I started my own private practice because I wanted to practice autonomously. I knew what I wanted to do, with whom I wanted to practice, what patients I wanted to serve and in what community I wanted to serve. If we don't continue to develop our professional practice autonomy, my fear is we're going to be dictated to by other organizations; they will tell us how to practice (through "top-down" directives).

When we started our private practice, we had to create a business plan. I did not have the business acumen or financial literacy that I needed to start a business. *I had to learn on the fly!* Luckily, I knew a good tax accountant who I could trust and who literally would walk us through how to start our business. Our business model relied on health insurance (100%). This required us to negotiate managed care contracts, understand what it meant to

DOI: 10.4324/9781003524250-13

have limitations on access to physical therapy and limits on the number of visits, and to understand that health insurance companies could *reduce* our reimbursement rate each year.

Physical therapists will encounter various financial challenges during the term of their professional life, and personal life for that matter. If we don't understand basic business and financial concepts, we're not going to be "at the table" – as clinicians or managers, with other health care executives – especially in interdisciplinary venues. We need to be able to communicate in the "same language" used in the *business of health care* so that we are included (not excluded) from those critical conversations in which we need to be involved. We need to be able to have intelligent financial conversations with political leaders to advocate for policy changes.

Business models in health care and physical therapy need to change. Nowadays everything is about big data. We've got to know where our data is and what it stands for. It's all about artificial intelligence, or AI, making sense of the data, and making it meaningful to improve clinical practice operationally, improve efficiency for the end user clinicians, make it safer for the patients, and hopefully make it more cost-effective for the entire health care system. We must code our patients appropriately. We're treating complicated patients with complicated diagnosis codes; they have comorbidities and social determinants of health. Only 1.7% of Medicare claims have social determinants of health diagnosis codes included because we don't use them effectively enough.

Physical therapists are still conservative in their approach to business modeling. People don't like change; we're afraid of new models. It's been the *fee for service* world for so long (which we understand), but how do we move forward into the vision of value-based care and "what's next"? How do we get into more of a wellness model/approach? How do we negotiate contracts better? We need to value (and charge appropriately for) our services. Many therapists are practicing in cash-based models now, but we remain concerned about our patients' pockets, always wondering, "are we charging them too much money for their copays?" Our education is extensive and we're providing great value. I also hope that therapists embrace technology more. The technology movement in health care presents us with new opportunities.

Bottom Line!

"We can't stay where we're at today to serve tomorrow's patients. We must change; we must keep up and move forward (ahead of the change). Regulations are going to change; technology is going to change. Our consumers are going to change. If I had my practice today, I would operate it in a very different manner. It would be totally upside down."

Karen M. Hughes

Chapter Introduction

The purpose of this chapter is to continue to help you to practice innovative and possibility thinking. We structured this chapter to share stories (business model case examples) of real-world experiences. We hope that these authentic narratives will help to inspire and guide you when you hit the ground running in professional practice. We also hope that by sharing these real-world experiences, you can start to pull together pieces of the "practice management puzzle." You can do this by continuing to build your list of successful and unsuccessful management and business practices (i.e., some dos and don'ts).

What Is Business Modeling?

From a big picture perspective, the term **business model** refers to an organization's plan for making a **profit** or for achieving their financial goals (i.e., a solid financial bottom line).[1] A business model identifies the products/services that the business plans to sell, its identified target market(s), and any anticipated expenses (i.e., possibly to start *and* run/operate the business over time). In chapter 11, **business planning** will be discussed in detail. Through business planning, an organization will clarify its business model explicitly – a critical practice needed for both new and established businesses. Over time, businesses may revise or update their business models to reflect changing business (internal) environments and external market demands/needs, and in response to anticipated trends and future challenges.

Aha!

Some Advice for Assessing Business Models

"Know what your daily schedule will look like. Assess if you have complete control or no control over deciding the frequency and duration of your patients' schedules. Determine ahead of time if you can flex your schedule when/if you want to bring someone in at a time when it may look like you're not available on the schedule. The surprise that I've heard from people is that they didn't realize they were going to oversee two or three people every 30 minutes."

Dr. Sandra Norby, PT

Activity 10.1 Why Do We Resist Talking about Money?

Recall from chapters 3 and 7 the discussions about the resistance from physical therapists in talking about money. Yet a fundamental part of envisioning a business model is to determine how revenue can be generated (where revenue is the total amount of money generated from a business's primary operations) and how "the business" can ensure a successful and sustainable financial bottom line (i.e., net income or the company's total earnings after deducting expenses).[2]

Reflect on the following questions:

Why do you think physical therapists resist integrating or learning about the financial aspects of clinical practice?

____

____

How comfortable are *you* in integrating or talking about the financial aspects of physical therapist practice? Circle the best option.

Not at all! *Somewhat comfortable* *Very comfortable*

Review some of the possible reasons why physical therapists resist the financial realities of practice. Check all that you think apply.

- ☐ It's because we went to physical therapy school to help people to feel/get better.
- ☐ It's because we don't understand the business aspect of physical therapy.
- ☐ We resist the reality that physical therapy is a business.
- ☐ We don't connect the dots between billing, coding, payment and being paid (i.e., earning our paycheck, earning our living).
- ☐ It's because we recruit people into physical therapy who are not interested in business.
- ☐ We think a not-for-profit business is a business model that doesn't focus on the financial bottom line.

Bottom Line!

When evaluating an organization or practice as a place in which to practice, you might want to find out how it makes its money (not just what it sells but how it sells it). That's its business model.

Business Models: Key Components and Decisions

Though business models vary in form and function, they all feature the same essential components. While all business models aim to increase revenue, they include many other factors outside of income. The main components of a business model include value proposition, target market(s), demand analysis (i.e., target market needs), startup costs, competitive advantage, cost structure (fixed and variable), key metrics for measuring success, resources (tangible and intangible), and its revenue model (framework for how an organization plans to generate revenue/income). Hopefully, some of these terms and concepts are becoming more familiar to you. Many/most of these components are discussed throughout this book, especially in chapter 11. For now, priority is given to examining the concept of value applied to business models in physical therapy. Recall in chapter 3 that we discussed the shift to value-based care. Understanding and demonstrating "value" is critical in current and future health care and physical therapy practices. The **value proposition**, a primary component of the business model, is a succinct description of the products/services that a company offers and why they are desirable to customers or clients, ideally stated in a way that differentiates the products/services from those of its competitors.

Creating Value in Physical Therapy: Successful Practices

We asked a few colleagues, "How is your business model demonstrating value in your community?" These are their responses.

Response 1: Dr. Fred Gilbert

Most of what we look at from an outcome standpoint and from a value-generation standpoint is focused on the provider. As a business, we view our providers as having a life and thriving in a way in which they can impact their community. If you think about a "typical" setup right now, physical therapy clinics are looking mostly at patient outcomes. Patient outcomes drive reimbursement and national (patient) outcomes drive our profession. But it's an issue if you're doing that at the expense of not looking at the people delivering the care (the providers). Providers need to have the emotional space and the mental energy to be able to engage with their patients. You can't ignore the provider-side. Providers get really burnt out treating a ton of patients every day, repeatedly. Part of what drives our (company) outcomes is that our providers set their own schedules, they set their own prices, and they decide the communities in which they want to work. The outcome that we measure is a Thriving Index.[3] We have this fundamental belief that *if a provider is thriving then the patient will thrive.*

Response 2: Dr. Ryan Wood

Immensely and I say this with confidence! We give back. We provide pro bono/free service(s) for individuals living with homelessness because sometimes somebody's down on their luck. We're not going to turn them away in that instance. We have sliding fee scale programs based on federal poverty guidelines and that includes the members of a household. We also offer many community education programs. We did an opioid symposium to educate providers on different types of non-pharmacological interventions and strategies. My wife, an occupational therapist, is educating teachers on ADHD, sensory processing disorders, lowering medication intake, and creating better learning experiences. We get creative in partnering with other organizations. We do a lot for the community; it's been a blessing and it's really helped us to grow.

We also asked some physical therapist practice owners: "How could/should physical therapists create value in the future?" These real-world responses are captured below.

Response 3: Karen M. Hughes

We must fit into the larger community and think further upstream about keeping people healthier, reducing hospital readmissions, helping with the root causes of social determinants of health, preventing falls, and the discussions about nutrition and sleeping habits. People can't heal, they can't reduce their pain if they aren't eating or sleeping adequately. We can't just think about musculoskeletal injuries, sprains, and strains. We must think of our patients holistically and be prepared for those larger, valuable conversations.

Response 4: Dr. Barb Tschoepe

You must be confident in yourself, who you are as a practitioner. Be confident in your potential value to the entire health system – whether it's an organization, or a group of people or a community. You must have enough confidence to say "This is what I *can* offer. This is what I *can't* offer." Then after you identify what you can and can't do, figure out with whom you want to partner to achieve your goals. Our original business model focused on employers but ten years later, the focus was on the community. It was about direct access and private pay clients. We let others know what physical therapy should and could be by applying the basic foundations of business.

Response 5: Dr. Sandra Norby

The value proposition is established now through APTA's published report on the economical value of physical therapy. This study shows the financial benefit or economic value of physical therapy versus from anecdotal perspectives. We must understand that there is no other health professional that has our entire skill set – our range of diagnostic and assessment abilities. When a patient comes to you, you're the "smartest person they've ever seen." Everyone must understand that we're so unique that people need to see us! It doesn't mean that we can diagnose and treat everything, but we can assess and formulate a plan; the plan may mean that patients stay with us (full-time or part-time), or the plan might mean we refer them to another health professional who can take better care of them.

Individually, we've got to take responsibility to let our communities know who we are as professionals and what we do. We can't keep grumbling because people go to the chiropractor or the massage therapist rather than to us. We've got to take ownership. As an individual, you've got to participate in the conversations to let people know who you are and what we can do for them.

Activity 10.2 How Do You Explain the Value of Physical Therapy?

Developing your talking points or your elevator pitch in advance will prepare you for future conversations. Answer the following questions in the space provided.

How would you explain the value of physical therapy to a patient? Draft your script (i.e., talking points).

____

____

____

Would you say there is added value in seeing *you* as their physical therapist? Draft your script (i.e., talking points).

____

____

____

How would you tell your family, friends, and neighbors about "what they can expect" in value from seeing a physical therapist. Draft your script (i.e., talking points).

____

____

____

Would you tell your family, friends, and neighbors that there is added value in seeing *you* as their physical therapist? Draft your script (i.e., talking points).

____

____

____

Practice saying your responses out loud!

Dispelling the Myth of the Not-For-Profit Business Model

Earlier in this chapter, we mentioned that physical therapists tend to shy away from and resist learning or talking about the financial aspects of clinical practice. There also seems to be a misunderstanding (or myth) that non-profit organizations do not need to care about finances (as much as for-profit ones do). Overall, as a physical therapist, it may seem or feel easier to align with the mission of a not-for-profit organization, but it is important to clarify that *all* organizations – even not-for-profit ones – still need to manage the financial bottom line if they want to be successful at building a sustainable business model.

According to the Council of Nonprofits, the term "non-profit" is misleading. Non-profits can make a profit, should try to generate positive revenue streams, and build reserve funds for sustainability. The key difference between non-profits and for-profits is that a non-profit organization cannot distribute its profits to any private individual (i.e., shareholder).[4] This (private or individual) benefit is prohibited because tax-exempt charitable non-profits are formed to benefit public rather than private interests (although non-profits may pay reasonable compensation to those providing services).[4]

Business Models Driving Social Change: Social Entrepreneurship[5]

In chapter 9, entrepreneurship was discussed. Social entrepreneurship extends beyond the traditional boundaries of for-profit and non-profit business models by employing innovative business models and technologies to solve social issues.

> TOMS (https://www.toms.com/us/impact.html) is an example of a business model that embraces social entrepreneurship. This company started giving away one pair of shoes for each pair it sold and has given shoes to more than 100 million underprivileged children.

These social enterprises must generate enough revenue to cover their costs (i.e., achieve financial sustainability) while staying dedicated to their mission. Hybrid models, which combine for-profit and non-profit elements, offer flexibility in funding and operations, enable these organizations to pursue their goals without compromising their values.

Aha!

Socially Responsible Entrepreneurship Matters!

Social entrepreneurship inspires individuals (i.e., entrepreneurs and intrapreneurs) and organizations to rethink the role of business in society.[5]

Bottom Line!

The boundary between making a profit and making a difference is becoming intertwined, signaling a future where the success of a business is measured, not just by its financial performance but by its contribution to society.[5]

Business Model or Business Plan? (Both!)

By now, you may be starting to discover that there are grey areas or areas of overlap between the terms business model, business modeling, and business planning. It can be confusing. A business model is a foundational part of the company and expresses the primary method through which the company generates its profit (or revenue), its value, and hopefully its plans for new growth though innovation. The business plan is a detailed explanation that includes specific goals, strategies, and resources. Business models and business plans are essential tools for creating a successful company. Business models and business plans may differ somewhat, but both are useful and fundamental for successful business management especially when these tools are used as living "roadmaps" to guide decision-making and resource allocation.

Different Types of Business Models in Physical Therapy

There are several different types of business models in physical therapy,[6,7] and new models are constantly emerging. An overview of a few common business models is provided in box 10.1. These models include:

- In-network (i.e., health insurance);
- Out-of-network;
- Cash-based practice;
- Health and wellness partnership;
- Workplace-based physical therapy; and
- Concierge services.

Box 10.1 Characteristics of Common Business Models in Physical Therapy

In-network (health insurance)

- Most common model in physical therapy.
- Physical therapy practice accepts health insurance (payor mix varies by practice).

- Requires providers to complete contracting process (time-consuming) to negotiate reimbursement rates.
- Patients referred from within established networks (in-network referrals from providers practicing within network).
- Less burden for patients due to in-network accessibility and ease of payment.
- Practice absorbs the administrative burden associated with billing and payment (i.e., authorizations, denials, appeals, etc.).
- Practice accepts lower reimbursement rates (i.e., contracted rates with insurers).
- Restrictions on patient care are imposed by health insurers and may impact quality of care negatively (i.e., volume-based care).
- Possible increased risk of provider burnout (i.e., volume-based care).

Out-of-Network

- Practice does not belong to (health insurance) networks (to avoid low reimbursement rates, closed/limited provider panels, and patient care restrictions).
- Patients are billed when services provided or physical therapy practice bills patient's health insurance company directly (patient responsible for any unpaid portions).
    - Health insurance companies may limit out-of-network coverage.
- Allows greater autonomy over treatment options.
- Positive impact on quality care.
    - Practice not restricted by rules and regulations imposed by health insurance companies.
- Higher profit margins possible.
- Marketing costs and efforts are needed to attract/persuade "in-network" patients and referrers to seek services 'out-of-network': (i.e., in-network providers more likely to refer patients to in-network physical therapists).

Cash-Based Practice

- Similar to out-of-network model but different.
- Patient responsible for the full cost of physical therapy.
- All services are rendered on a cash basis.
- Practice does not request payments from health insurance companies.
- Higher quality of care possible (less restrictions).
- Less administration burden, lower overhead.
- Reduced risk of provider burnout.
- Not ideal for Medicare patients.

- Marketing costs and efforts to persuade patients of the benefits of high-quality care (i.e., value).
    - May need training in marketing to be able to sell the idea of paying fully "out of pocket".
- Access may be limited to a certain demographic(s).

Health and Wellness Partnership(s)

- Attract broader range of patients.
- Expansion possible to provide a variety of specialties/services.

    Possible partners include:

    - physicians, chiropractors, massage therapists;
    - gyms/fitness clubs, yoga/Pilates studios, sporting equipment stores; and
    - assisted living facilities.
- Easier access to (mutual) referrals.
- Possible market share growth possible.

Workplace-Based (On-site) Physical Therapy

- Physical therapists partner directly with companies – i.e., on-site physical therapy.
- Prevention/treatment of job-related injuries.
    - Examples: corporate ergonomics, injury prevention, work readiness testing, telehealth physical therapy for remote employees.
- "Corporate physical therapy" can be added to clinic by contracting (with companies) to offer discounts/full payment for their employees.
- Reduced costs (i.e., on-site location).
- Improved injury prevention/treatment.

Concierge Services

- Services offered on a *subscription basis* or as part of a package that treats specific ailments (i.e., ACL injury).
- Beneficial model for patients with recurring symptoms; can access physical therapy frequently.
- Predictable income (i.e., prepaid subscriptions): generates steady revenue.
- Better long-term patient/client relationships.
- Flexibility to align with mobile physical therapy model (i.e., offer home/work visits).
- Limited usage for Medicare patients.
- May lead to patient/client dependence.

Ultimately, your business model depends on your goals, passions, and the needs of your patients/community along with your team's unique specialties. Partnering with different companies may allow you to provide physical therapy on-site, in a mobile format, virtually/remotely, or possibly using a cash-based model.

Real-World Business Models in Physical Therapy: Case Scenarios

The following real-world examples (case scenarios) capture authentic stories about different business models in physical therapy. We've attempted to highlight both successful and unsuccessful practices (lessons learned) from these stories.

Activity 10.3 Successful and Unsuccessful Business Models and Practices

If you were to start your own practice, what would you be most passionate about?

___

___

After you review each case scenario, create a list of ideas (what to do or what not to do) using table 10.1.

Table 10.1 Ideas!

Description of Business Model (Case Scenario 1)	*Successful Practices What to Do*	*Unsuccessful Practices What NOT to Do or What to Avoid*
Example: For-profit *and* not-for-profit business models	Business plan (personal *and* professional financial planning) Organizational culture (intentional priority) Community engagement (i.e., educational programs/outreach) Role diversification (lowers burnout)	Incompatible culture (i.e., "mill model")
Description of Business Model (Case Scenario 2)	*Successful Practices What to Do*	*Unsuccessful Practices What NOT to Do or What to Avoid*
Description of Business Model (Case Scenario 3)	*Successful Practices What to Do*	*Unsuccessful Practices What NOT to Do or What to Avoid*

(*Continued*)

Table 10.1 (Continued)

Description of Business Model (Case Scenario 4)	*Successful Practices What to Do*	*Unsuccessful Practices What NOT to Do or What to Avoid*
Description of Business Model (Case Scenario 5)	*Successful Practices What to Do*	*Unsuccessful Practices What NOT to Do or What to Avoid*

Case Scenario 1: Dr. Ryan Wood, CEO and Co-Founder of Forefront Therapy and Forefront Community Therapy

When we moved back to my wife's hometown, I could not find a culture in an organization that I could "buy into." I couldn't find organizations in my area that had the *right* practice model or the *right* culture for me to practice in. Initially, I chose a practice opportunity 40 minutes away from where I lived to find the culture in which I could treat one-on-one because the "mill model" is not a business model that I can support. From an outpatient model perspective, there's nothing worse than the "mill model"; it lowers quality, it increases burnout; it serves the owner(s). But after two years of this long daily commute (and after finally listening to my wife who kept telling me, "You need to start a business"!), I slowly started to engage in the idea of practice ownership. I never wanted to start my own private practice. I started the process of business planning while completing a Master of Health Administration (MHA) degree. We planned for nine months before we "pulled the trigger." It was not a whimsical decision. We started the private practice because I could not find an organization with which I was content.

The business plan is as important as it gets. When we started our private practice, we had a 56-page, single-spaced 10 font business plan full of market analyses. The business plan provides an entire foundation of everything from which you are going to work (i.e., from a financial projection perspective) and which you're able to fall back on when things get hard. As I built this plan, I had to create a personal financial plan as well as a business plan (i.e., what if I needed to take a low salary for a few years, could I/we afford to do so?). It lets you be in a position where you're not as fearful. Embracing risk is part of the business planning process. It's always scary to start something like this; it's intimidating – total imposter syndrome all the time!

At the start, our business model was for-profit because we had no idea about the non-profit world. In our for-profit practice, we have our three core pillars. Our first core pillar is one-on-one patient care; no overlapping (i.e., double-booking) or sharing of patients (i.e., with techs) unless specialty necessitates. Our second core pillar is education and research because we love learning and growing. Our third core pillar is accessibility for all. These core pillars reflect the culture I can support. Initially as a for-profit company, we would take pro bono cases because there is an immense need and a social responsibility to do things differently in our area and in our practice. We slowly started growing organically, and as we grew, we spent time thinking about alternative business models – how to execute our mission differently to minimize risk, and how to provide these services to *everybody*, get paid well for it *and* support our team's growth. I remembered reading about non-profit hospital organizations (from the MHA program) that on average make 18% more than for-profit organizations. Non-profit does not mean no profit; it's a tax-exempt organization. We added the not-for-profit aspect to our business model as a way to serve our mission, not go broke nor expect the team that we're building to take substantial salary cuts to help to fulfill our mission as well.

The ability to grow community health became an additional huge benefit to our new business model. As a profession, we are more than just *clinical.* Through our non-profit, we offer a great deal of community education and programming that is now grant-supported and we're partnering with other agencies and organizations to do so. For example, we're partnering with an arthritis foundation to offer a cooking class that is supported by a grant. We're providing healthy cooking for individuals with arthritis, teaching them strategies. Our not-for-profit provides a cool platform for creativity.

Diversification of roles is another benefit we gained from our expanded business model. By having our 501(c)(3) organization where we can apply for grants and then do financially supported community work, we can also allow our team to have diversification in their roles to hopefully lower burnout. We can support someone on our team who is passionate about serving individuals (i.e., older adults) with arthritis. There's a lot of benefit in that role diversification.

Bottom Line!

"We must get innovative. Hopefully sharing my business model can inspire others. The only model that's bad for our profession is the 'mill model.' Cash-based practice is not *bad* but it doesn't change policy. It doesn't allow service for your entire community because you're still only serving people one-on-one."

Dr. Ryan Wood

Aha!

Ideas about Business Models

After reading the first case scenario, list the ideas you gained about starting your own private practice (what to do and what not to do) by reflecting on ideas about different business models. Continue to add to your list as you read on.

Case Scenario 2: Dr. Fred Gilbert, Chief People Officer at MovementX

Our current business model has three pillars: delivery of care; health tech (support/platform); and coaching (financial and clinical). Our business model was designed primarily around giving providers the tools to be able to practice as out-of-network providers and create viable businesses. Our business plan is tech-focused (i.e., lead generation with a focus on helping to find patients), but it's also heavily coaching-focused. We're developing people into business practitioners. We teach our providers how to run their small businesses, operate within a larger ecosystem, and build sustainable business practices.

Our providers go to people's homes, to their offices, and to their gyms. They treat people where people move, where movement matters the most. Most of our providers practice in a mobile fashion, particularly in-home. They're providing physical therapy services in these locations as out-of-network or cash-based practices.

We focus on helping our providers to thrive. We help them to thrive financially; we help people to manage their personal finances. We help them to thrive personally, physically, and emotionally as well. Most of our providers treat about 20 patients a week compared to what we're used to in a clinic, which is 12 to 15 patients per day – a vastly different caseload. We've always believed that if we can take care of providers then the providers will take great care of their patients.

Case Scenario 3: Dr. Sandra Norby, CEO and Co-Founder of Home Town Physical Therapy

I created a business plan when I started my own private practice. We determined that our "hometown" community could benefit from a free-standing private practice clinic. I went online to download business plan software and calculated our projections. In prior management roles, I knew about the contracted rates for reimbursement and how many visits we needed to cover our expenses. We went through the SBA loan process for our first clinic. We live in the community in which I grew up and we wanted to make a statement to this community right from the very beginning that we were going to be there for a long time. Therefore, we constructed a building right from the start (most of our loan was for the building). In the other communities in which we later expanded, we rented a storefront for our clinic, but in this case we did not want to rent.

Our company is called Home Town Physical Therapy (the name is on target especially when someone has a connection with in that community). We started the practice with me as the physical therapist and a friend of mine who knew rehab billing payors. We opened in June and by November I had a full caseload. The speed of the growth for a startup was a lot quicker than if someone who grew up somewhere else decided to enter this market. Some growth also has to do with personality and the ability for that person to get into the community. It's our responsibility to connect with people in our communities by leveraging multiple touchpoints. If we only *practice* when the patient is in front of us for an hour, then we might be missing some opportunities to connect in other ways.

In developing our business model initially, we knew that going fully cash-based in our area wasn't going to be an option, especially because this was our primary business income (i.e., we needed to support our family). We became fully enrolled in all payors that individuals in our community would need for access to care. We aim for a payor mix: 25% workers' compensation, 50% commercial insurance, and 25% government payors (Medicare, Medicaid); it fluctuates depending on which community people are in.

Our business model is unique because we grew our company by helping others to open their clinics in other hometown communities by leveraging our established administrative processes to streamline their ability to open their practices. We formed a separate administration company to provide ongoing administrative support for billing, compliance, payroll, and HR functions. We have been involved in four startups and two acquisitions.

Bottom Line!

"Physical therapists *leave money on the table* because they don't understand coding and they've been told somewhere to be careful to not go a minute over because then they will be audited. We must teach our physical therapists to know their value, and not give things away for free."

Dr. Sandra Norby

Case Scenario 4: Dr. Barb Tschoepe, Co-Founder of Waldron's Peak Physical Therapy

I'm all about the community need and how we engage with community members. I started consulting (30 years ago!) on injury prevention, particularly in large companies (high-tech and R&D organizations such as IBM and the drug manufacturers) in the Boulder, Colorado, area and in the region. We were promoting health and wellness, physical activity, and appropriate movement as it related to what the employees were doing in their various roles at work. By promoting this health and wellness concept, not so much pathology management, the focus became, "How do we prevent the injuries from happening?"

We were challenged to identify practices to which we could refer clients because they were still practicing "traditional episodic care"; they weren't tying their practice to the overall health of that individual or to how we could promote a healthier workforce. I started the private practice because of that clear market need. We didn't call ourselves *movement experts* at the time, we said *movement was our expertise*. Basically, we set up a wellness model where we contracted directly with these R&D companies so they could send their employees to us if they were having challenges. We set up screening models; we wanted to see their employees before they were hurt (or barely hurt), or at the point when they had a significant pathology.

We contracted directly with the self-pay employers – they had their own health insurance (i.e., they were self-insured), they could designate funds how they wanted or needed, and controlled how and where they were going to spend their dollars. They were also about wellness and health promotion and not treating the pathology.

Our practice grew faster than I expected. We expanded to private pay clients because once individuals got to know us, they realized "the value" of our business model, that it was different from what they were experiencing with other physical therapists in the community.

Bottom Line!

"We are bigger than treating the illness, the patient, and the body part. We are here to promote the health of the individual."

Dr. Barb Tschoepe

Case Scenario 5: Dr. Jennifer Brown, CEO of Dynamic Home Therapy & Neurofit

I did not have a business plan when I started my private practice because I didn't intend to start a business. I was working for a great health system that I loved for most of my career, but I noticed that there was a lot of "red tape." I would "get spoken to" for spending too long with my neuro clients or for not discharging patients quickly enough; I didn't understand "the why" behind those conversations. I started seeing clients privately when they were discharged, if they wanted a few extra visits (i.e., for wellness).

My practice kind of fell into my lap. I applied for Medicare B and saw some people on my own. My practice started with just me and then suddenly there were so many referrals that the practice took off quickly! I didn't anticipate that happening. I didn't know what a business plan was; I didn't know anything about business. I knew I disliked billing and the numbers. I wanted to treat and give really good quality care – that's how it happened. Eventually I hired a few contract therapists to help with some of the visits.

My practice started as just physical therapy for geriatrics, but then it became more of a niche neuro practice. We were the only neuro specialized outpatient at home model (not home care) in the Philadelphia area. We just kept growing until we had to hire more people. We also needed a multidisciplinary practice to really serve this population (that found us), so we hired people (physical therapists, occupational therapists, and speech therapists). We grew because of our passion and because we found the *right* team that shared this passion. We grew because there was a big need from people with chronic neurological disease and not a lot of options for them when they were discharged from one level of care. My practice ended up being a great match and filling a need for this population.

About two and a half years later, I learned about SCORE (https://www.score.org/), I was assigned a mentor and we started working on our business plan. When I went through the business planning process, I learned that I really knew nothing about business planning or business practices from school or from other work experiences. I learned that I had to think more strategically. I didn't realize how much I had to consider from legal and compliance standpoints. We started as a Medicare part B provider, and we were out-of-network with all the other insurance providers. I realized that I had to have a plan to determine my vision. It's changed over the years, but it's always to help people with neurological disorders live their best lives possible –for them and their caregivers. The business planning process helped to push me to think more. I don't want to just see people in their homes. I want to grow my service area geographically. I became excited to add more of a wellness component and that excitement guided us into another division of our practice. We started wellness classes and Rock Steady Boxing for Parkinson's. It got me thinking that eventually we will need a "brick and mortar" practice too.

I still don't like business and business planning, but I have learned what works and what's working. I've learned that the companies that have so much red tape or who are not thinking "outside of the box" about other revenue streams, especially with all of challenges associated with health insurance, they're missing out. You can really grow if you think outside of the box these days. A year ago, we switched EMRs, our marketing strategies, we rebranded, we redid our website, it was almost like a whole new business, but it had to happen. This new growth is helping us to be at the front line of all these changes in health care. I'm learning that it's huge to have more options to serve our clients and our communities.

Business Models for Physical Therapists: A Few More Ideas for Success

We asked a few physical therapist practice owners the following question, "How could/should physical therapists change their business models?" These real-world responses are captured below.

Response 1: Dr. Barb Tschoepe

We need to build the mindset of the whole professional being part of the health care industry. I would use health system, instead of health care system, to include wellness, prevention, health promotion, and the community. Health care is saying you need something. We must be savvier because other health professionals are coming "into our space." We must have a sense of our value and then ask, "what can we do differently to develop a business model?" That business model could have a traditional approach to it, but it needs to have an outreach strategy, possibly a non-profit design, and various outlets that come together to make the enterprise successful. We could collaborate more. Mental health is a prevalent critical challenge in our communities and money is supporting mental health now. Are we collaborating with behavioral health professionals to support the needs of individuals whose primary need is mental health? We know if we keep people physically active, monitor, and support them, it's going to improve their mental health.

Response 2: Dr. Fred Gilbert

The traditional business model is where you have three, five, or seven clinicians in a clinic and they each see 12 to 15 patients per day depending on the type of clinic. The traditional model is "stable," but there's not a lot of schedule or patient flexibility to it. The traditional model is a good business model in which to learn, particularly for newer graduates, but it tends to be one in which your earnings, your ability to get to the community, and your ability to try out new ideas are limited or restricted.

If you look at the newer innovative models, these practices leverage technology well (i.e., Luna Physical Therapy). They're predominantly run by technology groups. But they don't really train their employees to be independent or autonomous – they train them to do a task. You're delivering a service but there's little or no personal development.

What we've tried to hit with our business model is the best of both worlds. We're helping you to create viable businesses that are stable, we're putting you in an environment that's supported by technology, *and* we're also coaching/teaching you, so that you become this independent person within a bigger community. It's this balance of innovation versus stability and how to find that middle ground. I see "traditional models" as being too rigid, while newer models are not personal (i.e., not connected) enough. We're trying to win right in the middle of that. Right now, we're working on how to scale *culture*. Culture is the business model for us, and we layer everything from it. Who you are, how you lead, how you facilitate, how you empower. It all reinforces and builds culture.

Bottom Line!

A business is an ecosystem that must have a plan: who to sell to, what to sell, what to charge, and what value it is creating. A business model describes what an organization does to systematically create long-term value for its customers.[1]

Suggested Readings

Alter A. *Anatomy of a Breakthrough: How to Get Unstuck When It Matters Most*. Simon & Schuster; 2023.

References

1. Kopp CM. Learn to understand a company's profit-making plan. Investopedia. Updated February 19, 2024. Accessed March 17, 2024. https://www.investopedia.com/terms/b/businessmodel.asp
2. Boyte-White C. Revenue vs. income: What's the difference? Investopedia. Updated February 23, 2024. Accessed May 4, 2024. https ://www.investopedia.com/ask/answers/122214/what-difference-between-revenue-and-income.asp#:~:text=Revenue%20is%20the%20total%20amount,the%20number%20of%20units%20sold
3. Life evaluation index. Gallup. Accessed May 4, 2024. https://www.gallup.com/394505/indicator-life-evaluation-index.aspx
4. Myths about nonprofits. National Council of Nonprofits. Accessed May 4, 2024. https://www.councilofnonprofits.org/about-americas-nonprofits/myths-about-nonprofits
5. Miller J. The rise of social entrepreneurship: Business models for social change LinkedIn. March 14, 2024. https://www.linkedin.com/pulse/rise-social-entrepreneurship-business-models-change-jason-miller-ciuac/
6. Comparing physical therapy business models for your practice. MEG Business. March 2, 2021. Updated March, 2024. https://www.megbusiness.com/comparing-physical-therapy-business-models-for-your-practice/
7. Shanahan D. 7 physical therapy business models you should consider. Exer Labs, Inc. July 12, 2022. https://www.exer.ai/posts/physical-therapy-business-models

11 Getting Started

Planning for the Future

Kristin Schweizer and Chris Petrosino

No matter the size of the organization, no matter the industry, no matter the product or the service, if we all take some responsibility to start with WHY and inspire others to do the same, then, together, we can change the world.

Simon Sinek, author and speaker on leadership[1]

Chapter Objectives

1. Explain the purpose of a business plan.
2. Describe the components of a business plan.
3. Discuss the purpose of each element of the business plan.
4. Differentiate between the emphasis of a business plan for an outpatient practice setting versus an inpatient practice setting.
5. Explore how the business plan process can be applied to a new physical therapy practice.

Management Vignette

Patrick Buckley PT, DPT, Pn1

When I was at physical therapy school learning about business planning and management, I did not fully appreciate the importance of the content. With the NPTE looming and the excitement of starting a career working with patients, the material did not seem as relevant to me as the clinical skills we were learning. But when it came to the moment that I was gearing up for my own business venture, the first place I looked were my notes from school. The business plan that we developed in physical therapy school came in very handy when trying to put together my very own plan.

Looking back on how things started for me, it was a blessing in disguise. An opportunity arose, and I could not say no. I had a wife, a one-and-a half-year-old daughter, a dog, and a 30-year mortgage at the time and was

DOI: 10.4324/9781003524250-14

exiting my cushy clinical director position to start my own thing. Was it a good time? Is there ever a good time? What my supportive wife told me was, "If you wait for the perfect time to do this, you're going to wait forever." So there really is no perfect time to start a business. But the best way to ease fear and anxiety around the business venture is the creation of the business plan.

One thing that I've learned along the way is that I am *not* the only physical therapy entrepreneur out there. There is quite a large group of private practice business owners who have been doing this much longer than I have. I've learned that reaching out to them, even sometimes cold calling them, has been immensely helpful. At first, I kept saying to myself, "Figure it out, Patrick! Look it up! There's got to be a book on this somewhere." Going it alone was the worst idea and easily the biggest mistake in my career, and the opposite of what we were taught at school. When I finally reached out and started "picking the brains" of other physical therapy owners, and even owners of other industries, my mind exploded. They showed me that there are various business standards and indicators to track, among other important things.

I started to realize the importance of certain aspects of business management, business planning, marketing, finances, and scaling/growth. Keeping a finger on the pulse of the business is so important, the pulse being the key performance indicators (KPIs). There are so many key indicators that can be tracked to give owners the overview of the business, and those markers need to be tracked. If it's important, you're going to track it. If you want to lose weight, you're going to track your weight loss. It's the same for the business indicators.

Some of the most difficult challenges as a small business private practice owner is competing with the large corporations, hospitals, and physician-owned practices. Those practices have much stronger negotiation powers with health insurance companies and can receive much higher reimbursement rates than the small practice for providing the same (or even better) services. The revenue isn't as robust; therefore, I must track those important KPIs with much more detail. This contributes to the obstacle of hiring physical therapists. It's hard to compete with the large pay scales that hospitals and large physical therapy corporations can provide, so it requires a little extra work to negotiate these obstacles. Small private practices can provide plenty of other "benefits" that those larger practices just can't provide.

I've been a business owner for quite a few years now, and I still feel that I am learning every day. I take courses on business and even some of my continuing education units are business-related. I love being a physical therapist and I love helping and providing excellent physical therapy services to people. By having a business, I can provide more excellent physical therapy services to more people. Everyone who goes into the physical therapy field does it for pretty much the same reason ... the money, right? Ha, no! We do it because we are good people and want to help others. This is what I tell people when they ask me to describe my business to them, "We are a group of great people doing great things for our community."

Introduction to Planning as a Management Practice

Planning is the process by which we establish goals and design strategies to achieve them. Effective planning projects the resources, such as time, skills, money, and equipment, needed to achieve the desired outcome. Planning also considers potential hazards that may derail progress towards goals.

We plan most aspects of our daily lives, and it is a critical element of management. Business planning helps an organization to define its goals clearly and what it will take to get there. The development of a plan guides the prioritization of resources and informs decision-making within a business.

Activity 11.1 You and Planning

Consider a time when you needed to develop a plan. Perhaps you were planning a vacation, applying to colleges or graduate schools, or studying for final exams. Reflect upon your process of planning. (See also the discussions and activities from chapter 2.)

How did you structure your plan?

____

Were tasks broken down into smaller, more achievable goals?

____

Were your plans organized by day, week, or longer?

____

What did you find successful about how you planned?

____

The Business Plan

Have you ever thought about starting a physical therapy practice or developing a program within an existing business to provide care to a specific patient population? Often physical therapists begin to consider these options when they have a passion for a certain patient population, discover a need in a defined community, or desire to provide care in a specific manner. The business planning process facilitates turning these ideas into reality.

A **business plan** is a formal document that outlines the scope of a developing business. It charts the course of the business, defines the strategy, and establishes targets. The business plan contains research about the needs of the target market(s), a description of the services provided by the business, how these services will meet the needs of the consumer and how they differ from the competition, the resources needed to operate, how the business will be marketed and financial projections for the business. These projections are necessary when requesting funds for the business start-up. Each element of the business plan will be discussed in further detail in this section.

Box 11.1 Suggested Table of Contents for Business Plan

1. Executive Summary
2. Business Description
   a. Mission
   b. Vision
   c. Values
   d. Description of Services
3. Market Analysis
   a. Strengths
   b. Weaknesses
   c. Opportunities
   d. Threats
4. Operations Plan
   a. Facilities and Equipment Plan
   b. Human Resources Plan
5. Marketing Plan
6. Financial Plan/Projections

Executive Summary

The executive summary contains a high-level overview of the key elements outlined in the business plan. Although it is the first item in the business plan, it is often written last, summarizing the key points that are elaborated in the document. The executive summary should be written in a way that excites and intrigues the reader, or at least makes them interested in delving deeper into the business plan.

Business Description

In his book, *Start with Why*, Simon Sinek states that businesses that focus on the "Golden Circle" can differentiate their value from the competition.[1] The model of the Golden Circle starts with the business clearly articulating "why" they do what they do. The "why" represents the passion behind the business. It is what will motivate customers to stay loyal and what will attract and retain employees. Next, the business describes "how" they do it. And finally, they describe "what" they do.

The business description captures the "why" and begins to describe the "how" by outlining the organization's vision, mission, and values (see also table 11.1).

Vision

According to Collins and Porras, a vision statement comprises two critical elements: the organization's core ideology and the envisioned future.[2] In line with Sinek's Golden Circle, the vision describes the "why" of the business and represents the direction of the future.

> **Tool**
>
> Refer to Simon Sinek's TED talk for additional information and inspiration: https://www.ted.com/talks/simon_sinek_how_great_leaders_inspire_action

Mission Statement

In contrast to the vision statement, the mission is in the present. It succinctly states "how" the company will accomplish its vision. The mission statement may include who the company is, what services it offers, and to whom it will provide these services.

Values

An organization's values are a set of core beliefs foundational to achieving the mission and vision. Values should be palpable in the culture of the workplace and may be used in employee selection or employee recognition programs. Recall the discussions about culture from chapter 4.

Diversity, Equity, Inclusion and Belonging (DEIB) Statement

An organization's DEIB statement demonstrates its commitment to a workplace that is supportive of individual differences and steadfast in creating an inclusive environment.

Table 11.1 Example of Vision, Mission, and Values

Organization	*Vision Statement*	*Mission Statement*	*Values*
Mary Free Bed Rehabilitation	To be the national leader in high-value rehabilitation and post-acute care, and to develop an integrated system of care.	Restoring hope and freedom through rehabilitation.	Restore hope and freedom with joy. Together, we • work collaboratively and with innovation; • include people whose diversity reflects all those we serve; • are truthful and respectful; • heal with our hands and treat with our hearts; and • approach our work with joy.

Activity 11.2 Find the Purpose of a Health Care Provider

Search for the mission, vision, and value statements of a health care provider that you would select to care for you or your loved one. Can you identify the provider's "why," "how," and "what" they do?

The business description also identifies the target population and the services offered by the business. The target population is the group of potential customers the business is planning to serve. Examples in a physical therapy practice setting may include children with developmental disabilities, adolescents and young adults with orthopedic conditions, and older adults with neurologic diagnoses. By understanding the needs of the target population, the business is designed to offer services that meet the needs of the potential consumers. Thus, the practice description defines the services that will be offered by the organization. In a rehabilitation practice, the services offered would include services such as physical therapy, occupational therapy, dry needling, sports performance, neurologic rehabilitation, or work hardening. This describes "what" the company does to complete the elements of Sinek's Golden Circle. Target markets were discussed in detail in chapter 8.

Market Analysis

In business planning, the market analysis includes a thorough evaluation of the environment in which the business intends to operate. This includes a detailed understanding of the target population, competitors, referral sources and external environmental factors, also referred to as market drivers.

Analysis of Target Population

It is essential to know whether the potential customers exist in the geographic region in which the business will be located. For example, developing a pediatric practice in a region heavily populated with retirement communities may not be viable. First, the business developers need to determine the radius from which they will be drawing consumers. The radius may be smaller or larger depending on factors such as whether the facility is in an urban, suburban, or rural area, traffic patterns, use of mass transit, consumer convenience, among others. Within the established radius, the business developers must understand the demographic makeup of the population. The US Census Bureau is a resource that provides information about the population of individuals within a community in terms of age, gender, and socioeconomic factors including employment, income, and health care coverage.

Activity 11.3 Discover a Target Population

Using the US Census Bureau weblink available at https://www.census.gov/, answer the following questions about your hometown. What impact do these findings have on a potential physical therapy practice?

How many people over the age of 65 live in your community?

____

What is the average household income in your community?

____

What percentage of individuals in your community are without health care coverage?

____

Furthermore, the incidence of the primary conditions the business is targeting will help you with projections of patient volume. For example, a practice that intends to target patients with musculoskeletal conditions would want to investigate the incidence of new musculoskeletal injuries and apply that rate to the population of the community it intends to serve. Sources such as the Centers for Disease Control, the National Institutes of Health, and the World Health Organization are invaluable as are research articles discussing the epidemiology of various injuries and illnesses.

Activity 11.4 Define a Target Population

Discover the incidence of the following pathologies in your hometown community using the sources listed above.

Musculoskeletal conditions

____

Parkinson's disease

____

Long COVID

____

The primary goal of the research regarding the target market is to determine whether there is a need for the services the business provides in the geographic market being researched. The projected volume of clients that the clinic may see is a function of the demographic features of the market, incidence of the conditions the clinic wishes to target and the number of competitors in the area. A clinic will have a higher projected volume of patients if the business is located in an area that has a large number of people at risk for developing a common injury or illness with very few competitors.

A secondary goal of understanding the target population is to evaluate the services they require, who provides these services, what equipment, supplies, or training would be necessary, and when the clients access the services. For example, the needs of an adolescent population with musculoskeletal conditions compared to an older adult population with neurologic conditions would vary in terms of the skills of the providers, hours of operation, and equipment. The needs of the target population can be obtained through multiple sources including the clinician's understanding and experience of the population, the best available evidence about the optimal treatment approach, and surveys or focus groups with representatives from the target population. This information will be used in the business planning process when determining facility and human resource needs.

Finally, a thorough assessment of the target population results in a profile of potential payor sources for the services that the business is planning to provide. Whether the business model is health insurance based or cash based (out-of-network), ensuring a viable payor source is of critical importance to the success of the business.

Analysis of Competitors

Within the defined radius, potential competitors are evaluated. Competitors can be classified as either primary or secondary. Primary competitors provide the same services as the business that is being developed and targets the same population. Secondary competitors are in the same category but offer different services. For example, if the developing business plans to provide physical therapy services to individuals with low back pain, primary competitors will include other physical therapy practices in the radius. Secondary competitors may include chiropractic practices and massage therapy providers in the area. When analyzing competitors, it is important to evaluate the services they are providing, hours of operation, location, ease of access, specialized equipment or technology they are using. In this same example, it would be important to know if competitors are using dry needling or low-level laser therapy, if their providers are specialized in manual therapy techniques, if their hours of operation are limited or more expansive, if their clinic has sufficient parking or proximity to public transportation, or if they accept a range of insurances for payment. The findings can be organized in a table format and information used to inform decisions made throughout the business planning process.

Aha!

Scheduling for Whose Convenience?

Do you set the hours of operation of your clinic that so they are convenient for the clinical team, or to accommodate patients/consumers, or both? Consider the impact on multiple constituents.

Analysis of Referral Sources

Another component of the market analysis is identifying potential referral sources. Depending on the target population, referral sources may be other health care providers such as physicians and other non-physician providers. These are considered primary referral sources. It is important to consider the types of providers that would be most likely to refer to your business. For example, if the business is intending to provide care to patients with musculoskeletal conditions, then orthopedists and physiatrists may be primary referral sources, whereas if the practice intends to treat patients with pelvic pain and incontinence, then gynecologists and urologists may be the primary referral sources. Secondary referral sources may include non-health care professionals. For example, if the business is specializing in working with performing artists, then dance studios and dance companies may be secondary referral sources. The analysis of referral sources should include a comprehensive review of both primary and secondary referral sources. Consideration must also be given to clients who may be accessing physical therapy services via direct access. In this case, clients are significantly more involved in the decision-making about where they will access their care and organizations need to tailor their practices, including marketing strategies, directly to the client.

Analysis of the External Environment

In addition to the market factors, target population, competition and referral source analysis, other market drivers that may be analyzed include:

- economic factors such as the real estate market and its impact on rental property costs, changes to reimbursement rates or interest rates;
- the political climate including potential changes to scope of practice and payment policies and regulations; and
- ecological influences such as seasonal impact on patient volume and the likelihood of natural disasters.

Each of these factors and trends may influence decision-making for the business and thus need to be taken into consideration in the planning process.

Organizational Analysis

In addition to evaluating the external environment, a business must self-evaluate its own performance. In doing so, the organization identifies strengths that it can leverage and weaknesses that it can try to mitigate. The following factors should be considered in an assessment of the internal environment of the organization:

- Whether the organization's practices align with its mission, vision and values.
- Human resources such as staffing levels, staffing mix, staff expertise, employment law, and retention rate.
- Facility resources such as specialized equipment and sufficient space.
- Geographic location such as proximity to referral sources, adequate parking and accessibility.
- Established relationships with referral sources.
- Organizational practices such as policies and procedures.
- Compliance with federal, state, and regulatory agency guidelines.
- Financial health including health insurance contracts, reimbursement rates, revenue cycle, referral sources, length of stay, readmission rates, case and payor mix. Depending on the medical record and billing systems the facility uses, reports may be generated to provide this information. Alternatively, these data may be collected manually.
- The quality of care delivered and clinical outcomes such as goal attainment, and change in outcome measurement scores.
- Stakeholder perception including patient experience of care, employee satisfaction, and referral source satisfaction.

SWOT Analysis

The SWOT (Strengths, Weaknesses, Opportunities and Threats) analysis is a commonly used tool used to organize the results of this analysis and presents factors that will impact the success of the business achieving its mission and vision. The outcome of the analyses of the internal and external environmental factors is to determine the competitive advantages and disadvantages of the business. The internal environment is scanned for strengths and weaknesses. Identified strengths are leveraged to set the business apart from competitors. Weaknesses are analyzed and rectified or mitigated. The external environment is assessed by evaluating opportunities and threats outside of the organization. Opportunities can be capitalized on by the business, whereas threats may be mitigated. The SWOT analysis is conducted during various phases in the life cycle of a business, beginning with the business planning process. The SWOT analysis is typically depicted as a matrix.

The research conducted at this point in the process is referred to as a **feasibility study**. The purpose of the feasibility study is to determine whether the business concept or model is a viable option. If the target population exists and the market conditions are favorable, then the business is considered feasible, and the remaining elements of the business plan are developed. This includes the organization's operations plan, marketing plan, and financial projections.

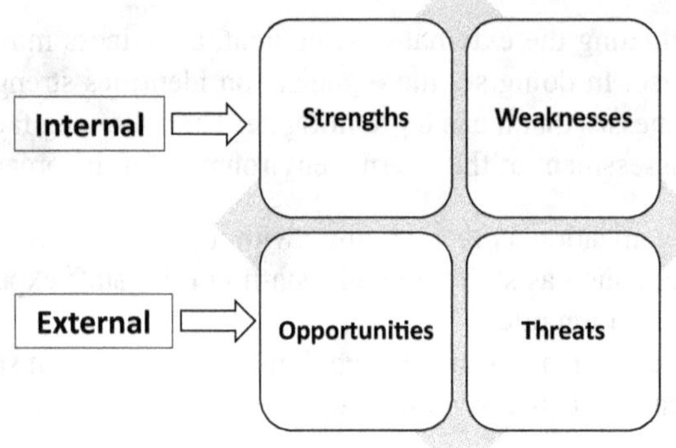

Figure 11.1 SWOT Matrix

Operations Plan

The operations plan details the organization's requirements to deliver the services outlined in the business description. It takes into consideration the physical plant, that is, the brick-and-mortar structure, equipment and supplies, as well as the providers needed to deliver the services.

Facilities Plan

Location, Location, Location!

The common cliché that "location, location, location" is the most important thing to consider when selecting a property holds true in determining the location of a physical therapy practice. Visibility and convenience are of chief importance when selecting a property. Ideal clinic spaces are visible from the street and located in an area frequently accessed by potential consumers. Depending on the target population, clinic spaces in medical office buildings, retail plazas or industrial parks may be appropriate. Consideration should be given to the ease of access from the street and into the building. Spaces on the first floor or with elevator access are optimal. The property must also have sufficient parking spaces conveniently located near the entrance of the building as well as adequate interior and exterior lighting to ensure patient and staff safety.

Activity 11.5 From Brick and Mortar to Screens and Modems

Answer the following questions in the spaces provided.

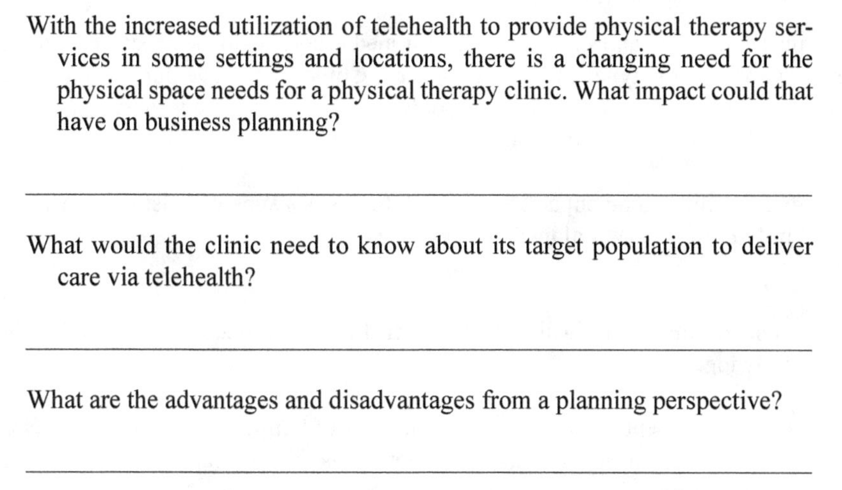

With the increased utilization of telehealth to provide physical therapy services in some settings and locations, there is a changing need for the physical space needs for a physical therapy clinic. What impact could that have on business planning?

What would the clinic need to know about its target population to deliver care via telehealth?

What are the advantages and disadvantages from a planning perspective?

Cost, Layout, and Design

The terms of lease agreements are evaluated for numerous factors, with primacy given to price per square foot and build-out needs. Tenant build-out needs include the construction required to make the space ready to house the clinic. This may include adding or moving walls or doors, electrical outlets and lighting, and the installation of flooring, cabinets, or specialized equipment.

The size of the clinic space depends on a range of factors that are largely influenced by the target population. The projected volume of patients, specifically the number of weekly patient visits, can be used to estimate a clinic's square footage needs. The American Physical Therapy Association's Private Practice Section suggests that space capacity will be reached when the number of weekly visits reaches 15% of the clinic's square footage.[3] For example, if the clinic measures 1,500 square feet, it will reach capacity when there are 225 patient visits per week. This calculation serves as a starting point for determining a new clinic's space needs.

The needs of the clients determine how the practice will be structured, which then determines how the space will be designed. For example, if the target population is elite athletes and the clinic plans to focus on sports performance, then the clinic would likely need to plan for multiple pieces of equipment and perhaps a turf field. Comparatively, if the target population is individuals with complex neurological conditions, the clinic will need to accommodate wheelchairs and may consider an overhead lift system. If clients with pelvic health conditions are the target population, private treatment spaces are necessary. Additionally, a dedicated waiting room, office, staff room/kitchenette, bathrooms and locker or changing rooms may be designed.

Equipment and Supplies

Clinical equipment and supplies are determined according to the needs of the target population and the types of services offered. Clinics may have purchasing agreements with specific vendors and may obtain a discounted rate to purchase equipment and supplies through them. Examples of such vendors include:

- SunMedical Equipment and Supplies (https://www.sunmedicalstore.com/);
- AliMed (https://www.alimed.com/); and even
- Amazon (https://www.amazon.com/).

In a general outpatient physical therapy practice, typical equipment may include the following:

- General treatment equipment: treatment tables/plinths, low mat tables, practice stairs, steps of varying heights, treatment stools, parallel bars, assistive devices, rolling mirror.
- Tools for tests and measures: blood pressure cuff and stethoscope, pulse oximeter, goniometers, dynamometers, reflex hammer, sensory testing kit, inclinometer.
- Modalities: hydrocollator, freezer, compression devices, ultrasound, electrical stimulation device, biofeedback unit.
- Exercise equipment: treadmills, bikes, weights (dumbbell and ankle weights), leg press, pulleys, medicine balls, physioballs, foam rollers, wedges, rocker boards, airex pads.
- Safety equipment: gait belt, AED, first aid kit.

Each target population may have its own needs in terms of equipment. For example, if the patient population is primarily neurologic, having a body weight support harness system that can be used over ground and/or over a treadmill would be valuable. Consideration should be given to the lowest speed and increments of speed of the treadmills, the ease with which parallel bars can be adjusted, the need for standing frames or transfer devices. If the clinic serves a pediatric population, having age-appropriate toys, climbing structures, floor mats, and pediatric height table and chairs would be necessary.

Special consideration may be given to equipment that is more costly. Equipment that costs greater than a set dollar amount established by the business, for example, $5,000, and has a life expectancy of greater than one year, is referred to as capital equipment. **Capital equipment** is accounted for differently in the budgeting process than operational expenses that would typically be used within the budget year. Another factor to consider is whether to lease or purchase equipment. It may be better to lease equipment that depreciates quickly over its useful years or that relies on evolving technology, whereas it may be better to purchase equipment that retains its value and has a reasonable maintenance program.

Equipment for the administrative duties of the clinic is also necessary. Basic office equipment would include desk, chairs, computers, furniture for the waiting room, garbage cans, copier/scanner/fax machine, phones, and file cabinets. Other non-clinical equipment may include washer/dryer, breakroom refrigerator, table and chairs, coffee pot, and microwave. Of critical importance to the business is the purchase of software for the following services: electronic medical record, scheduling, billing and claims management. There are integrated systems that can serve all functions as well as generate detailed reports to track trends and outcomes. Prior to selecting the electronic medical record system or program management systems, organizational leadership should obtain demonstrations of the systems and speak with current customers of the system providers to obtain user feedback.

Activity 11.6 Building a Practice for Your Target Population

Reflect on the following questions and jot your answers in the spaces provided.

What patient population are you most excited to work with and why?

____

____

What does the evidence suggest are the most effective treatment approaches?

____

____

How would you design a space to provide optimal care to these individuals?

____

____

What equipment or supplies would you need to provide optimal care?

____

____

Human Resources Plan

The human resources plan includes designing the complement of people performing the work of the organization. Recall that there are distinct legal considerations and nuances around employee selection, training, and compensation that were discussed in chapter 6. This section focuses on the structure and composition of the people needed to provide the services to the target population. In the broadest context, the human resources of a physical therapy clinic can be categorized as either clinical or administrative. The clinical staff provide patient care while the administrative staff provide support with tasks such as scheduling, insurance verification, collection of copays, data entry, correspondence, and report generation. Both clinical and administrative staff are vitally important to the success of the business. Respecting each other's roles and contributions is foundational to effective teamwork which then positively impacts the culture of the organization.

Staffing Mix

The determination of the staffing mix is driven by the needs of the target population. The staffing mix of a physical therapy clinic refers to the balance of providers that an organization chooses to employ in terms of their scope of practice and level of expertise. For example, a clinic that provides sports performance may choose to hire exercise physiologists, athletic trainers, certified personal trainers, and physical therapists. The training and expertise of providers may also be considered. If the clinic specializes in certain niche practice areas, selecting providers with board certification or advanced training in these areas is beneficial. For example, a clinic specializing in treating the older adult population may seek to hire a physical therapist who holds Board Certification in Geriatrics or is a Certified Exercise Expert for the Aging Adult. A comprehensive understanding of the optimal treatment approaches and best practice guidelines for the target population guides the decision-making process for staffing composition.

Activity 11.7 Developing Your Expertise

What special education, training, or certifications are available to physical therapists to enhance the care provided to the patient population with whom you are most interested in working?

____

Is there a Board Certification in your area of interest and, if so, what are the requirements to earn the certification?

____

Administrative staff are often the face of the business, and as such they must have exceptional customer service and communication skills. Administrative staff should have high levels of computer literacy as they will interface with various program management systems including scheduling and billing/claims management.

Additional training and expertise that would add value to the organization include experience with insurance verification and knowledge of medical terminology.

Staffing Levels

In addition to the composition of the staff, the number of providers needed to deliver the care is calculated. A **full-time equivalent** (FTE) is a unit of measurement that expresses the number of full-time employees needed to perform the work of a business. The composition of the staff performing the responsibilities may be full-time or part-time. For example, an organization's work week is 40 hours, and they have two employees who each work 40 hours per week and two employees who each work 20 hours per week. The organization's total number of FTEs is three. This was calculated by adding the total number of hours per week (40+40+20+20 = 120) and dividing that by the number of hours worked per week by one full-time employee (40). So 120/40 = 3.

Aha!

Dispelling the Myth of Productivity

Productivity is the amount of work that an employee is expected to perform during each period. Recall from chapter 3 when productivity was discussed. In physical therapy practice, productivity is often represented by the number of patients seen or number of units billed per number of hours worked. For example, an organization may expect a physical therapist to be 75% productive. This means if the physical therapist works an eight-hour day, they would be expected to have produced six billable units of physical therapy service. Considering multiple stakeholders' perspectives, what are the potential advantages and disadvantages of using productivity as a measure of value of one's work?

Determining the total number of worked hours required to meet the needs of the projected volume of patients assists in staffing projections. To calculate the projected number of FTEs for the business, the business leaders determine the number of visits that one FTE is expected to provide. Then the projected total number of visits is divided by this number to determine the number of FTEs needed. For example, if one FTE is expected to provide 60 visits per week, or 3,120 visits per year, and the business is projecting that they will have 120 visits per week, or 6,240 visits per year, then the business would need two FTEs to provide the projected number of visits. This process is repeated for each type of service offered by the business; for example, physical therapy, athletic training, occupational therapy.

When forecasting human resource needs for a new business, it is important to account for the ramp-up period. The ramp-up period is the time it will take the new business to provide care to its projected volume of patients. Just because a new physical therapy clinic opens its doors does not mean it will see its projected volume of patients immediately. It will take time to build its referral base, market to the community, and build its reputation. Therefore, human resources need to grow over time. It would not be feasible to hire the full complement of staff needed to care for the projected volume of patients on the day the business opens. The business leadership needs to make strategic decisions about how and when to hire.

An important aspect of human resources planning is ensuring sustainability in providing the critical work of the company. For example, if a physical therapy practice is known for providing care to children, it is essential that the organization continues to provide those services even if the individuals who initially provided the care leave the organization. This is referred to as succession planning. Succession planning may include developing existing personnel in new skills or hiring new staff members with the expertise needed to ensure continuity.

Marketing Plan

The marketing plan provides an overview of the strategies that the business will use to market its services. Recall from chapter 8 the detailed discussions related to various marketing practices. The goal of marketing is to persuade potential customers to become actual customers. An outcome or goal for a marketing strategy, such as an increase in new patients or a certain number of new referrals from a new referral source, should be established prior to initiating the plan. When developing the marketing plan, the business managers must consider several key factors: the audience, the message, the strategies and the desired outcomes of the marketing plan relative to the cost of the marketing strategy.

A business markets to a range of stakeholders who become the audience for the marketing plan. Stakeholders include potential patients, their families, referral sources, payors or insurance companies, potential employees and the community, among others. Each stakeholder has a different need that the business is trying to fulfill. A patient and their family members' goal is for their symptoms to improve as quickly as possible. The health insurance companies or payors are looking to save money by reducing utilization. Potential employees want a supportive work environment. Understanding the interests of each stakeholder helps to shape the message that is delivered through the marketing strategy.

The message of a marketing plan conveys the value of the business to each of the stakeholders. Value is a function of quality (objective improvements and the experience of care) and cost (financial, time, and risks). The message is designed to convince the stakeholders that services provided by this physical therapy practice provide greater value than the alternative, whether that is another physical therapy clinic or alternative treatment approach. The message may be tailored to address the specific aims of each stakeholder.

The marketing plan also includes the strategy to be used for delivering the message. Chapter 8 discusses a range of marketing strategies, including direct marketing, promotion, and the use of social media. The choice of strategy is dependent on the audience that the marketing plan is targeting. For example, use of social media may not be an optimal choice if the audience is an older adult potential patient population; however, if the business is targeting the children of the older adults who may be involved in the decision-making process with their parents, then social media may be an appropriate choice. In this case, the message would be directed at the value of the service to an older adult parent. The timing and cost of the marketing plan are also factors that influence the strategy.

Finally, the marketing plan includes a process to measure the outcomes of the strategy used. It is important to know whether the marketing strategy and message used accomplished the objectives of gaining more customers or an increase in the number of referrals from a provider. This will inform future marketing strategies.

Financial Plan

The financial plan summarizes the financial projections of the proposed business. The goal of the business planning process is to determine whether the proposed business will be financially viable. This relies on the revenue, i.e., the money coming into the business, being greater than the money being spent, i.e., the business's expenses. Both revenue sources and expenses should have been evaluated throughout the previous phases of the business plan. Sources of revenue such as the projected volume of patients, types of services that will be provided, and the payors/insurance companies need to be considered in the market analysis. The expenses, or costs to the business, include the resources required to operate the business. Examples of expenses include rent, equipment, human resources, and the marketing needs that have been detailed in the operations and marketing plans.

The financial plan assigns monetary value to the revenue and expenses, allowing the financial health of the business to be evaluated. This information is used to make decisions about the business. Understanding the revenue stream helps business owners to determine what the business can afford in much the same way that monitoring your personal bank account informs whether you can afford to go on vacation or out to dinner. If you could not afford the trip or dinner, you would have several options. The first is decreasing expenses by finding a less expensive vacation spot or restaurant or evaluating the level of importance of other items you would spend money on like a new outfit for the vacation. The second option is increasing revenue by picking up an extra shift at work or asking a loved one for a loan. Businesses have similar decisions to make regarding their finances and need to have the data available to make these important decisions.

At the start of a business, there are expenses that need to be spent prior to the business bringing in revenue from delivering the service. In a physical therapy practice, the clinic space needs to be rented, equipment purchased, staff hired, and marketing strategies employed prior to treating the first patient. These expenses that are needed to open the business are called **start-up costs**. There are several options to secure funds to pay for start-up costs. Many business owners use their personal savings to invest in their business. A second source of start-up funds is loans. Loans may be obtained from family or friends of the business owner or from a bank, credit union or microlender. Consideration must be given to the terms of the loan including interest rate, repayment period and penalties. Other options for funding of start-up costs include crowdsourcing or grants.

Several budgeting tools are used in the financial planning process. The pro-forma budget projects the business's revenue and expenses monthly for the first several years of the business's existence. It accounts for a ramp-up period in patient visits, projected payments from patients or insurance companies, as well as the costs of providing these services. Completion of a pro-forma budget projects the start-up costs as well as the point at which the company's revenues should exceed its expenses. This is called the **break-even point**, the point at which the business becomes profitable. Employee salaries and benefits factor significantly into the break-even analysis. This information is critically important to the business owner as it indicates the number of patient visits needed to cover the cost of providing the visits. It is also important to potential investors or lenders to gauge the safety of their loan or investment. Regardless of whether a business is considered for-profit or non-profit, the business needs to have financial reserves to cover their costs and plan for fluctuations in the market.

The fiscal health of a business is expressed by various financial measures. Operating gain represents the profit generated by the business and is calculated by subtracting total expenses from the total revenue. Operating margin represents the percentage of the revenue that is profit and is a more robust measure of fiscal health than operating gain alone. It is calculated by dividing the operating gain by the total revenue and is expressed as a percentage (see box 11.2). Financial management was discussed in chapter 7.

Box 11.2 Example of Operating Gain and Operating Margin Calculation

A business's revenue = $300,000 and its expenses = $260,000
Operating gain = revenue minus expenses or $300,000–$260,00 = $40,000
Operating margin = operating gain divided by revenue or $40,000/$300,000 =.13 or 13%

Activity 11.8 The Financial Conundrum

Most physical therapists do not go into the profession to think about budgeting and finance; however, as discussed in chapter 3, health care is a business and without generating revenue, we cannot practice our profession.

How will you continue to handle this internal conflict? How can we look at numbers as symbols representing patients whose lives we get to impact and improvements we help to facilitate?

How can you develop financial literacy to advocate for your patients and the profession? (Recall the discussions related to financial literacy in chapter 7.)

Having a financially profitable business is a key organizational goal of any physical therapy practice. Organizational goals set the long-term expectations of a business. They are typically expected to be achieved in three to five years. Organizational goals represent the priorities of the business and set the strategy for the organization. Organizational goals should answer the question, "What does success look like?" If organizational goals are achieved, the business is making progress towards realizing the vision of the organization. Organizational goals tend to be broad, with specific, measurable objectives that target levels of performance.

Key performance indicators (KPIs) are measures used to assess an organization's progress towards achieving critical business objectives. KPIs can be compared to the short-term goals in a plan of care for a patient. If a patient meets a short-term goal, it is likely that they will progress to achieving a long-term goal. If the patient is not making progress towards the short-term goal, it indicates that a change needs to be made in their plan of care. The same is true in managing a business. Failure to achieve KPIs suggests that the organization may not achieve critically important organizational goals.

Organizational goals and their KPIs represent the priority areas of the business. In his book, *Hardwiring Excellence: Purpose, Worthwhile Work, Making a Difference*, health care consultant Quint Studer suggests that goals should be set in the following priority areas referred to as pillars: service, quality, financial, people and growth.[4] Studer's pillars align with the proposed Quintuple Aim,[5] an extension of the Institute of Healthcare Improvement's original Triple Aim.[6] The Quintuple Aim framework, intended to set goals to advance health care delivery, emphasizes the importance of improving the health of a population, reducing expenditures, promoting quality services, caring for the health provider and fostering health equity.

Special Considerations for Other Practice Settings

The emphasis in this chapter has been on building an outpatient physical therapy practice. This is in large part due to the current payment models for physical therapy services that are different in each practice setting. In outpatient settings, payment is primarily volume-based, meaning that the more services that are delivered,

Table 11.2 Examples of Organizational Goals and KPIs for Each Pillar

Pillar	*Organizational Goal*	*KPIs*
Service	Be the physical therapy provider of choice for patients with musculoskeletal conditions	Patient satisfaction scores Patient experience Referral source satisfaction scores
Quality	Provide evidence-based care to achieve high quality outcomes	Goal attainment rate Percent achievement of minimal clinically important difference on select outcome measures
People	Recruit and retain employees who embody the mission, vision, and values of the organization	Employee engagement survey results Retention rates Participation rates in employee wellness programs Provider experience Employee satisfaction
Financial	Increase revenue by 5%	Payment per visit Cost per visit Number of new referrals Average number of visits per episode of care Average number of units billed per patient visit No show and cancellation rates Denial rates Payor mix
Growth	Develop a concussion rehabilitation program	Number of new referrals for concussion rehabilitation

Note: Specific targets, or objectives, would be set for each KPI.

the more the organization gets paid. Therefore, in this model, physical therapy services are revenue generating.

In other practice settings, such as acute care or rehabilitation, the facilities are paid on either a per diem or per discharge basis. The payment is intended to cover all the costs of caring for the patient (consider room and board, nursing care, rehabilitation services, etc.). The payments, while weighted for the complexity of the patient, are not directly connected to the number of services provided. Thus, the facilities are financially incentivized to provide as few services as necessary to meet the needs of the patient while maintaining quality of care. In these settings, physical therapy services are a cost to the organization; thus, managers need to organize the practice or department for efficiency to be cost-effective.

When developing new programs in these settings, less emphasis is placed on revenue generation and more on decreasing expenses or defining the value to the patients, organization, and community. For example, the rehabilitation department in an acute care hospital may want to develop an early mobility program for patients in the intensive care unit. Establishing this program may necessitate the hospital hiring an additional physical therapist and purchasing several pieces of equipment. The hospital will not get paid more for these services. However, early mobility programs have been associated with enhanced patient outcomes such as decreased length of stay and fewer complications.[7] Both of these outcomes are better for the patient and are financially advantageous to the hospital. Thus, when developing a proposal for a program such as this, these points need to be illustrated and measured.

Planning for the Future: The Strategic Planning Process

The complexity of the health care industry, with its multiple competing stakeholders, changing payment landscape, technological advances, aging population, provider burnout rates, and unprecedented events such as the COVID-19 pandemic, necessitates planning, forecasting, and adaptability. This is accomplished through a dynamic and evolving strategic plan that is aligned with the organization's mission, vision, and values. The mission, vision, and values are the compass that an organization uses to chart its course in the ever-evolving health care environment.

A strategic plan charts the course of a health care organization or business, or a program or service line within a health care system or business. The strategic planning process for an organization mirrors in many ways the American Physical Therapy Association's patient and client management model in patient care.[8] The organization begins by assessing the internal and external factors that impact the viability of the program or business in achieving its mission and vision by conducting a SWOT analysis. The assessment of these factors leads to the development of organizational goals and KPIs. From thereon, the organization develops its plan of operations, or specific action steps it will take to achieve its goals. Next, the outcomes are monitored and compared to the established goals. If progress is being made towards the goals, strategies are maintained or refined. If there is no progress being made the action steps should be reconsidered. Quality improvement strategies were addressed in chapter 5.

While the strategic plan charts the course of an organization, it must stay responsive to change in both the internal and external environments. Engaging key stakeholders and integrating the strategic planning process into the culture of an organization promotes a more thorough assessment of the organization's performance, generates buy-in, and enhances stakeholders' ability to contribute positively to the organization. By maintaining a pulse on both the internal and external environments, an organization can readily leverage organizational strengths, capitalize on potential opportunities, and mitigate threats. The need to harness an entrepreneurial spirit and foster a culture of innovation was discussed in greater detail in chapter 9.

Table 11.3 Parallels between Strategic Planning and Patient/Client Management Model

Patient/Client Management Model	*Strategic Planning*
Reason for Referral	Mission/Vision/Values
Examination	SWOT Analysis
Evaluation/Diagnosis/Prognosis/Goals	Organizational Goals and KPIs
Intervention/Plan of Care	Plan of Operation
Outcome Assessment	Outcome Assessment

Aha!

Three Perspectives of Strategic Planning

"When it comes to the future, there are three kinds of people: those who let it happen, those who make it happen, and those who wonder what happened."

John M. Richardson Jr., American academic and author, lecturer, and consultant in applied systems analysis, international development, and the sustainability/resilience of political-economic social institutions

Activity 11.9 Planning Your Future

What role does strategic planning play in helping you to craft the vision for *your* future?

___

___

___

Case Study: Management Case Scenario

ABC PT and Wellness recently developed its mission and vision statements after careful consideration of its core values and the needs of the community. It conducted a market analysis and SWOT analysis to determine the landscape of outpatient physical therapy services in the area and to assess the physical therapy needs of the community. The result of the market analysis indicated a gap in services for the neurologic patient populations, specifically those with stroke, brain injury, and spinal cord injury.

What additional information would you need to know about the target population?

___

Where would you obtain that information?

___

How would this inform decisions about the care offered to the target population?

The SWOT analysis revealed several strengths of ABC PT and Wellness including having a board certified physical therapist in neurologic physical therapy. However, one of the organization's weaknesses is a lack of a defined referral source and the need to obtain equipment. An opportunity is a new neurologist who recently joined a local practice; however, a threat is a new outpatient physical therapy practice that has just opened in the area.

What additional information would you want to know about the internal and external factors that might influence the decision to develop a neurologic physical therapy service line at ABC PT and Wellness?

Is there additional information you would want to know about your competition?

How would you seek this information?

ABC PT and Wellness determines that developing a neurologic physical therapy program is a feasible venture.

What resources would be necessary in terms of staff, equipment, and facility design to implement this program?

What value would this program offer the target population?

To whom would you market the program?

How would the message differ based on the stakeholder?

ABC PT and Wellness develops the following operational goals:

1. Provide high-quality health care to the community.
2. Increase revenue generating service lines.
3. Recruit and retain talented health care providers.

What KPIs would you measure to assess the success of the business?

Suggested Readings

Brown B. *Dare to Lead: Brave Work, Tough Conversation, Whole Hearts.* Random House; 2018.

Harvard Business Review. HBR IdeaCast. https://hbr.org/2018/01/podcast-ideacast

Sinek S. *Start with Why: How Great Leaders Inspire Everyone to Take Action.* Portfolio/Penguin; 2009, p. 250.

Studer Q. *Hardwiring Excellence: Purpose, Worthwhile Work, Making a Difference.* Fire Starter Publishing; 2003.

References

1. Sinek S. *Start with Why: How Great Leaders Inspire Everyone to Take Action.* Portfolio/Penguin; 2009.
2. Collins JC, Porras JI. Building Your Company's Vision. Harvard Business Publishing. September 1, 1996. Accessed March 6, 2023. https://hbsp.harvard.edu/product/96501-PDF-ENG
3. Martin P. Select and design a practice site: Use a competitive marketing analysis to guide your decision. In: Sanders JS, ed. *Private Practice: The How to Manual.* 2nd ed. APTA Private Practice; 2014.
4. Studer Q. *Hardwiring Excellence: Purpose, Worthwhile Work, Making a Difference.* Firestarter Publishing; 2003.
5. Nundy S, Cooper LA, Mate KS. The quintuple aim for health care improvement: A new imperative to advance health equity. *JAMA.* 2022; 327(6): 521–522. doi:10.1001/jama.2021.25181
6. Institute for Healthcare Improvement. Triple aim and population health. Accessed March 21, 2023. https://www.ihi.org:443/Topics/TripleAim/Pages/default.aspx
7. Zang K, Chen B, Wang M, et al. The effect of early mobilization in critically ill patients: A meta-analysis. *Nurs Crit Care.* 2020; 25(6): 360–367. doi:10.1111/nicc.12455
8. American Physical Therapy Association. APTA Guide to Physical Therapist Practice: Chapter 2. Accessed March 21, 2023. https://guide.apta.org/chapters/chapter-2

Index

Note: Bold page numbers refer to tables; *italic* page numbers refer to figures.

abusive environments 99–100
accessibility 260
accuracy, and precision *115*
action domains 22–3
action plans 38–40, **39–40**, **43**, **48–9**, 142, 160–1, 191
acute care 10, 288
administrative burden 13, 257
administrative staff 282–3
administrators 7
adoption of innovations 243–6
advertising options, local 214
Affordable Care Act 78, 154
Age Discrimination in Employment Act 153
aging population 77, 289
Alter, Adam 164
AMA (American Medical Association) 182
Americans with Disabilities Act (ADA) 153–5, 221
AOC (Add on Code) 186
AOPT (Academy of Orthopedics) 245
APTA (American Physical Therapy Association) 4, 82; and direct-to-employer services 242–3, 245; on economic value of physical therapy 253; and financial literacy 171; patient and client management model **289**; PPS (Private Practice Section) 245, 279; *Standards of Practice for Physical Therapy* 12–13; on student debt 168
Aristotle 116
artificial intelligence 79, 197–8, 249
authorization/pre-certification 180–1
autonomy 25, 35, 79, 238, 248, 257

B2B (business to business) 210
B2C (business to consumer) 210
balance billing 175
Balanced Scorecard 130
Baldwin, Andrew 31–4, 37, 46
basic skills *7*, **8**
Baylor University Medical Center 134
behavior change, personal 52
behavioral interviewing 146
behavioral management theory 18
benchmarked outcomes 129
Bennis, Warren 9
Berl, Jason 140–2, 154
best practices 95, 122; identifying 24, 129
billing xxiv, 11, 64, 170, 184–7; dysfunctional 117; incorrect 179
billing software 221
blogs 204–5, 211
board certification 4–5, 282
body language 141, 147
bottom lines 75–6; financial 64, 108, 251
bottom-up management 14–16, 20
boundaries: setting 48, 54; spanning 22, 53–4
Boyd, John 233–4
brand identity 206–8, 210, 212–13
break-even point 175–6, **176**, 286
Brown, Jennifer 108, 264–5
Buckley, Patrick 268–9
budgeting 166–7, 169–71; tools 286
bullying 99–101
bureaucratic management theory 18
burnout 36, 57, 289; and business of health care 78; and management style 25; and organizational culture 89, 94; and retention strategies 145
business, use of term 67–8
business description 271–3, 278
business failure 196
Business Focus 206

business fundamentals 62, 68–9
business literacy xvii, xxiv, 1–2, 24, 63–6, 79, 219; assessing 69–70
business management 2, 63, 74, 175, 256
business models 66, 171–2, 249; assessing 250; and business plans 256; demonstrating value 252–4; key components and decisions 251–2; not-for-profit 255; in physical therapy **256–8**, 259–66, **259**; use of term 250
business plans xvii, 250, 256, 270–1; and business models 259–60, 262, 264–5; making 270; suggested table of contents 271–87
business skills, need for 64
business terminology 64, **83–4**
buying decisions 71–4

capital equipment 280
care model transformation 78
career development 147, 158
career management and planning 160–1
cash-based business model **257–8**, 259, 261–3
Cates, Sara 169
centralized management 18
chain of command 14
Challenger Safety 104
change management 11, 22, 50–3, 57–8, 219, 223–5, 241
chaos theory 19–20
charge capture 178, 182–3
charge codes 121, 126
charges: in health care finance 173, **174**; reviewing 175
charity care 118, 176
Chimenti, Chris 154–5
chronic diseases 66, 77, 198
Civil Rights Act 154–5
civility 19, 101
Clark, Diane 10, 61–4, 75
classical management 18
clinic spaces 278–9, 285
clinical care documentation 181–2
clinical microsystems 36
clinical staff 190, 282
CMS (Centers for Medicare and Medicaid Services) 77, 182–5
coding 64, 170, 182–4, 188
collection and denials 179, 186–7
communication, bottom-up and top-down 97–8
communication management 22
communication skills 56, 282
the community, being in 89
community health 36, 261
compensation packages 64, 148–50; common terms and definitions **149**; finding benchmarks 150
competency domains *21*
competition, unfriendly 98
competitive advantage 252, 277
competitor analysis 273, 275
compliance 133, 142, 153–4, 263, 265, 277; regulatory 179, 198
conceptual skills 7–8
concierge services **258**
conflict management 6, 11, 54–5, 134–5, 236–7
connectedness, perceptions of 95–6
Consolidated Omnibus Budget Reconciliation Act (COBRA) 154
consumer behavior 71–4, 200–3
consumer-directed health care 78–9
consumers 67; patients as 73–4; use of term 71
contingency management theory 19
contract negotiations 66
Contributor Safety 104
core values 4, 89; alignment on 107; and organizational culture 94, 98
cost shifting 176–7
cost structure 252
costs, in health care finance 173–6, **174**
countercultures 96
COVID-19 pandemic 79; and marketing 201, 211
CPT (current procedural terminology) 182–4, **183**, 186
creative conflict 89
culture: definition of 90; discovering 108; and employee experience 144; *see also* organizational culture
customer service 186
customers 67; use of term 71
cutthroat environments 98–100

dashboards **131**, 133, 135
Davids, Keith 233
debt 164, 166, 168–70; bad 173, 176
decisional roles 8
decision-making: decentralized 20; financial 191–2; and leadership style 133; shared 35, 170
deep change 52
defining your business **208**

DEIB (Diversity, Equity, Inclusion and Belonging) 107, 272
delegation xxiv, 32–3, 46–7, 133
demand analysis 252
Denmark 36
developmental change 52
diffusion of innovation 243–4
direct access xxiv, 80–1, 241, 253, 276
direct-to-employer services 242–3, 245–6
Disciplines of Execution 4
disrespectful environment 99
disruptive innovation 239–43
diversity, equity, and inclusion *see* DEIB
division of labor 18
DMAIC (define, measure, analyze, improve, and control) 123–4, **124**, 136
dominant culture 90, 95–6
Drucker, Peter 220, 222
dumping 47

earned media 211
economic value 80, 82
education, clinical 221
efficiency 6
8 Minute Rule 183
Eight Step Change Model 241
Einstein, Albert 132
Electronic Health Record (EHR) 121, 124, 183
elevator pitch xvii, 254
emergency care 174, 220
emotional intelligence 34, 151
employee engagement 24–5
employee experience 106–7, 140, 142–5, 149
employee life cycle 142–4, *143*; stages of **143**
Employee Retirement Income Security Act (ERISA) 154
employee satisfaction 277, 288
empowerment 5, 16
EMR (electronic medical records) 80, 197, 265, 281
enabling domains 22–3
energy management 11, 47–50
entrepreneurial culture 241
entrepreneurial spirit 222, 229–31, 234
entrepreneurship 222–3; and innovation 228–9, 235–9; recognizing opportunities 233–4; social 219, 255, 267; and SWOT 231–2
episodic care, traditional 263
Equal Pay Act 153, 155
equipment plan 280–1
ethical behavior 99
evidence-based practice 13, 112
evidence-informed practice (EIP) protocols 121, 126–9, 136
evidence-informed practice management 13–14
executive summary 271
expense variance 191–2
external environment, analysis of 231, 276–7, 289

facilities plan 278–9
failure 51; accepting 5; fear of 52; learning from 132; managing 223–5
Fair Labor Standards Act (FLSA) 153–4
faith 33, 89
Family and Medical Leave Act (FMLA) 153–4
family feel, culture of 89
fear, culture of 98
feasibility study 277
fee for service 118, 249
feedback 62, 151; soliciting 102, 227
filers 42
financial conundrum 286–7
financial counseling 180–1
financial goals 170, 250
financial health 171, 189, 277, 285
financial health literacy 170–1
financial literacy 64, 164–8, 170–1, 192; apps for 167; developing 287
financial management xviii, 170; jargon of 172, **173**
financial performance 188–91, 256; review **188–90**
financial plan 285–7; personal 260
financial skills 23–4, 166
first principle 113, 116–20, 126, 132
first-time managers 31–3
fiscal health 286
fit, self-assessment of *159*
Five Whys 133
fixed costs 175–6, 191–2
focus 43–5
for-profit entities 67, 118
Foster, Steve 88–91, 94
Four-Frame Model 104
FranklinCovey Time Matrix 40, **41**
FTEs (full-time equivalents) 283

Gawande, Atul 126
Gemba walks 126

generation-defining characteristics 201–3, *201*
Gilbert, Fred 36, 65–6, 252, 262, 266
goal setting 4, 35, 37–40, 52–3, 151, 160, 287; principled 118–19
goals: and entrepreneurial opportunities 233; in practice marketing 207
Golden Circle 271–3 Goleman, Daniel 44
gossip 54, 98, 107
growth and development, investing in 143, 158
growth evaluation 192
guidance and control, implicit 233

Hamel, Gary P. 248
hand hygiene policy 122–3
Hansen, Morten 116
Harris, Hilary 111–12
HCPCS (healthcare common procedure coding system) 182–3, **183**, 186
health and wellness partnership **258**
health care: as a business 24, 63, 73, 75–9, 249; future landscape 197–201, 216; and wellness 265–6
health care coding *see* coding
health care consumers 73; changing 77–9
health care dysfunction 113, 117–18
health care environment 22, 289
health care waste 125–6
health insurance: administrative burden of 13; and business literacy 66–7; in compensation package 149; in United States 77, 79
health insurance reimbursement: decline in 81, 165, 168, 249; maximizing 118; negotiating for 170, 269; prices for 174
health system performance, optimizing 77–8
Heraclitus 222
HFMA (Healthcare Financial Management Association) 171, 173
hierarchy 9, 18
HIPAA (Health Insurance Portability and Accountability Act 57, 154, 182
historic visits 181
hopeful vision for the future 36
Hospital Price Transparency Rule 174–5
hours of operation 275–6
HR *see* human resources management
HR compliance 153
Hughes, Karen M. 58, 248–9, 253
Hull, Brian 154
human factors 6
human relations management theory 19
human resources xxiii; in organizational analysis 275, 277
human resources management (HRM) 87, 142, 144–7, 153; and business literacy 63, 70; categories of laws **153–5**; essential processes **144**; and leadership 154–9; in NCHL model 23–4; strategic 145
human resources plan 281–4
human skills 7–8

ICD-10 codes 182–3
Immigration and Nationality Act (INA) 154
immigration laws 154
incivility 100–1
Inclusion Safety 104
inclusive environment 99, 101, 103, 272
information, accessibility and credibility 201
information flows 14
information sharing 66, 95
informational roles 8
inner focus 44
in-network business model **256–7**
innovation xviii; championing 243–6; and conflict 55; disruptive and sustaining 239–43; and employee experience 107; and entrepreneurship 226, 228–9, 235–6; in health care 77, 79; improvement without 238; and leadership 4; and management 6; and organizational behavior 16; and stability 266; as a value 207
insurance verification 181, 283
integrated health systems 81
interest rates 169, 276, 286
Intermountain Healthcare 127, *127–8*
internet search topics 201, *202*
interpersonal relationships 142
interpersonal roles 8
interprofessional organizations 129, 131
interviewing 141, 145–6; common questions 148; preparing for 147–8; STAR model of 147
intrapreneurship 219–20, 226–8, 255

Jensen, Gail 233
job descriptions 145, 148, 151–2, 226
job satisfaction 24, 66; and management style 24–5; and organizational culture 108, 156

Kennedy, John F. 116
knee arthroplasty 127, *128*

knowledge sharing 98
Kotter, John 241
Kouly, Michael 96
KPIs (key performance indicators) 64, 115, 121, 130–1, 190–1; in business planning 269, 287–9, **288**; for marketing 215
Kraybill Conflict Style Inventory 55

labor specialization 18
laggards 245–6
LAMP Leadership Program 4
leadership 22; and management 3–6, 9–12, 133, 154–5; skills xviii, 10, 12, 155; styles 133
Leadership Competencies for Health Services Managers 21
lean activities, examples **126**
lean management 112–13, 123–5, 127–8, 131; categories of **124–5**
Learner Safety 104
learning organizations 16–18, 106, 161, 241
lease agreements 279
Lencioni, Patrick 106
liability insurance 57, 65
loan repayments 169
longevity 196, 200
low back pain, classification of *127*, 127

machine xxiv
macromanagement 27
maintenance xxiv
Malmgren, Pippa 171
management: as a subset of business 62; use of term 6–9
management development 16, 159
management levels 7–8, 14–15, *15*; in classical management 18
management problems 141
management skills xvii–xviii, 5, 11, 219; and management level 15; and management style 21; and supervision 27
management structure 68–9
management styles 6, 15, 95, 135; developing your own 21–7; ineffective 98; and theories 18–19
management theories 17–21
management vignette: Baldwin 31; Berl 140–2; Buckley 268–9; Chimenti 155; Clark 61, 63; Foster 88–9; Harris 111–12; Hughes 248–9; Pearlmutter 164–6; Petrosino 220–2; Sher 195–6; van den Bent 3–5
managerial roles *8*, 112
managerial work 5–7, *7*, 9, 87
managing people *see* human resources management
market analysis 273–7
market drivers 64, 77–80, 273, 276
market forces 82, 228
market share 80, 203, 228, 231, 238–41, 246
market value 66
marketing xxiv; digital 202; three Ps for physical therapy practices 206–9, *206*, 211–12, 216; traditional four Ps of 205, 209–12, *209*, 216
marketing innovation 228–9
marketing management 196–7
marketing plan *211*, 212–16, **212–15**, 284–5
marketing spending 198
marketing strategies 203–4, 228, 265, 276; and marketing plan *211*, **212–15**, 216, 284–5
markets, use of term 68
material xxiv
Maxwell, John C. 155, 223
media coverage 205, 211
Medicaid 66–7, 77, 173, 177, 182, 263
medical error 126
Medicare 13, 66–7, 173–4, 177; in business models 263–5; coding for 182–3, 185; for physical therapy 81; and social determinants of health 249; spending on 77; therapy cap 114; and value-based care 78
Medicare Advantage plans 242
Medicare patients 183
mental health 198, 266
methods xxiv
microaggressions 100–1
microcultures 95–6
micromanagement 25–6, 47; and organizational culture 93, 97, 101, 107
Microsoft 157
middle management 9, 14–15
mill model 259–61
mindfulness 45, 49
MIPS (Merit Based Incentive Payment System) 81
mission, in practice marketing 207–8
mission statement 13, 272, **272**
modifiers 184–5, 187–8
money xxiv; talking about 250–1
motivation: intrinsic 4, 11, 24, 45; perceived levels of 19; sources of 119

MOTM (Man on the Moon) Statement 119–21, 123, 129, 133, 136
Motorola 113, 123
MUEs (medically unlikely edits) 185, **186**
multitasking 18, 33, 44–5
Musk, Elon 116

narratives, authentic 219, 250
National Aeronautics and Space Administration (NASA) 116
NCCI (National Correct Coding Initiative) 184–5, 187
NCHL (National Center for Healthcare Leadership), Health Leadership Competency Model 3.0 22–4, *23*
negotiation 56, 148
newsjacking 205
Newton, Isaac 120
NHE (National Health Expenditures) 77
9 Box Grid 158, *159*
No Surprises Medical Billing Act 174–5
Norby, Sandra 66, 81, 250, 253, 262–3
not-for-profit businesses 65, 67, 74, 118, 169; model of 251, 255, 261, 266
nursing groups, community-based 36

occupational health services 241–3
Occupational Safety and Health Act (OSHA) 154
office politics 54, 105
onboarding 141, 143–4, 147, 151–2
online indexes 214
online services 201
OODA (Observe, Orient, Decide, and Act) 233–4, *234*, 237
open-door policy 156
operating gain and operating margin 286
operational definitions 172–3, **173**
operational efficiency 108, 179
operational goals 120–1, 291
operational structures 111, 113, 116, 122, 125
operations management xviii, 9, 113–14, 116–17, 125–6, 135; pragmatic 131–2
operations plan 277–84, 289
organization style 42–3
organizational analysis 277
organizational behavior 16–17
organizational chart *14*
organizational climate 23, 96–7, 102, 107
organizational culture 4, 64, 88–94; assessment 104, **105**; change in 107; entrepreneurial 241; learning in 106; negative or "toxic" 97–101; positive and supportive 96, 101–4; strategic planning in 289; sub-and micro-95–6
organizational goals 7, 83, 105, 123, 287–9
organizational health 106
organizational innovation 103, 229
organizational purpose 116
organizational structure 14, 18, 96, 229, 240
organizational trust 102
organizations, use of term 68
other focus 44
outcome measurements 113, 116, 121, 124, 129–30, 277
outer focus 44
out-of-network business model **257**, 262, 265
outpatient settings 31, 287–8

Pareto charts *129*, 136
patient access 80, 180–1
patient care, one-on-one 260
patient engagement, digital tools 81
patient experience xxiii, 74; and burnout 25; and business of health care 75, 78–9; evaluating **199**
patient experience economy 201
patient interactions 75, 107
patient outcomes 25, 36, 124, 171, 198, 252, 288
patient responsibility 173, 178, 180–1
patient safety xxiii, 25
patient volume 189–92, 202; projected 228, 274–6, 279, 283–4
patient-centered care 64, 198
patient/client management 1, 11
payment transformation 78
payment variances 186–7
payor mix 173, 177, 191–2, 256, 263, 277, 288
PDSA (Plan, Do, Study, Act) cycle 131–2, *132*
Pearlmutter, Lori 164–6
people skills 53
performance management 35, 141–2
perseverance 89, 248
personal finances 166, 262
personal growth 51
personalized care 197–8, 200–1
personas 210, 212
Petrosino, Chris 220–2
physical therapy: as a business 65–6, 76, 80–2; dimensions of expert practice 233; economic value of 82, 252–4; and management 1; other practice settings 287–9

pilers 42
pillars 262, 287–8, **288**
planned change 52, 106
planning: as management practice 270; *see also* business plans
point of service collection 180, 191–2
policy creation 122–3
population health, improving 78, 126
Porter, Michael 121
possibility thinking 250
practice management 3, 12–14, 63
precision 114–15, *115*
Pregnancy Discrimination Act 153
pre-registration/registration 180
preventive care 198
price shopping 173–5
price transparency 170, 201
prices, in health care finance 173, **174**
pricing, in marketing 210–11
primary competitors 275
principles: in practice marketing 207; *see also* first principle
prioritization 33, 37–42, 270
private practice, commitment to 88–9
pro bono services xviii, 173, 252, 260
process flow 125
process improvement training 112
process innovation 228
procrastination 34, 37, 45–6
product or service innovation 228
productivity 62, 65; and employee experience 107; and financial decision-making 191–2; and management theories 18–19; myth of 283–4; and organizational climate 96; and organizational culture 94; physical therapy and 242
professional development 47, 129, 160, 231
professional responsibility 22
profit, net 175–6, 189, 192
pro-forma budget 286
project plan 45–6
promotions 210–11
provider experiences xviii, 25, 66, 75, 78, 288
psychological safety 102–4, **104**
PTP (Procedure to Procedure) 185
public speaking 205
purpose 14; accuracy of 113–17, 120; commonality of 89; and operational success 118–21, 126–9; and organizational culture 90; in practice marketing 207; sense of 95, 229; shared 74, 134–5; *see also* MOTM
Quadruple Aim 78
quality improvement 113, 123–9, 131, 135, 289
quality measurement 113
quality of care 25, 118–19, 124–5, 241–2, 277, 288
Quintuple Aim 77–8, 115, 118, 287

RACI Matrix 237, **238**
ramp-up period 283–4, 286
RCA (root cause analysis) 126, 130, 131–3
readiness for change 52
recruiting 145–6; successful strategies 146–7
referral sources 89, 228, 273, 276–7, 284, 288
refueling 48
registration process 180
regulatory compliance requirements 129
rehabilitation 187, 288
relationship building 53, 64, 105, 151, 156
relationship management 1, 11, 22, 53–4
relative advantage 244
resilience 107, 152, 222, 225
resistance to change 52, 97–8, 106
resource management 33
retention 143–5; and connectedness 95; and work culture 101, 107
revenue: in health care finance 173, 175–6, 286; KPIs for 190
revenue cycle 64, 170, 173–4, 177–88, 277; key steps in **179**; operational definitions **178**
revenue model 252
revenue sources 173, 226, 285
revenue variance 191
Richardson, John M. 290
risk, and entrepreneurship 222–3, 227
risk management 57
risk-taking, interpersonal 102–3
Rogers, Everett 243
role diversification 260–1
role modeling 23
Rosenthal, Elizabeth 117–18
rounding for outcomes 123
rural areas 202, 273

SBAR (situation, background, assessment, recommendation) 134
scheduling 79, 180
Schein, Edgar 90
scientific management theory 18
SCORE 265
scorecards 130, 133

screening models 264
search engine optimization (SEO) 207
secondary competitors 275
self-awareness 5, 23; and focus 44
self-care 48–50; action plan for **49**
self-change 51
self-control 49
self-improvement 51
self-leadership 11, 53, 151
self-managed teams 35–6
self-management 4–5, 11, 27; and conflict management 56–7; and employee life cycle 142; and organizational culture 90, 107; and personal change 53; practices and strategies 33–5; and team building 151
self-motivation *see* motivation, intrinsic
self-reliance 49
self-renewal 48
self-understanding 55
selling yourself 64
The Seven Habits of Highly Effective People 48
shared interests 134
Sher, Tracy 195–6, 204
shrinkflation 171
SHRM *see* human resources management, strategic
silos, breaking down 54, 242
Sinek, Simon 61, 80, 88, 104, 268, 271–2
Six Sigma 113, 123–4, 130, 136
skills-based approach 7
SMART goal-setting 37–8, 152
social determinants of health 234, 249, 253
social entrepreneurship 219, 255
social media 196–8, 205; in marketing plan 284–5; organic mentions on 211; turning off 44–5; and websites 207
social media analytics 214
social responsibility 22, 261
socialization 200, 205
software: for business planning 262; as capital equipment 281; for clinical education 221; and financial decision-making 176; innovation in 228; and virtual care delivery 198–9
SpaceX 116
spaghetti diagrams 126
staffing levels 277, 283
staffing mix 277, 282
stakeholders 77, 113; communication with 22; internal 102; in marketing plan 284; value created for 113, 121, 123–4
start-up costs 252, 285–6
strategic planning 289–90, **289**
stress management 1, 11, 49–50
Studer, Quint 287
subcultures 95–6
succession planning 158–60, 284
surprise bills 174–5
sustainability 77, 236, 255, 284
sustaining innovation 239–43
SWOT (strengths, weaknesses, opportunities, and threats) 231–2, **232**, 277–8, *278*, 289–91
systems management theory 19

target audiences 197–8, 205, 207–13, 215; identifying 201–3
target markets 250, 252, 270, 273, 275
target population 273–7, 282, 290–1; analysis of 273; building a practice for 281; defining 274–5; and facilities and equipment 278–80
Taylor, Frederick Winslow 113
team building 151–3, 237–8
team communication 134
team-based skills 62
teamwork xviii, 107, 135, 151, 156, 282
tech-driven practice solutions 199
technical skills 7–8
technology, evolving impact of 79
telehealth 79, 134, 197–9, 201–2, 258, 279
telemedicine *see* telehealth
therapist productivity rates 191
TherapySouth 90–1
third-party payers 242, 246
30 minute rule 44, 46
Thomas-Kilmann Conflict Mode Instrument (TKI) 55
thought leadership positioning 204–5, 216
Thriving Index 252
time management 1, 11, 37–47, 152, 216; and focus 43; four categories of **41**
TOMS 255
top-down management 14–16, 18
total expenses 175, 189, 191, 286
total mind and body wellness *see* wellness
total revenue 175, 188, 286
Total Worker Health 241–3, 245
toxic work cultures 97–101
Toyoda, Sakichi 133
Toyota 113, 125
Traction 4
Tracy, Brian 46
transparency 98, 152

trialability 244
Triple Aim 77–8, 287
triple focus 44
Tschoepe, Barbara 58, 66, 76, 241, 253, 263–6
tuition reimbursement 149
turnover 93, 119, 123, 145–6

unethical behavior 99
United States: health care system of 67, 77, 118; hopeful vision for the future 36; medical error in 126
US Census Bureau 273–4

value 80; creating 252–4; in marketing plan 284
value proposition 252–3
value-based care 78, 192, 249
values: in business plan 272, **272**; in practice marketing 207–8
van den Bent, Jerre 3–6, 11, 16, 20, 27, 154
variable costs 175–6, 191–2
variance 112; decreasing 125; unwarranted 114, 129
violence, workplace 57
virtual care delivery 198
vision: in business plan 272; clarifying 157; in practice marketing 207–8
vision statement 207, 272, **272**
visualized goals *120*
volume-based care 78, 113–15

wage compression 81–2
wage incentives 18
website design 206–7
wellness 66, 81, 199–200, **200**
wellness model 249, 264–5
Wood, Ryan 65, 252–3, 259–61
work cultures 98–101; establishing 156
work environment 23; and organizational culture 93–4, 96, 98; supportive 284
work hardening 220, 273
work relationships 93, 145
work style 93, 108
workers compensation laws 154
workplace bullying *see* bullying
workplace drama 98, 102
workplace stress, chronic 25
workplace-based business model **258**

X & Y management theory 19

For Product Safety Concerns and Information please contact our EU
representative GPSR@taylorandfrancis.com
Taylor & Francis Verlag GmbH, Kaufingerstraße 24, 80331 München, Germany

www.ingramcontent.com/pod-product-compliance
Lightning Source LLC
Chambersburg PA
CBHW052119230326
41598CB00080B/3876

* 9 7 8 1 6 3 8 2 2 0 8 7 9 *